Tackling Causes and Consequences of Health Inequalities

A Practical Guide

Tackling Causes and Consequences of Health Inequalities

A Practical Guide

James Matheson
with thanks to John Patterson and Laura Neilson

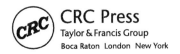

CRC Press
Taylor & Francis Group
Boca Raton London New York

CRC Press is an imprint of the
Taylor & Francis Group, an **informa** business

CRC Press
Taylor & Francis Group
6000 Broken Sound Parkway NW, Suite 300
Boca Raton, FL 33487-2742

© 2020 by Taylor & Francis Group, LLC
CRC Press is an imprint of Taylor & Francis Group, an Informa business

No claim to original U.S. Government works

International Standard Book Number-13: 978-1-138-49988-1 (Hardback)
International Standard Book Number-13: 978-1-138-49986-7 (Paperback)

Library of Congress Cataloging-in-Publication Data

Names: Matheson, James, author. | Patterson, John, Dr., author. | Neilson, Laura, author.
Title: Tackling causes and consequences of health inequalities : a practical guide / by James Matheson, John Patterson, Laura Neilson.
Description: Boca Raton : CRC Press [2020] | Includes bibliographical references and index. | Summary: "Addressing health inequalities is a key focus for health and social care organizations, yet this is the first book to explore how best frontline health workers in areas of deprivation can address these problems. This book offers a concise but comprehensive overview of the key issues in health inequalities and how practically to address them"-- Provided by publisher.
Identifiers: LCCN 2019045426 (print) | LCCN 2019045427 (ebook) | ISBN 9781138499867 (paperback) | ISBN 9781138499881 (hardback) | ISBN 9781351013918 (ebook)
Subjects: MESH: Healthcare Disparities | Health Services Accessibility | Social Determinants of Health | United Kingdom
Classification: LCC RA418 (print) | LCC RA418 (ebook) | NLM W 76.1 FA1 | DDC 362.1089--dc23
LC record available at https://lccn.loc.gov/2019045426
LC ebook record available at https://lccn.loc.gov/2019045427

Visit the Taylor & Francis Web site at
http://www.taylorandfrancis.com

and the CRC Press Web site at
http://www.crcpress.com

Dedication

To all the people who should have lived longer

Contents

Foreword

MICHAEL MARMOT

This book is an antidote to learned helplessness. The opening line of my book *The Health Gap* was 'Why treat people and send them back to the conditions that made them sick?' A clinician, faced with overwhelming evidence that social conditions had made her patient sick, might be tempted to throw up her hands – what is she, or he, to do about those conditions. The mission of this book is to provide an answer, many answers.

When I began as chair of the WHO Commission on Social Determinants of Health I said that we wanted to foster a social movement for health equity achieved through action on the social determinants of health. The argument was that all social change came through social movements: universal suffrage, civil rights, women's rights, improvements of working conditions. So, too, with health equity – reducing those social inequalities in health that could be remedied and were hence unfair.

Not being expert in social movements, I emphasised two components: a commitment to social justice and taking the practical steps necessary to achieve change. The purpose of the WHO Commission report was to do both of these. Laying out a commitment to social justice is one thing; generating practical advice for the whole world is another. How could we recommend practical steps that would at the same time be appropriate for sub-Saharan African countries, South Asia, Latin America, North America, Australasia and Europe? Hence, I welcomed the invitation of the British Government to translate the findings and recommendations of the global commission for one country, England. The result was the Marmot Review, *Fair Society Healthy Lives*. We laid out six domains of recommendations: equity from the start; education and lifelong learning; employment and working conditions; having enough money to afford to live a healthy life; healthy and sustainable places to live and work; taking a social determinants approach to prevention.

Two linked thoughts about that list, relevant to the present volume: we didn't mention healthcare; nor did we address the question of what clinicians can do about the social determinants of health.

We didn't address healthcare, not because it is unimportant, but because I take it as unarguable that the whole population should have universal access to healthcare, free at the point of use – the NHS, in other words. The second is more challenging: the role of clinicians. Even if clinicians recognise the importance of social determinants of health in their individual patients' patterns of health and disease, what can they do about them?

In answering that question, the present volume represents an important link in the chain from evidence to action. After the WHO Commission report a common question was: OK, but what should actually happen now? One answer was the British Government commissioned a report, *Fair Society Healthy Lives,* precisely to address that. OK, but your recommendations were somewhat general; who is going to do what?

The answer to that question is that one set of actors, not the only ones, are clinicians at the front line. A clinician who asks the question can read this book to find out how it is possible to take action on social determinants of health. By laying out what can be done, this book gives doctors the opportunity not only to fulfil their obligation to treat the sick but also to address the causes of health inequalities and thereby improve population health and health equity. It thus embodies both the moral cause of social justice and health and the practical steps necessary to achieve it.

Editors

Dr James Matheson graduated from St George's, University of London in 2009. He trained in Lancashire and Cumbria before moving to work with Hope Citadel Healthcare, a community interest company which provides primary care in areas of concentrated disadvantage. He has worked overseas and has been published in the area of humanitarian disaster response, teaching around this subject at St George's, and holds a diploma in the medical care of catastrophes.

Dr Matheson is passionate about addressing causes and consequences of health inequalities, working as a general practitioner and teaching and training the next generation of GPs to guard the health of our patients. He is a visiting senior lecturer at Manchester Metropolitan University and, through the Shared Health Foundation, teaches a number of courses from undergraduate to postgraduate level on subjects around deprivation medicine, health inequalities and the social determinants of health.

Dr Laura Neilson works in Greater Manchester trying to reduce health inequalities. She set up Hope Citadel Healthcare ten years ago when she was a medical student. Hope Citadel provides GP services in areas of deprivation, currently holding three CQC outstanding awards and running nine practices.

Dr Neilson also runs the Shared Health Foundation, an organisation funded through philanthropic donations. Shared Health Foundation pilots innovative approaches to reduce harm from health inequalities and currently delivers work for young people who are self-harming, families living in temporary accommodation, health literacy for parents of under five's and advocacy for young carers. Together with a great team with which she works she developed Focused Care, a project based in 50 GP practices in Greater Manchester that makes invisible patients visible, unpicks the story behind the story and allows our hard-pressed households to thrive.

Dr Neilson also works in A&E as a regular doctor. She won the Health Service Journal (HSJ) Rising Star Award in 2016 for her 'inspirational style' and teaches on health inequalities. She has three boys and is therefore somewhat of an expert by experience in Minecraft and Harry Potter.

Dr John Patterson is medical director of Hope Citadel Healthcare, a social enterprise working within the NHS, overseeing practices and walk-in centres in hard-pressed neighbourhoods around Greater Manchester. They currently run nine practices serving a population of 31,000. Dr Patterson is lead for Focused Care, which supports the most vulnerable and needy households.

Dr Patterson also works within Oldham Clinical Commissioning Group (CCG). His role initially concentrated on quality, innovation, productivity and prevention (QIPP) and medicines optimisation. Building on previous successful projects and working with an exceptional team, the CCG has seen a reversal of the largest per capita prescribing spend in the country as well as significant improvement in the quality of prescribing. From 2018 he has taken over the role of chief clinical officer.

When not at work he is busy getting in trouble with his wife by re-enacting famous Irish rugby victories with their four willing children.

Contributors

Tim Anfilogoff
NHS England
East of England, UK

Gemma Ashwell
Bevan Healthcare CIC
West Yorkshire, UK

Charlotte Auty
University of Manchester
Manchester, UK

Anna Bailey
University of Manchester
Manchester, UK

Peter Baker
Global Action on Men's Health
Brighton, UK

Helen Barclay
Bevan Healthcare CIC
West Yorkshire, UK

Gary Bloch
University of Toronto
Toronto, Canada

Michael Brookes
Reeth Medical Centre
North Yorkshire, UK

Paul Bywaters
University of Huddersfield
Huddersfield, UK

Lisa Chattington
Focused Care CIC
Greater Manchester, UK

Bushera Choudry
Walkden Medical and AskDoc
Greater Manchester, UK

Charlotte Cockman
Shared Health Foundation CIC
Greater Manchester, UK

Sarah Cockman
Shared Health Foundation CIC
Greater Manchester, UK

Ann Marie Connolly
Formerly of Public Health England
London, UK

Cathy Cullen
North Dublin City GP Training Programme
Dublin, Republic of Ireland

Catherine Cutt
IRIS Specialist Domestic Violence and Abuse Service
Manchester, UK

Marian Davies
Chair of Adolescent Health Group, Royal College
of General Practitioners
London, UK

Jenny Drife
START Homeless Outreach Team
London, UK

Deena El-Shirbiny
Person-Centred Care Network of Champions
Royal College of General Practitioners
London, UK

Rebecca Farrington
Specialist Asylum Seeker Service
Greater Manchester Mental Health Trust
Greater Manchester, UK

Riya E. George
Queen Mary's University of London
London, UK

Ritika Goel
University of Toronto
Toronto, Canada

Enam-ul Haque
University of Manchester and AskDoc
Manchester, UK

Susan Harris
Psychological Medicine in Primary Care
Oldham, UK

Phil Harris
Developing Effective Services for Adolescents,
Families and Adults
Bristol, UK

Clarissa Hemmingsen
University of Manchester
Manchester, UK

Julia Hose
Psychological Medicine in Primary Care
Oldham, UK

Ben Jackson
Sheffield Medical School
Sheffield, UK

Helen Jones
Leeds Gypsy and Traveller Exchange
Leeds, UK

Elizabeth Keat
Homeless and Health Inclusion Team
Leeds, UK

Jessie Keeble
Bevan Healthcare CIC
West Yorkshire, UK

Jessica Lee
University of Manchester
Manchester, UK

Michael Marmot
Institute of Health Equity
London, UK

Milena Marszalek
Queen Mary's University of London
London, UK

James Matheson
Shared Health Foundation CIC
Greater Manchester, UK

Camran Miah
University of Manchester
Manchester, UK

Dot Mundt-Leach
University of Manchester
Manchester, UK

Laura Neilson
Shared Health Foundation CIC and Hope
Citadel CIC
Greater Manchester, UK

Austin O'Carroll
North Dublin City GP Training Programme
Dublin, Republic of Ireland

Dominic Patterson
Fairhealth
Yorkshire and Humber, UK

Anna Pratt
Hope Citadel Healthcare CIC
Greater Manchester, UK

Mark Purvis
Sheffield Medical School
Sheffield, UK

Tom Ratcliffe
Fairhealth,
Yorkshire and Humber, UK

Ming Rawat
North Dublin City GP Training Programme
Dublin, Republic of Ireland

Clare Ronalds
IRIS Specialist Domestic Violence and Abuse
Service
Manchester, UK

Jamie-Leigh Ruse
National Energy Action
Newcastle-upon-Tyne, UK

Rachel Steen
Health Education England
London, UK

Ruth Thompson
Manchester Health and Care Commissioning
Manchester, UK

Hannah Thompson
Signpost Young Carers
Stockport, UK

Louise Tomkow
Humanitarian and Conflict Response Institute,
University of Manchester
Manchester, UK

Caroline Watson
Secure Environments Group
Royal College of General Practitioners, UK

Gabi Woolf
Health Inequalities Standing Group
Royal College of General Practitioners
London, UK

Introduction

JAMES MATHESON

This book is inspired by those dedicated volunteers and professionals who have gone the extra mile to create health, happiness and well-being for those most in need. It aims to share their methods and achievements so that they may be more broadly applied, for the benefit of all.

'Of all the forms of inequality, injustice in healthcare is the most shocking and inhumane'

Martin Luther King Jr

We live in an unfair society within an unfair world, where unequal distribution of wealth contributes to dramatic inequalities in morbidity and mortality between those who have, those who have less and those who have not. Within our country's boundaries, a baby born into deprivation can be expected to die up to 15 years sooner and spend up to 17 more years in poor health than a baby born into wealth. Every year between 1.3 and 2.5 million years of life are lost to the premature deaths caused by health inequalities, along with all the social, financial and emotional devastation that those lost years carry with them.

As clinicians we have long been aware that many of the medical or medically framed problems our patients bring to us have their origins in factors much deeper and broader than simple medical pathology – that behind the first line of the story lies the history of a life, from childhood traumas and upbringing, education, social norms and individual habits, work or lack of work, emotion, mood and the feeling of control over one's life, or lack of it. All of this ends up in a consultation in our surgeries. These, the real social determinants of health, have often been regarded as outside the domain of healthcare and considered areas that busy doctors and their wider teams would lack the time, resources and often inclination to address. Those who have inspired this book have, through their work, shown that the truth is otherwise and that primary care is perfectly placed to make the interventions that can change, for the better, the

lives of those whom society has allowed to fail. We look to share their knowledge and experience with you through the chapters which follow.

Many of the papers and reports have been focused at the societal level and the interventions proposed have been at the strategic, national or regional level. The introductory chapters of this book will provide an overview of the literature and then reframe it with a focus on the issues faced by our patients and by ourselves in our work alongside them.

Section II of the book encompasses the knowledge and skills required to provide quality care in a safe and sustainable manner in the highly challenging environment of deprivation. Some of these skills will be specific to certain situations or populations but many are the generic skills applicable by GPs working alongside patients to provide personalised, continuous care for all their patients. The Royal College of General Practitioners has researched the learning needs reported by GPs working in deprived areas to formulate a health inequalities curriculum and this, together with feedback from those working and training in deprivation and social medicine, have guided the content. Whilst no single tome is likely to be fully comprehensive of the rich array of experience, the chapter contents are based on the real-world recommendations of doctors already doing the job, so we trust it will be both sufficiently broad-ranging and with adequate depth, without overloading the reader. Whilst the cutting edge of scientific progress advances apace, sadly, the issues of deprivation are likely to persist in similar fashion for many years so, whilst some medical textbooks will quickly become outdated, we anticipate the learning in this book will remain relevant for a long time to come.

The knowledge and skills section includes chapters on issues prevalent in areas of deprivation such as smoking and drug misuse, with a practical focus on approaches and useful interventions to address the problems. Complex mental health issues are common presentations in areas of concentrated disadvantage and, living the chaotic lifestyles which often accompany such conditions, patients can struggle to engage with psychiatric services. Advice on strategies to manage complex psychiatric illness and support patients through crises, short and long term, are included. Safeguarding is a regular and frequent concern and is covered along with guides to adult and child social services written by the people who work in those agencies with advice on how to ensure joined-up teamworking in areas of concern. Safety can be a concern when working with medical and social complexity and there is expert advice on prescribing issues in difficult areas, medico-legal issues and safety in practice. At a time when doctor burnout is a headline issue in medicine, resilience has become a central theme to deprivation-focused medical training. To work effectively in this emotionally-charged and stressful field, with the additional pressures of deprivation, requires a commitment not just to patients but also to self-care. This section includes advice on how to look after yourself so you can best look after your patients, your family and the life outside work to which you are also entitled.

Section III looks at populations and groups affected by health inequalities. Traditionally there has been a perception that health inequalities relate to marginalised and excluded groups within society and, indeed, excessive disease burdens are still very much manifest in these populations.

There are, however, huge numbers of people whose health outcomes are poor, who do not fall into one of these recognised groups but whose ill health stems from poverty and the environment and life implications that poverty brings with it. For this reason, this section includes work on addressing the health consequences of deprivation generally and specifically through all ages; from ensuring a good start in early life, to the prevention, postponement or mitigation of the effects of disease in later life.

The expanding literature and research into health inequalities has so far identified interventions which can be effective at the policy level, but there remains a dearth of evidence as to what works in terms of interventions at the practice level. As that evidence base starts to be assembled, Section IV aims to share evidence of good practice as to what innovative groups have been doing to address causes and consequences. Great work has been done by practices or services in certain areas in identifying unmet healthcare needs in specific marginalised populations. These organisations have highlighted holes in service provision which they have then gone on to fill but, of course, in a more perfect world, that need would not be there if mainstream services were able to cater for all parts of society with a medical and social need. A concept of inclusive health has developed which encourages health and social services to ensure that no group or individual is excluded from health and well-being due to their life circumstances. Examples of inclusion health in practice, and its successes, are included in this section.

This book will equip you and your team with the knowledge and practical advice needed to work in areas of deprivation and shares the skills and experience of those working in this environment to advance the cause of social justice and best help patients in this challenging and exciting area of practice.

PART 1

Setting the Scene

An Insight from the Front Line

LAURA NEILSON

It doesn't take into account the vulnerability, the trauma, the deficit of love, the overwhelming need for acceptance, the potent power of being totally broke. It is more than choice.

I'm guessing that if you are reading this book, then you already have a passing interest in health inequalities and know some of the topics mentioned here, but recaps can never hurt.

On a simple level, health inequalities are simply the difference in health outcomes, the morbidity or mortality of one population compared to another, usually comparing richer demographics with those less well off. The beginning of this thinking really emerged with Tudor Hart and his inverse care law, published in 1971 in *The Lancet*:

> The availability of good medical care tends to vary inversely with the need for it in the population served. This inverse care law operates more completely where medical care is most exposed to market forces, and less so where such exposure is reduced.

This idea landed in the medical community like a firecracker. If Twitter in the digital world is harsh, then it pales when reading the comments and letters from fellow medics sent to *The Lancet* from 1971 onwards. Black, Acheson and Whitehall all contributed to a growing understanding of inequalities. More recently heroes such as Marmot, Wilkinson, Pickett and Watt have picked up the mantle. These giants of academic research, detailed analytics, critical and forensic thinking, continue to describe and prove health inequalities are prevalent and present. They continue to call out the injustice and refuse to allow the establishment and the individual to deceive themselves that all is right. The inconvenient truth is that all is not alright.

In the UK there is potent inequality. Within all areas of the country there is a gradient along income levels. Those with the most money have the healthiest, happiest, most secure lives with the most years of disease-free living *and* they live longer. Those who are poorest have shorter lives with more disease and more burdens. You can see the difference in life expectancy of over 10 years across one area or even one town. In parts of London the differences are evident across the distance of three tube stops. Or even more soberingly, in one tower block. We see inequality by ethnicity, by education, by access to green space, by type of job. The academics can show us whatever way we ask for. The inequality is still there.

THEORY OF INEQUALITY

How these inequalities come to be so great, is the debate of many a clever thinker. The life-course theory suggests that they notch up over the course of a life. Those born into poverty often go on to experience poverty. We know that antenatal health has a huge impact on the foetus and child at birth. The impact of the first 1,000 days on life outcomes is a key piece of academic work that should shape our policies and investment. The impact of childhood trauma is only just being fully realised, and the newly emerging field of epigenetics is both thrilling and terrifying at the same time. Life events often throw people into poverty and there is increasing work describing the importance of resilience and social networks as buffers for the effects of life events. Simple explanations of choice and behaviour are usually popular with politicians, but they don't quite cut the mustard in the real world; think about the woman who has gotten out of one domestic violent relationship only to get into another. Choice isn't quite the right understanding of the situation. It doesn't take into account the vulnerability, the trauma, the deficit of love, the overwhelming need for acceptance, the potent power of being totally broke. It is more than choice. Other theories of economic or political empowerment explain some inequalities: social determinants of health offer the most all-encompassing evidence base for consideration and pscyho-social theories give insight to individual or family stories. Macroeconomics, structural injustice, reduction in social mobility – there are papers upon papers listing theories and evidence. All interesting, all useful, all have their place. But, the pervasive, persistent plod of poverty is still there and what do you do as a practitioner in the field?

THE CAKE APPROACH

During the first few years of my working in deprivation, interventions to tackle health inequalities were aimed at specific groups of people. These usually covered groups like the homeless, travelling communities, sex workers, refugees and asylum seekers, perhaps people with learning disabilities and more recently veterans.

Indeed, I had set up and continue to run work for these groups of people and there is nothing wrong with them; they are needed and do great work. And yet when I looked at the estate I lived and worked on, even if I did an intervention for each category of people, it did not touch the majority of the population. It did not shift our health outcomes. It was like having a massive cake and slicing off a piece for asylum seekers, sex workers, travellers. Once you had finished slicing you assumed there would be no cake left. Only you realised there was still a massive hunk on the plate. Where we lived and worked there was just a whole load of people in poverty and that was the defining characteristic. So, we started to think about the cake differently.

In fact we started to think about a bubble.

THE INEQUALITY BUBBLE

We took diabetes and started to look at health outcomes. In Manchester there are an estimated 150,000 people with diabetes. Of these, 18,000 have high HBA1c levels so they are outside the target, a further 10,000 are 'exceptioned' by general practice. Patients can be 'exceptioned' because they are terminally ill, in prison or other reasons. Whatever the reason, they are unlikely to have well controlled diabetes. No one 'exceptions' patients who hit the target! And then there are approximately an extra 23,000 patients who had diabetes but are not yet diagnosed. In total in Greater Manchester there are 51,000 diabetics who do not have a working care plan for diabetes (Figure 1.1).

What puts you into this 51,000 people is interesting. It seems you got into this bubble if you were poor, if you were in a domestic violent (DV) relationship, if you were known to the law, if you were an immigrant, if you had a learning disability, an addiction, mental health problem, if you had temporary housing or no housing. In summary you got into this bubble if you had a factor of inequality, and the fact you are in the bubble perpetuates the inequality.

Think of it like a football with a massive rip in it (Figure 1.2).

No wonder we never seemed to hit the goal of meeting health targets, or reducing inequalities. That football is never going to score a goal.

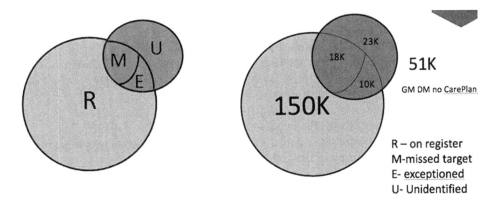

Figure 1.1 The inequality bubble.

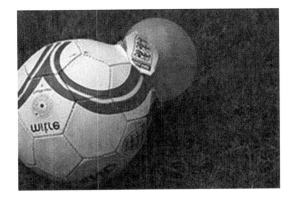

Figure 1.2 The football.

Turns out the bubble is the same whatever the chronic disease, and the things that put you in the bubble are the same. We started thinking of health inequalities as:

$$HI = \left(FTT \times B^{US} \right)^{SD}$$

Health inequalities is 'failure to thrive' multiplied by 'barriers to universal services' exacerbated by 'social determinants of health' (verbally said as Fit Bus SD)

Suddenly health inequalities weren't about groups of people and a deficit fixed with simple solutions. It was about engagement, complexity and unpicking situations to enable thriving to occur.

FAILURE TO THRIVE

'Failure to thrive' is a term from paediatrics for babies and children who do not grow as they should. The reasons children do not grow are vast and varied from the one in a million diagnosis to the complex interplay of social factors. Failure to thrive is a narrative description that allows clinicians and others to gently and collectively unpick the often interplaying issues. When we looked at our patients, failure to thrive seemed to fit as a description of what we actually saw.

BARRIERS TO UNIVERSAL SERVICES

Many of our patients had medical conditions, but medical diagnosis alone would not lead to thriving. Many of them struggled to navigate the services there to help. Sometimes, this was because of the complexity of using the service, the hoops you have to jump through or the cultural differences at play (incidentally, the biggest of which for our estate is the concept of a diary). Other times people struggle to engage because of their own behaviour which might be a bit aggressive, or their short attention span, or their perception that they don't fit. If we are honest our public sector services are not always best placed to deal with people with multiple complex issues; there is often a referral roulette between or across services.

SOCIAL DETERMINANTS OF HEALTH

These are hugely at play in our patients. Maslow's hierarchy of needs is potently demonstrated. Who cares about a smear test or hypertension if you can't pay your rent or have no school uniforms?

Gradually, over the years we have shifted our approach with the mantra of 'Fit Bus SD' in our heads. We have tried to build trust and deepen relationships with patients and the community. Instead of co-producing treatment plans with patients, a method so often taught at medical school, we have bartered plans. Quid pro quo. Housing letter for a smear. Disability appeal for coming to the gardening group. Party at the practice if you actually go ahead with the bypass surgery. Stars on the chart if you don't call the ambulance service every day but go to the coffee group.

The model of engagement, trust building and unpicking has led us into territory we would not have imagined. Providing food while patients are waiting for universal credit, partnerships with school holiday clubs, Christmas hampers, gardening groups run by alcoholics who aren't ready to stop drinking. It has made us aware of the price of benzodiazepine on our estate and the link with our prescribing (that's an uncomfortable thought). Advocating to housing associations – these patients in rent arrears are not naughty, they are needy.

GENUINELY A GENERALIST

As we have continued we have become more generalist. The general of general practice is not general enough. The lines blur further. As a group we are now equally fluent in the language of cancer diagnosis and the benefits system as to how you can get hold of a fridge or carpet. Our medicine has got deeper too. If your patients won't or don't go to secondary care appointments you can either re-refer and play referral roulette again *or* learn more medicine, find comrades along the way who will give you plans over the phone, see the patient at the beginning of clinic before they 'lose the plot' and let the specialist nurse come to your little GP clinic. We've got bolder at calling things out – adults with learning disabilities never diagnosed, adults with ADHD, post-traumatic stress caused by rape, attachment disorders from a life of neglect. As one patient neatly put it, 'I know here my shit is your shit. We're all in the shit together'.

The aim of this book is to pull together the lessons, learning and experience of a collective who are currently working in deprivation medicine and they themselves are thriving. Which might sound odd if you've got this far in reading.

You see there is hope to be found in
deprivation.
And there is beauty,
And there is joy, and hilarity,
And deep relationships,
And triumph,
And pride,

There are the best of people having the
worst of times.
And the worst people surprising you by
turning around and being their best.

There is great medicine,
Prescribing that stretches the brain,
Relationships that stretch...
And then restore the soul.

There is creativity,
Solution finding,
Endless learning,
And never a wasted skill.

There is truly opportunity to see people
freed,
To see people put back together,
To see restoration come.

And you will be told some of the
dirtiest jokes ever.

Working in areas of deprivation is
addictive.
As one of my colleagues said, 'Surfing
is more fun when the waves are
highest'.

Our hope is that more of us go surfing.

TOP TIPS TO SURF IN DEPRIVATION

1. Look for the story behind the story. Presenting symptoms are often not purely medical and there is likely much more to the presentation, don't be afraid to delve.
2. Build trust. Sort the small things that the patient asks you to sort first and build trust – write the letter to housing, sign forms (you may be the only person they can ask to sign them). Don't be tight and charge; instead build up a bank of good will and trust, then spend it on

the things you want your patients to do but they are reluctant to. Spend it getting the smear test done, the dementia assessment, the childhood vaccinations, etc.

3. Work in partnership. Your patients are complicated – they and you need help and support, with anything and everything. Find out who the workers are, find out where the local debt advice centre is, find out what voluntary sector organisations are around and what they do. Where is the food bank, how can you get a fridge, a buggy – you need all the help you can get.

4. Don't underestimate the power of social contact. Encourage patients to make friends. Do something at your surgery to help foster friendships, be it a monthly coffee morning, a choir, a nit, natter and chatter group.

5. Look for the invisible. Start with the computer – search for those who have not been seen for years, search for those who have not had a smear, or vaccinations. Look for households with multiple people living in them or addresses with multiple people; these are likely to be probation, homeless or temporary housing addresses.

6. Find the other professionals in the area. The head teacher, the PCSO, the housing officer you will share common patients with and get a fuller picture.

7. Bend mainstream services to meet your patient's needs. Many services are commissioned to do domiciliary visits or offer alternative access. Find out if they do and ask it for your patients.

8. Be the best doctor you can be. Learn more medicine, create good relationships with consultants so you can get good advice, accept your patients will DNA outpatient appointments and agree a plan with secondary care for when this happens.

9. Remember your patients are expert survivalists. Use this attribute to bring behaviour change. Praise the good. Celebrate progress, however small. Shower them in positivity. Use the tactic of 'I had a patient who once…'.

10. Have a holiday! Take a break! Keep a hobby! Have a laugh! Find a friend to walk the path with you. Remember working in deprivation is a marathon not a sprint. Keep yourself and your team well.

2

An Introduction to Health Inequalities

ANN MARIE CONNOLLY

Good fortune in health is more often by design than by accident.

Health is usually the outcome of the lives people lead and the conditions into which they are born and grow. Health inequalities mean that if you are poor you may become ill at a younger age, suffer more years in poor health and die earlier than those with more resources.

Health inequalities have been defined as 'systematic differences in health status between different socioeconomic groups. These inequities are socially produced (and therefore modifiable) and unfair' [1]. This definition recognises that the differences in outcomes for people are not random but result from the very fabric of the social and economic context that shape people's lives.

Patterns of inequalities in health are usually shown as the differences in measures of diseases and deaths between the people living in areas with different levels of deprivation. More deprived areas experience higher death rates, higher disease rates and earlier onset of disease compared with more affluent areas. For instance, life expectancy for men living in the most deprived areas of the UK is 9.3 years lower than for those living in the most affluent areas [2]. The gradient in self-reported poor health is even steeper with a gap of 19.1 years for both men and women between the richest and poorer areas. Areas of deprivation are not evenly distributed across the country but are concentrated in certain regions: north-east and north-west of

England, parts of London, some coastal towns and Glasgow city, Scotland [3]. The south Wales valleys and large cities, with some north Wales coastal and border towns rank as the most deprived areas in Wales [4].

The gradient in disease and mortality rates is seen across a full range of mental and physical health problems. Rates of cardiovascular disease show an inequalities gradient internationally [5, 6] as well as in this country where rates of premature mortality can be up to 3.5 times as high in the most deprived decile compared with the least deprived [7]. COPD rates show marked inequalities with particularly high incidence and mortality rates in the northeast and northwest of England and in Scotland, while the gap in incidence between the most and least deprived quintile varies almost threefold [8]. Inequalities are also in evidence in mental health problems. For instance, there were twice as many GP consultations for anxiety in areas of deprivation than in affluent areas in Scotland [9] and people living with severe mental illness experience some of the worst inequalities with a life expectancy of up to 20 years less than the general population [10].

What is particularly notable is that for those in the most deprived decile of areas in the country, healthy life expectancy (the average number of years that an individual is expected to live in a state of self-assessed good health) is only about 52 years whereas in the least deprived areas of the country people can expect to have a healthy life until the age of 70. Not only does disease onset start at a younger age, people in poorer areas are more likely to have multiple morbidities starting at a younger age and tend to have a greater number of disorders compared to those in more advantaged areas [11].

Some of this early onset of disease can be attributed to well known risk factors such as smoking. Although smoking rates are declining for all groups, there remain differences in rates of smoking between different parts of the country; rates are higher in more deprived communities [12, 13]. The gradient also demonstrated lower rates of physical activity and dietary intake of fruit and vegetables in areas of deprivation [14]. But differences in behaviours only partly explain different health outcomes. For instance, there are higher levels of alcohol consumption amongst more affluent groups, but the harm related to alcohol consumption, as measured in alcohol-related hospital admissions and mortality rates, is higher in more deprived groups [15, 16].

Beyond individual biology and behaviours there are many other factors impacting on health and illness experienced by individuals. Inequalities in health start before birth. This is evident in the fact that stillbirth rates are almost twice as high in deprived areas compared with the least deprived areas [17]. This pattern can also be seen with infant mortality, with rates more than twice as high in the most deprived areas [18]. This excess mortality varies depending on ethnicity with significantly higher rates for Pakistani and Black African/Caribbean babies [19].

Over the course of people's lives, the places they grow up in, the homes they live in, the jobs they have access to and the wealth they acquire all play a part in their chances of good health [20]. These experiences are cumulative across a lifetime. The influences are at their most important in childhood and are often transmitted from generation to generation. In Scotland, more than a third of children in the most deprived quintile live in low-income households compared to fewer than 1 in 20 in the least deprived quintile [21]. In the UK there were 4.1 million children living in poverty in 2016–2017, approximately 30% of children, or 9 in a classroom of 30 [22]. Child poverty can blight childhood with impacts extending into adulthood.

It has long-lasting effects, for example, by GCSEs, there is a 28% gap between children receiving free school meals and their wealthier peers in terms of the number achieving at least 5 A*–C grades. Growing up in poverty can mean being cold, going hungry and not being able to join in activities with friends. Long term, it influences earnings as well as overall quality and length of life.

Living in cold homes, living with damp or mould, coping with overcrowding or overcoming unsafe homes affect people's health [23]. Cold homes cause cardiovascular disease and mental health problems and exacerbate COPD and other health disorders [24]. Growing up in a cold or overcrowded home affects both mental and physical health and the ability to study and attain at school. People living in greater deprivation are more likely to have health hazards in the home [25]. Unsafe homes affect the likelihood of injuries, especially for frail older people or for infants or young children. The cost to the NHS of poor housing is estimated to be £1.4bn, particularly relating to the impact of cold homes and fall hazards [26]. About 20% of homes in the country do not meet the government's decent homes standard [27].

The quality of neighbourhoods, in terms of access to green spaces, a sense of safety and community, nearby services such as shops and transport, can all affect people's opportunity to partake in physical and social activity impacting their sense of well-being and mental health [28]. Most importantly, having a job is good for your health; providing income, a sense of purpose and social connections. However, not all jobs are equal and insecure, low paid employment without much prospect for progression is associated with poorer physical and mental health [29].

These multiple and complex interactions throughout a life can occur in different proportions, leading different individuals and families to have greater or lesser numbers of protective factors or experience greater or lesser degrees of adversity. Difficult early experiences are more likely to affect each further step of life, predicting greater chances of poorer education, lower pay and worse living conditions.

Adversity can be ongoing or recurrent with periods of relative security interspersed with times of challenge and stress across the life course. These patterns in turn affect the risk of disease and the capacity to manage behavioural risk factors.

Mullainathan and Shaffir describe how scarcity (of money, food or time) affects mental processes, in effect narrowing the mental 'bandwidth' [30]. This leads to coping in the short term rather than planning for the future, so those experiencing economic adversity are less likely to adopt health-related behaviours, mainly because their whole attention is focused on dealing with their poverty and adversity. This narrowing of the mental bandwidth can affect parenting skills and management of household finances.

The consequences that we see in the statistics and in surgeries get expressed in many ways. They seem unique to each individual but are part of wider epidemiological patterns that show people in poorer circumstances experiencing worse health at younger ages. Chronic inflammation plays a significant role in the association between socioeconomic position and health inequalities, with markers such as C-reactive protein being higher in those with lower socioeconomic means [31]. Clinical staff serving poorer areas are working against the impact of living conditions on their patients' health. This amounts to people living in poorer areas and poorer conditions ageing quicker than those in more affluent areas. This premature ageing process represented by earlier onset of disease is shown in biological markers (epigenetic ageing) [32] with impacts as great as many of the behavioural risk factors. This premature ageing process has the potential to be reversed, with that potential being greatest in the early phases of life. There is growing evidence about intergenerational transmission of environmental effects, for example, food consumption, on individual epigenetics whereby the exposure of parents or grandparents to certain conditions seem to lead to specific health outcomes for children not yet born [33, 34].

Ethnic differences in health vary across different health indicators. Bangladeshi and Pakistani groups were more likely to report limiting long-term illness, among both men and women at age 65 [35]. In the 2011 census, Gypsies and Irish Travellers had the highest prevalence of 'not good' general health [36]. Some ethnic groups are far more likely to live in deprived areas than others, for example 71% of Bangladeshi and 65% of Pakistani ethnic groups live in the 30% of the country considered most deprived.

Beyond those in the most deprived communities, there are specific groups within the population facing additional barriers to good health. Research suggests socially excluded populations, including homeless individuals, sex workers, prisoners and those with substance use disorders, have a mortality rate 8 times higher for men, and 12 times higher for women, than the average [36].

What does this mean for clinicians serving challenged areas?

People from poorer communities are more likely to end up presenting at A&E with acute problems rather than presenting at primary care with earlier symptoms of diseases such as cancer. Clinicians can support patients to have a greater understanding of the meaning of some symptoms and of how their bodies work, to aid earlier diagnosis.

Patients' presenting problems may just be the tip of an iceberg of difficult personal circumstances, some intermittent or temporary, some cumulative and long-standing. Patients may need additional services beyond clinical care if the stresses of their personal lives make it more difficult for them to cope with managing their illness or treatment. Ultimately, supportive advice to deal with housing, poverty, debt or relationship difficulties may be a prerequisite for being able to engage with prevention advice or to manage a prolonged treatment regime successfully.

Preventative efforts to support behaviour change are important especially when they relate to factors such as smoking. When supporting a patient to reduce behavioural risk factors in poorer communities it is important to recognise they are more likely to have multiple behavioural risk factors [37] and preventative support may need to be more intensive. An example of this is smoking cessation, as it is more difficult to stop smoking when coping with multiple challenges and stress.

Local clinical commissioning can be an opportunity to orientate clinical services towards the greater needs of those from poorer communities in terms of accessibility, intensity or design. It also allows for commissioning of services which provide wider support, such as citizens advice bureau (CAB) services [38], joint commissioning of housing advice with councils, commissioning of voluntary sector for community navigators and provision of social support projects. Community-based and owned activities can be effective and cost-effective ways of enabling individuals and groups to take control of both their personal and health problems.

Finally, clinicians can be advocates for their patient population, working at local, regional or national level. More locally, engagement with the health and well-being boards can inform health and social care planning. Working with integrated care systems can help shape thinking and strategy to orientate services to those with the greatest needs. Getting involved with professional bodies to help development of appropriate policy recommendations [39] is a further opportunity to influence change outside of the consulting room.

REFERENCES

1. Whitehead M, Dahlgren G. Concepts and principles for tackling social inequities in health – Levelling up Part 1. WHO Europe 2006.
2. PHE. Health profile for England 2018. Chapter 5. Available from: https://www.gov.uk/government/publications/health-profile-for-england-2018/chapter-5-inequalities-in-health [Accessed 15th March 2019].
3. Scottish Government. Scottish Index of Multiple deprivation. Available from: https://www2.gov.scot/Resource/0050/00504809.pdf [Accessed 15th March 2019].
4. Welsh Government. Welsh Index of Multiple deprivation. Executive summary. 2015. Available from: https://gov.wales/docs/statistics/2015/150812-wimd-2014-summary-revised-en.pdf [Accessed 16th March 2019].
5. De Mestral C, Stringhini S. Socioeconomic Status and Cardiovascular Disease: an update. *Current Cardiology Reports*. 2017; 19: 115.
6. Næss Ø. What drives trends in inequalities of cardiovascular disease? *Trends in Cardiovascular Medicine*. 2019; 29(5): 304–305.
7. PHE. Health Equity in England, Indicator 3. Cardiovascular disease mortality under 75 years. London: Public Health England; 2017. Available from: https://assets.publishing.service.gov.uk/government/uploads/system/uploads/attachment_data/file/733093/PHOF_Health_Equity_Report.pdf [Accessed 19th March 2019].
8. British Lung Foundation. *COPD*. Available from: https://statistics.blf.org.uk/copd [Accessed 19th March 2019].
9. NHS Scotland. Mental Health. Inequality briefing 10. NHS Scotland. Available from: http://www.healthscotland.scot/media/1626/inequalities-briefing-10_mental-health_english_nov_2017.pdf [Accessed 29th May 2019].
10. PHE. Guidance. Health matters: reducing health inequalities in mental illness. 2018. Available from: https://www.gov.uk/government/publications/health-matters-reducing-health-inequalities-in-mental-illness/health-matters-reducing-health-inequalities-in-mental-illness [Accessed 19th March 2019].
11. Stafford M et al. Briefing. Understanding the health care needs of people with multiple health conditions. Health Foundation. November 2018. Available from: https://www.health.org.uk/publications/understanding-the-health-care-needs-of-people-with-multiple-health-conditions [Accessed 13th March 2019].
12. ASH. ASH Briefing. Health inequalities and smoking 2016. Available from: http://ash.org.uk/information-and-resources/briefings/ash-briefing-health-inequalities-and-smoking/ [Accessed 19th March 2019].
13. PHE. Health Equity in England. Indicator 10. Prevalence of smoking among persons aged 18 years and over. 2017. Available from: https://www.gov.uk/government/publications/health-equity-in-england [Accessed 19th March 2019].
14. PHE. Health profile for England 2017. Chapter 5. Available from: https://www.gov.uk/government/publications/health-profile-for-england/chapter-5-inequality-in-health [Accessed 9th March 2019].
15. Institute of Alcohol Studies. Alcohol, Health inequalities and the prevention paradox. Available from: http://www.ias.org.uk/uploads/pdf/IAS%20reports/IAS%20report%20Alcohol%20and%20health%20inequalities%20FULL.pdf [Accessed 19th March 2019].
16. PHE. Local Alcohol Profiles. Available from: https://fingertips.phe.org.uk/profile/local-alcohol-profiles/data#page/8/

gid/1938132984/pat/6/par/E12000004/
ati/102/are/E06000015/iid/91414/age/1/
sex/4 [Accessed 19th March 2019].

17. Houses of Parliament. *POSTnote 527 Infant Mortality and Stillbirth in the UK*. London: Houses of Parliament; 2016.

18. ONS. Child and infant mortality in England and Wales: 2016. Available from: https://www.ons.gov.uk/peoplepopulationandcommunity/birthsdeathsandmarriages/deaths/bulletins/childhoodinfantandperinatalmortalityinenglandandwales/2016 [Accessed 19th March 2019].

19. Health Equity in England. Indicator 5 Infant Mortality, 2017. Available from: https://assets.publishing.service.gov.uk/government/uploads/system/uploads/attachment_data/file/733093/PHOF_Health_Equity_Report.pdf [Accessed 19th March 2019].

20. Institute of Health Equity. Fair society, healthy lives (Marmot review) 2010. Available from: http://www.instituteofhealthequity.org/resources-reports/fair-society-healthy-lives-the-marmot-review [Accessed 13th March 2019].

21. NHS Scotland. Child Poverty in Scotland: Health impact and health inequalities 2018. Available from: http://www.healthscotland.scot/media/2186/child-poverty-impact-inequalities-2018.pdf [Accessed 29th May 2019].

22. Child Poverty Action Group. Child poverty facts and figures. Available from: http://www.cpag.org.uk/content/child-poverty-facts-and-figures [Accessed 19th March 2019].

23. PHE. Homes for health; infographics. 2017. Available from: https://app.box.com/s/4b5g55itg5d9by8dxun8j37mcbtokd2d [Accessed 14th March 2019].

24. Marmot Review Team. The health impacts of cold homes and fuel poverty. 2011. Available from: http://www.instituteofhealthequity.org/resources-reports/the-health-impacts-of-cold-homes-and-fuel-poverty [Accessed 15th March 2019].

25. WHO. Social inequalities and their influence on housing risk factors and health. 2009. Available from: http://www.euro.who.int/en/health-topics/environment-and-health/Housing-and-health/publications/2009/social-inequalities-and-their-influence-on-housing-risk-factors-and-health [Accessed 15th March 2019].

26. BRE. The cost of poor housing to the NHS. Available from: https://www.bregroup.com/bretrust/2017/08/21/real-cost-of-poor-housing/ [Accessed 15th March 2019].

27. NAO. Housing *in England: overview. A report by the Comptroller and Auditor General*. London: National Audit Office; 2017.

28. PHE. *Spatial Planning for Health. An Evidence Resource for Planning and Designing Healthier Places*. London: Public Health England; 2017. Available from: https://www.gov.uk/government/publications/spatial-planning-for-health-evidence-review [Accessed 19th March 2019].

29. Bambra C. *Work, Worklessness and the Political Economy of Health*. Oxford: Oxford University Press; 2011.

30. Mullainathan S, Shafir E. *Scarcity: Why Having Too Little Means So Much*. New York: Time Books, Henry Holt & Company LLC; 2013.

31. Layte R et al. A comparative analysis of the status anxiety hypothesis of socioeconomic inequalities in health based on 18,349 individuals in four countries and five cohort studies. *Scientific Reports*. 2019; 9: 796.

32. Fiorito G et al. Social adversity and epigenetic aging: A multi-cohort study on socioeconomic differences in peripheral blood DNA methylation. *Scientific Reports*. 7: 16266.

33. Brygen LO. Annual review of public health. 34: 49–60 (Volume publication date March 2013).

34. Loi M, Del Savio L, Stupka B. Social epigenetics and equality of opportunity. *Public Health Ethics*. 2013; 6(2): 142–153.

35. PHE. *Local Action on Health Inequalities Understanding and Reducing Ethnic Inequalities in Health*. London: Public Health England; 2018. Available from: https://assets.publishing.service.gov.uk/government/uploads/system/uploads/attachment_data/file/730917/local_action_on_health_inequalities.pdf [Accessed 14th March 2019].

36. Aldridge RW, Story A, Hwang SW et al. Morbidity and mortality in homeless individuals, prisoners, sex workers, and individuals with substance use disorders in high-income countries: A systematic review and meta-analysis. *The Lancet.* 2018; 391: 241–250.

37. Kings Fund. Tackling multiple unhealthy risk factors: Emerging lessons from practice. 2018. Available from: https://www.kings-fund.org.uk/publications/tackling-multiple-unhealthy-risk-factors [Accessed 19th March 2019].

38. Manchester Metropolitan University. *Saving Lives with Advice: The Impact of Advice on the Health and Wellbeing of Citizens.* Manchester: Advice Manchester Clients; 2015. Available from: https://www2.mmu.ac.uk/media/mmuacuk/content/images/qstep/Saving-Lives-With-Advice.pdf [Accessed 13th March 2019].

39. RCGP. *Health Inequalities.* London: Royal College of General Practitioners; 2015. Available from: https://www.rcgp.org.uk/policy/rcgp-policy-areas/health-inequalities.aspx [Accessed 19th March 2019].

3

A Multi-level Approach to Treating Social Risks to Health for Health Providers

GARY BLOCH AND RITIKA GOEL

If medicine is to fulfil her great task, then she must enter the political and social life.

Health providers have long recognized the link between poverty, social deprivation and adverse health outcomes. The most famous progenitor of this conversation in the modern era is the German pathologist Rudolph Virchow. He famously wrote, 'If medicine is to fulfil her great task, then she must enter the political and social life. Do we not always find the diseases of the populace traceable to defects in society?' [1].

The connection between poverty and poor health outcomes has been demonstrated across most chronic illnesses, acute illness, accidents and trauma. The connection is especially profound among children, who suffer from the negative health impacts of living in poverty from their time in the womb and into adulthood [2–5].

Poverty is intimately connected to other social determinants, such as housing, employment and identity-based determinants of health, such as race, gender and sexual orientation. People from groups impacted by intersecting determinants, such as racialized women, are disproportionately affected by the negative health impacts of poverty and social marginalization [6–7].

Lately, even large health organizations, including the British Medical Association, the Canadian Medical Association and the World Medical Association are increasingly focusing on a discussion of what front-line health providers can do to specifically address the social adversity their patients experience [8–10].

SETTING A FOUNDATION FOR ADDRESSING POVERTY

An anti-oppressive framework helps us to understand people's identities and experiences as shaped by broader social structures [24].

This approach directs us to understand the lived experiences of marginalized groups through working with marginalized communities and learning the history of marginalization in our societies and through literature, art, music and film.

Critical reflection pushes us to struggle with the existence of power structures in society, how they impact on health, practice and interventions [25]. This approach involves an examination of the role one plays in power structures and an examination of the specific power and privilege of health providers.

ADDRESSING POVERTY AT THE MICRO-LEVEL

Micro-level poverty interventions focus on how to address poverty in clinical practice [26].

Trauma-informed Care

Trauma-informed practice emphasizes creating physical and emotional safety for patients, especially in a care environment where power differentials between provider and patient are high [27]. This approach requires active listening, closely monitoring a patient's responses and ensuring the patient feels comfortable and empowered. The physical clinical environment can also signal safety through signage, art and a welcoming reception staff [26].

Individual Provider Interventions

A clinical tool on poverty (Figure 3.1) suggests using the question, 'Do you ever have difficulty making ends meet at the end of the month?' to screen for poverty [28]. The tool then guides providers to reduce risks, based on the evidence which links poverty with adverse health outcomes. It advises direct intervention into income by directing patients to high-yield income benefit programmes, for example, benefits for low-income families and people with disabilities.

Understanding a patient's background through a thorough social history is a crucial step towards addressing poverty and social determinants. The IF-IT-HELPS tool (Figure 3.2) provides a comprehensive approach [29]. Effective social history collection incorporates a narrative approach, using open-ended questions and a patient-directed structure.

Team-based Interventions

Interdisciplinary health teams can be oriented toward addressing social needs. Promising examples of team-based interventions include: income security specialists, medical-legal partnerships and food security programmes [30–31].

Successful team-based interventions often require strong partnerships with community organizations.

ADDRESSING POVERTY AT THE MESO-LEVEL

The meso-level of poverty intervention focuses on addressing poverty in our health care practice and in the communities in which we live and work.

The Collection and Use of Social Data

The collection and interpretation of data is foundational to any attempts at meso-level intervention.

Sociodemographic data can be used to understand the social risks facing individual and groups of patients, then to plan programmes and services targeting specific needs and to evaluate health and social outcomes of those programmes.

Data on community social profiles is often available through government-administered databases and public health units [11]. This has in some cases been gathered for specific use by health teams [12–13].

There is a growing movement among health teams to establish social profiles through direct questioning of patients using social risk assessment tools. When collection is adequate and accurate they offer insight into the social profile of a provider's practice [14]. Individual-level information can be made available to front-line health providers to aid in social intervention [15].

Equity-oriented Programme Evaluation

Applying an equity lens to programme planning and evaluation is necessary to ensure services

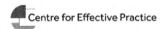 Centre for Effective Practice

Poverty: A Clinical Tool for Primary Care Providers

Poverty is not always apparent: In Ontario 20% of families live in poverty.[1]

(1) Screen Everyone

"Do you ever have difficulty making ends meet at the end of the month?"

(Sensitivity 98%, specificity 64% for living below the poverty line)[2]

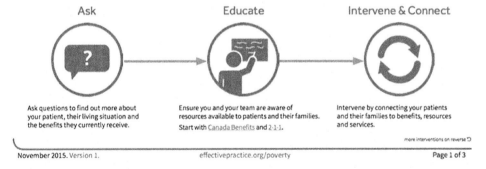

(2) Poverty is a Risk Factor

Consider:

New immigrants, Women, Aboriginals, and LGBTQ are among the highest risk groups.

Example 1:

If an otherwise healthy 35 year old comes to your office, without risk factors for diabetes other than living in poverty, you consider ordering a screening test for diabetes.

Example 2:

If an otherwise low risk patient who lives in poverty presents with chest pain, this elevates the pre-test probability of a cardiac source and helps determine how aggressive you are in ordering investigations.

Diabetes
Lower-income individuals are more likely to report having diabetes than higher-earning individuals (10% vs 5% in men, 8% vs. 3% in women).[3]

Cancer
Those in low income groups experience higher rates of lung, oral (OR 2.41) and cervical (RR 2.08) cancers.[5,10,13]

Chronic Disease
Individuals living in poverty experience an elevated risk of hypertension, arthritis, COPD, asthma, and having multiple chronic conditions.[1,4]

Poverty is a risk factor for many health conditions

Cardiovascular Disease
Those in the lowest income group experience circulatory conditions at a rate 17% higher than the Canadian average.[5]

Toxic Stress
Children from low income families are more likely to develop a condition that requires treatment by a physician later in life.[5]

Mental Illness
Those living below the poverty line experience depression at a rate 58% higher than the Canadian average.[6,7]

(3) Intervene

Ask Everyone: **"Have you filled out and sent in your tax forms?"**

- Ask questions to find out more about your patient, their employment, living situation, social supports and the benefits they receive. Tax returns are required to access many income security benefits: e.g. GST / HST credits, Child Benefits, working income tax benefits, and property tax credits. Connect your patients to Free Community Tax Clinics.
- Even people without official residency status can file returns.
- Drug Coverage: up to date tax filing required to access Trillium plan for those without Ontario Drug Benefits. Visit drugcoverage.ca for more options.

Ask	Educate	Intervene & Connect
Ask questions to find out more about your patient, their living situation and the benefits they currently receive.	Ensure you and your team are aware of resources available to patients and their families. Start with Canada Benefits and 2-1-1.	Intervene by connecting your patients and their families to benefits, resources and services.

more interventions on reverse ↻

November 2015. Version 1.   effectivepractice.org/poverty   Page 1 of 3

Figure 3.1 The clinical tool on poverty.

focus on the needs of the most socially vulnerable patients and community members.

Health equity impact assessment tools [16] guide providers through a step-by-step analysis of their community profile and the impact of their programmes on groups experiencing social vulnerability. The goal is to set a foundation for the development of programmes towards improving the outcomes of those most in need.

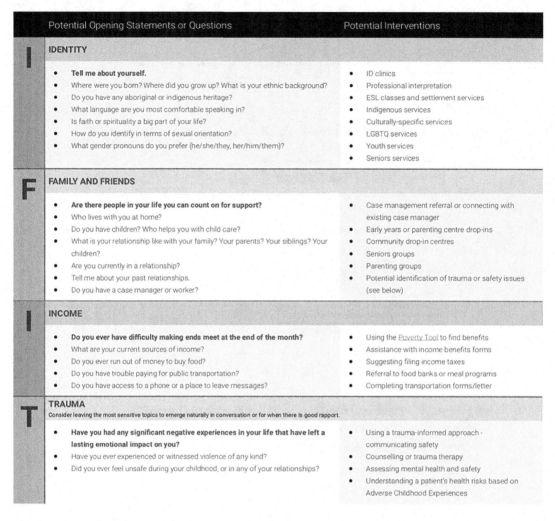

Potential Opening Statements or Questions	Potential Interventions
I — IDENTITY	
• **Tell me about yourself.** • Where were you born? Where did you grow up? What is your ethnic background? • Do you have any aboriginal or indigenous heritage? • What language are you most comfortable speaking in? • Is faith or spirituality a big part of your life? • How do you identify in terms of sexual orientation? • What gender pronouns do you prefer (he/she/they, her/him/them)?	• ID clinics • Professional interpretation • ESL classes and settlement services • Indigenous services • Culturally-specific services • LGBTQ services • Youth services • Seniors services
F — FAMILY AND FRIENDS	
• **Are there people in your life you can count on for support?** • Who lives with you at home? • Do you have children? Who helps you with child care? • What is your relationship like with your family? Your parents? Your siblings? Your children? • Are you currently in a relationship? • Tell me about your past relationships. • Do you have a case manager or worker?	• Case management referral or connecting with existing case manager • Early years or parenting centre drop-ins • Community drop-in centres • Seniors groups • Parenting groups • Potential identification of trauma or safety issues (see below)
I — INCOME	
• **Do you ever have difficulty making ends meet at the end of the month?** • What are your current sources of income? • Do you ever run out of money to buy food? • Do you have trouble paying for public transportation? • Do you have access to a phone or a place to leave messages?	• Using the Poverty Tool to find benefits • Assistance with income benefits forms • Suggesting filing income taxes • Referral to food banks or meal programs • Completing transportation forms/letter
T — TRAUMA Consider leaving the most sensitive topics to emerge naturally in conversation or for when there is good rapport.	
• **Have you had any significant negative experiences in your life that have left a lasting emotional impact on you?** • Have you ever experienced or witnessed violence of any kind? • Did you ever feel unsafe during your childhood, or in any of your relationships?	• Using a trauma-informed approach - communicating safety • Counselling or trauma therapy • Assessing mental health and safety • Understanding a patient's health risks based on Adverse Childhood Experiences

Figure 3.2 The IF-IT-HELPS framework.

Equity-oriented Community Engagement

The engagement of community members in health programme planning, evaluation and delivery is now considered essential to ensuring health services are focused on the most important community needs [17].

There are many ways in which community members' voices can be incorporated into health team planning and evaluation. These range from periodic consultation to incorporation of community members or patients into governance and decision-making structures (Table 3.1)

Community engagement needs to be sensitive to particularities of team structures and goals. A useful guide to incorporating a community engagement approach into health teams was developed by the Boston Public Health Commission [18].

ADDRESSING POVERTY AT THE MACRO-LEVEL

While the interventions above may directly improve the health of patients by addressing upstream social determinants, a true reduction in health inequities will require a change in the social policies and structures which allow those inequities to persist.

Primary care providers have a strong history of involvement in advocating for social policy. In

HOUSING

H

- **Where are you staying right now?**
- When did you last have a stable place to stay?
- Do you need help finding housing?
- What is your housing like?

- Referral to emergency shelter
- Drop-in services
- Housing worker
- Legal clinic
- Tailoring care to challenges of homelessness

EMPLOYMENT

E

- **Are you working right now?**
- What do you do for work? What other kinds of work have you done in the past?
- Do you have benefits such as drug coverage?

- Resume-writing services
- Employment counselling services
- Ensuring medications are covered or low-cost

EDUCATION

- **How far did you go in your education?**
- How did you do in school?
- Do you have any trouble reading or writing?

- Literacy classes
- Tailoring patient information and communication
- Developmental assessment and services

LEGAL

L

- **Do you have any legal issues you need help with?**
- What is your current immigration status in Canada?
- Have you had contact with the legal system?

- Legal clinics
- Immigration support services

PERSONAL SAFETY

P

- **Do you have any safety concerns?**
- Do you feel safe in your relationship?
- Has your partner ever hurt you? Your children?
- Do you feel safe in your home / neighbourhood?

- Violence Against Women services
- Crisis helplines
- Legal services
- Counselling
- Support groups

SUBSTANCES

S

- **Do you smoke? How many cigarettes a day?**
- How often do you drink alcohol? How many drinks on average?
- Do you use any recreational drugs? What about in the past?

- Motivational interviewing and pharmacological therapies
- Support groups and counselling
- Inpatient and outpatient rehab and programs
- Detox and harm reduction services

SEXUAL HEALTH

- **Are you sexually active?**
- How many sexual partners have you had in the past six months?
- What kinds of sexual activities do you usually engage in? Vaginal intercourse? Anal sex? Oral sex?
- Have you ever had any sexually transmitted infections?

- STI screening based on exposure history
- Contraceptive counselling
- Barrier protection counselling

Content by Dr. Ritika Goel, MD, MPH, CCFP

Figure 3.2 (Continued)

Canada, Health Providers Against Poverty [19] and the Decent Work and Health Network [20] were formed by health providers in collaboration with people with lived experience and advocacy organizations to address poverty and 'precarious work' as threats to health.

Health providers write newspaper articles, hold press conferences, sign open letters, lobby elected representatives, perform deputations to parliamentary committees, write policy papers, join rallies and engage in creative actions. One of the authors was invited to participate in a governmental working group to redesign the income security system in Ontario [21].

Health provider organizations also engage in systemic advocacy. The Ontario College of Family Physicians' Committee on Poverty and Health focused on educating primary care providers and medical trainees in addition to establishing partnerships with health and social service organizations. The College of Family Physicians of Canada's Social Accountability Working Group [22] seeks to bring social accountability to the core of family medicine [23].

Health providers bring an evidence-based health equity lens which assists in ongoing efforts to direct policy change toward improving the social determinants of health.

Table 3.1 Community-based Decision Making

	Inform	Consult	Involve	Collaborate	Empower
Public participation goal	To provide the public with balanced and objective information to assist them in understanding the problem, alternatives and/or solutions.	To obtain public feedback on analysis, alternatives and/or decisions.	To work directly with the public throughout the process to ensure that public concerns and aspirations are consistently understood and considered.	To partner with the public in each aspect of the decision-making process including the development of alternatives and the identification of the preferred solution.	To place final decision making in the hands of the public.
Promise to the public	We will keep you informed.	We will keep you informed, listen to and acknowledge concerns and aspirations and provide feedback on how public input influenced decisions.	We will work with you to ensure that your concerns and aspirations are directly reflected in the alternatives developed and provide feedback on how public input influenced decisions.	We will look to you for advice and innovation in formulating solutions and incorporate your advice and recommendations into decisions to the maximum extent possible.	We will implement what you decide.

REFERENCES

1. Virchow R. Report on the typhus epidemic in Upper Silesia. In Rather LJ (ed.), *Collected Essays by Rudolph Virchow on Public Health and Epidemiology*, Volume 1. Canton, MA: Science History Publications; 1848/1985, pp. 205–319.

2. Bierman AS, Ahman F, Angus J et al. Burden of illness. In Bierman AS (ed.), *Project for an Ontario Women's Health Evidence-Based Report: Volume 1*. Toronto; 2009.

3. Singh GK, Miller BA, Hankey BF, Edwards BK. *Area Socioeconomic Variations in US Cancer Incidence, Mortality, Stage, Treatment, and Survival, 1975–1999*. NCI Cancer Surveillance Monograph Series, No. 4. NIH Publication No. 03-5417. Bethesda, MD: National Cancer Institute; 2003.

4. Fryers T, Melzer D, Jenkins, R. Social inequalities and the common mental disorders: A systematic review of the evidence. *Soc Psychiatry Psychiatr Epidemiol*. 2003; 38: 229–237.

5. Lightman E, Mitchell A, Wilson B. *Poverty Is Making Us Sick: A Comprehensive Survey of Income and Health in Canada*. Wellesley Institute; 2008.

6. Canada Without Poverty. 2019. Available from: http://www.cwp-csp.ca/poverty/just-the-facts/#demo [Accessed 1st June 2019].

7. Williams Institute. New patterns of poverty in the lesbian, gay, and bisexual community. 2013. Available from: https://williamsinstitute.law.ucla.edu/research/census-lgbt-demographics-studies/lgbt-poverty-update-june-2013/ [Accessed 1st June 2019].

8. Canadian Medical Association. *Physicians and Health Equity: Opportunities in Practice*. Ottawa: Health Care Transformation in Canada; 2013. Available from: http://healthcaretransformation.ca/2013/03/physicians-and-health-equity-opportunities-in-practice/ [Accessed 1st June 2019].

9. *Social Determinants of Health — What Doctors Can Do*. London (UK): British Medical Association; 2011.

10. Institute of Health Equity and World Medical Association. Doctors for Health Equity. The role of the World Medical Association, national medical associations and doctors in addressing the social determinants of health and health equity. 2016. Available from: http://www.instituteofhealthequity.org/Content/FileManager/wma-ihe-report_-doctors-for-health-equity-2016.pdf [Accessed 1st June 2019].

11. See, for example: http://www.toronto-healthprofiles.ca.

12. Hughes LS, Phillips RL, DeVoe JE, Bazemore AW. Community vital signs: Taking the pulse of the community while caring for patients. *J Am Board Fam Med.* 2016; 29(3): 419–422.

13. Beck AF, Sandel MT, Ryan PH, Kahn RS. Mapping neighborhood health geomarkers to clinical care decisions to promote equity in child health. *Health Aff.* 2017; 36(6): 999–1005.

14. Pinto AD, Glattstein-Young G, Mohamed A, Bloch G, Leung FH, Glazier RH. Building a foundation to reduce health inequities: Routine collection of sociodemographic data in primary care. *J Am Board Fam Med.* 2016; 29(3): 348–355.

15. Gottlieb L, Sandel M, Adler NE. Collecting and applying data on social determinants of health in health care settings. *JAMA Int Med.* 2013; 173(11): 1017–1020; Ontario Ministry of Health and Long-Term Care. *Health Equity Impact Assessment Tool.* Toronto, ON: Author. 2012. Available from the MOHLTC website: http://www.health.gov.on.ca/en/pro/programs/heia/tool.aspx [Accessed 1st June 2019].

16. Kwon SC, Tandon SD, Islam N, Riley L, Trinh-Shevrin C. Applying a community-based participatory research framework to patient and family engagement in the development of patient-centered outcomes research and practice. *Transl Behav Med.* 2018; 8(5): 683–691.

17. Boston Public Health Commission. *Community Engagement Plan 2016–2019.* Boston, MA. 2016. Available from: http://www.bphc.org/aboutus/community-engagement/Documents/Boston%20 Public%20Health%20Commission%27s%20 Community%20Engagement%20Plan.Final.pdf [Accessed 1st June 2019].

18. See: www.healthprovidersagainstpoverty.ca

19. See: https://decentworkandhealth.org

20. Ontario Ministry of Community and Social Services. Income security: A roadmap for change. Toronto, ON. 2017. Available from: www.ontario.ca/insomesecurity. [Accessed 1st June 2019].

21. Meili R, Buchman S. Social accountability: At the heart of family medicine. *Can Fam Physician.* 2013; 59(4): 335–336.

22. Canadian Medical Association. *Health Care in Canada: What Makes Us Sick?.* Canadian Medical Association Town Hall Report. Ottawa (ON): Canadian Medical Association; 2013.

23. Nzira V, Williams P. Useful concepts in anti-oppression. In *Anti-oppressive Practice in Health and Social Care.* London: SAGE Publications; 2019, pp. 21–40. doi: 10.4135/9781446213759.n2.

24. Ng S, Kinsella A, Friesen F, Hodges B. Reclaiming a theoretical orientation to reflection in medical education research: A critical narrative review. *Med Educ.* 2015; 49(5): 461–475.

25. Goel R, Buchman S, Meili R, Woollard R. Social accountability at the micro level. One patient at a time. *Can Fam Physician* 2016; 62: 287–290. (Eng), 299–302 (Fr).

26. BC Provincial Mental Health and Substance Use Planning Council (May 2013). Trauma-informed practice guide. British Columbia. 2013. Available from: https://www.homelesshub.ca/resource/trauma-informed-practice-guide [Accessed 1st June 2019].

27. Bloch G. Poverty: A clinical tool for primary care providers. Centre for Effective Practice. 2016. Available from: https://cep.health/clinical-products/poverty-a-clinical-tool-for-primary-care-providers/ [Accessed 1st June 2019].

28. Goel R. A Social History Tool using the IF-IT-HELPS mnemonic. Centre for Effective Practice. 2018. Available from: https://cep.health/download-file/1542915867.061284-96/ [Accessed 1st June 2019].

29. Jones MK, Bloch G, Pinto AD. A novel income security intervention to address poverty in a primary care setting: A retrospective chart review. *BMJ Open*. 2017; 7(8): e014270.

30. Sandel M, Hansen M, Kahn R, Lawton E, Paul E, Parker V,... Zuckerman B. Medical-legal partnerships: Transforming primary care by addressing the legal needs of vulnerable populations. *Health Aff*. 2010; 29(9): 1697–1705.

31. Beck AF, Henize AW, Kahn RS, Reiber KL, Young JJ, Klein MD. Forging a pediatric primary care-community partnership to support food-insecure families. *Pediatrics*. peds-2014.

4

A Tale of Two Cities – Hull and York

BEN JACKSON AND MARK PURVIS

It's the workforce, stupid.

It's evident that the main factor sustaining any healthcare is the investment in the people that deliver care. Technology does not care for people, buildings do not care for people. People care for people. Inequities in workforce distribution contribute to inequities in access to healthcare. Such inequities matter to all of us, contributing to worsening health outcomes in mental health, obesity rates and overall life expectancy [1]. We know that roughly 70% of NHS investment goes on workforce [2]. How this gets spent matters!

In Bill Clinton's 1992 US presidential campaign he coined the phrase 'it's the economy, stupid' to underline the core importance of the economy to almost all other political issues and challenges. In health and social care, if we are talking about quality, outcomes, effectiveness, efficiency, patient satisfaction, safety, doing the right job, doing the job right, reducing iatrogenic harm, reducing costs, improving care, preserving dignity or being more kind, these discussions are all underpinned by 'getting the workforce right'. This is sometimes described as getting the right people in the right place with the right attributes at the right time to meet the needs of the population served. We cannot think of a meaningful health and social care topic that is not underpinned by workforce. The same holds true for health inequalities – 'It's the workforce, stupid' (Figure 4.1).

Good health outcomes find their foundations in good social care and self-care.

If health were a cake the big, fat base layers would be self-care and social care, with much of that social care made up by an unquantified volume delivered by an informal workforce of unpaid carers and relatives. Every morning the population gets up and pays attention to its health and care needs: from meeting essential needs like being fed and watered, through meeting mundane needs such as getting dressed, towards so called 'higher needs' such as finding fulfilment (or internet access). Often individuals need help and the vast majority of that help is delivered by these layers of our care cake. Without these first layers, there is no cake! (Figure 4.2)

The next tier of the cake is primary care: where people come to make sense of their health journey, for more help and support accessing care. Secondary care is the icing on our cake and tertiary care are the cherries.

Yet when baking the care cake, we often focus on the cherries and not the base of the cake. We often assume that as long as we have sufficient cherries, the base of the cake will look after itself. We were once told 'there will always be some people who don't want to work in hospitals', as if the primary and social care workforce is somehow an inevitable by-product of producing a secondary and tertiary care workforce.

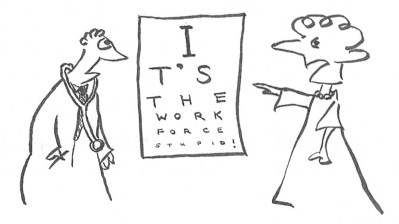

Figure 4.1 It's the workforce, stupid!

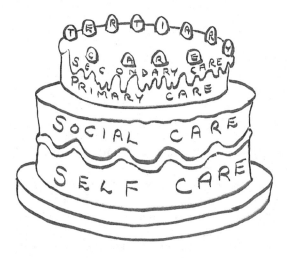

Figure 4.2 The healthcare cake.

That is not our perspective. Our perspective, as authors, is that of primary care clinicians; of course, this is a source of bias, our chapter is about primary care. Nevertheless, we believe that the cake needs to be baked from the base up.

WHY PRIMARY CARE?

There are compelling reasons why the primary care workforce is a key indicator of health inequalities. Evidence has shown for populations as a whole, improved primary care leads to improved quality of life and a reduction in hospitalisation for chronic health conditions [3, 4]. The rationale is that as general ill health is more prevalent in socio-economically deprived communities, healthcare

which focuses on populations rather than specific diseases and is accessible will more likely reduce overall health inequalities. An important additional factor here is that as primary care is also less costly than secondary care, making decisions to provide a more equitable distribution of services across wider geographical areas is easier for commissioners and providers of healthcare.

WORKFORCE CAPACITY, CAPABILITY AND ORGANISATIONAL RESILIENCE

Whether we look at the numbers of the workforce (capacity); the attributes of that workforce – their skills, knowledge, attitudes and other characteristics (capability); or the ability of the workforce to thrive in challenging and changing environments (organisational resilience), we find variation. This variation impacts most keenly on our areas with greatest healthcare needs, in particular in relation to comorbidities, as demonstrated by Mercer et al [5]. In the UK, we suggest that areas most affected are remote rural, deprived urban and coastal communities.

It is in these areas where despite greater needs and more complex work we have fewer staff [6, 7] that providers are more susceptible to workforce risks, particularly as it is often healthcare workers who have experienced least preparation who gravitate to these areas of greater risk and lower governance. The challenge in designing a system is to address all three of these workforce areas. It's not just about the numbers (Figure 4.3).

Imagine a primary care provider facing a challenge in all three areas [8]. Perhaps an organisation with an increasing list size in a deprived area which is unable to recruit or retain staff. This organisation develops a reliance on locum and agency staff. A knock-on effect is the diminution in the continuity of care provided. The high cost of these agency staff makes the practice less financially viable. A vicious spiral is created for existing staff with a predictable effect on retention throughout the whole practice team.

These vicious spirals can be contagious. Even a practice recruiting and retaining high quality and appropriate staff in sufficient numbers to meet the needs of the population it serves, and perceiving itself as resilient with a robust workforce succession plan, can quickly be caught up in this spiral if a nearby practice closes, displacing patients to them. Therefore, it's not just about supporting individual providers at risk but about supporting the whole landscape of provision. Once the dominoes start falling, it takes a lot more effort to recover the system than it would to prevent the first dominoes from falling.

THE RICH GET RICHER

Our perception as clinicians in Yorkshire and the Humber for the past two to three decades is that we have worked through two very different

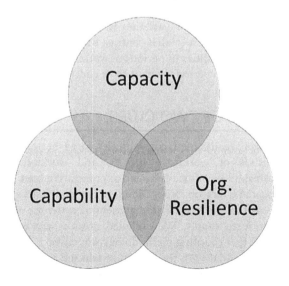

Figure 4.3 Capacity, capability and organisational resilience are interrelated and overlapping.

periods regarding investment in the primary care workforce. Following the 10-year period after the Labour election in 1997 there was a focus on building capacity and primary care workforce growth. After the crash in 2008, austerity measures led to a period of primary care workforce constraint.

The first period, from 1999 to 2008, was an era of investment in public services. Over this period NHS spending increased by around 4% per year with an emphasis on primary care. New contractual arrangements – Personal Medical Services (established in 2002) and Quality and Outcomes frameworks (established in 2004) – also provided overall extra investment in General Practice.

The second period following the financial crash of 2008 and the resulting austerity measures restricted public spending from 2009 to 2018. The graph below shows the significant differences in investment during these periods (Figure 4.4).

Nationally, the GP workforce grew in the decade up to 2009 with average UK numbers of patients per full-time equivalent (FTE) GP falling, between 1999 and 2009, from 1,791 to 1,684. From 2009 to 2018, however, the number of patients per FTE GP rose from 1,684 to 2,032. (Table 4.1)

WHY ONLY GP NUMBERS?

Quite apart from the difficulties of studying capability and organisational resilience, even studies limited to capacity (numbers of healthcare workers) of the primary care workforce are made more difficult by variations in skill mix between different provider organisations. Looking at single markers, such as the number of full-time equivalent GPs or family physicians per 1,000 patients can give an insight into the whole primary care workforce, but there is a high noise to signal ratio.

As a result, the complexity of the NHS as an organisation and the significant changes in the structures involved in co-ordinating services could make any investigation excessively complicated; we are not suggesting that we are providing a robust study that excludes the various possible confounding factors. In order to minimise such issues, we have kept our proxy measure of investment in GP teams serving primary care to that understood to be relatively robust: the number of patients per FTE fully registered GPs in the population described [9–11].

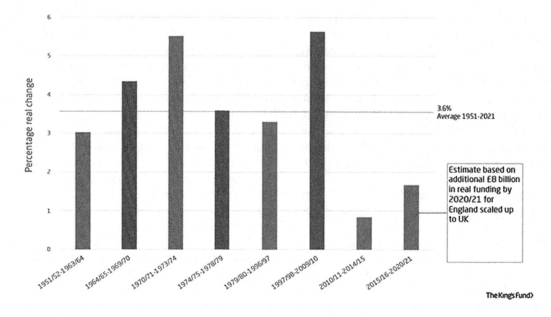

Figure 4.4 Real annual average changes in UK NHS spending, Kings fund.

Table 4.1 Average Numbers of Registered Patients per FTE GP

YEAR	Good times		Bad times
	1999	2009	2018
Registered patients per full-time equivalent GP (exc. registrars, retainers and locums).	1791	1684	2032

Source: NHS Digital – *full-time equivalent figures are used rather than headcount due to changes in participation over time.

We have deliberately excluded GP trainees, GP retainers and locums as the way these have been counted is likely to have varied and the substantive GP numbers better reflect the state of resilience and capability of the service provided to the community.

EXISTING EVIDENCE

Mercer et al. describe poorer access to care with less time to manage the increased burden of ill health and multimorbidity in poor communities [12]. Goddard et al. describe such inequalities increasing following changes to the regulations for new GPs in 2002 with new GPs settling in areas with clean air and easy access to public amenities [13]. Conversely Asaria et al. described how in a single geographical area there was a reduction in inequality from 2004–2005 to 2014–2015 in GP workforce [14].

Regarding investment and funding into primary care itself, more recent studies show us that the current funding arrangements in Scotland perpetuate the inverse care law rather than remediate it, and in England population health needs are poor predictors for variation in investment [15–17]. None of these studies contrast what happens to health inequalities in periods of workforce growth compared to periods of workforce constraint.

A TALE OF TWO CITIES

How have different communities fared between periods of workforce growth and workforce restraint? We took a Bayesian approach. We interrogated data from NHS Digital in two contrasting areas that we knew had experienced extremes of workforce supply. We excluded areas where we knew that counting methodology was suspect. We were familiar with the two areas selected through our work in postgraduate training in the region. One centred on Hull and the other on the Vale of York. Data was only available on NHS Digital from 2005 onwards so we were limited to examining 2005–2009 during the 'good times'. We recognised the smaller the area examined, the more marked the differences can be. For example, if you look at east Hull compared to central York the differences in workforce supply are greater, but we were constrained by NHS Digital data to look at larger areas due to the merger of PCTs into CCGs. There are pockets of relative affluence in Hull and relative deprivation in the Vale of York, but through personal knowledge of the areas themselves we feel these are minimal (Figure 4.5).

THE POOR GET POORER

Comparing Hull and York we found that in Hull the number of registered patients per FTE GPs per 1,000 registered patients rose slightly in 'the good times' (2005–2009), whilst in York the number of registered patients per FTE GPs fell slightly in the same period.

In 'the bad times' (2009–2018), as the number of patients per FTE GPs rose, both north Yorkshire and Hull experienced a rise in patients per FTE GP. However, whilst the average patients per FTE GP rose 16% in north Yorkshire, it rose 33% in Hull. There may be selection bias here, but if true across the UK we would conclude that in the good times

the rich get richer and in the bad times the poor get poorer. The data we examined does not shed light on the causes for the rich getting richer and the poor getting poorer. We do not know whether York was better at recruitment or retention or both (Table 4.2).

SOLUTIONS – DEEP, PERSISTENT, RELENTLESS

To counter such a profound divergence in resources, in order to not just mitigate, but to correct such inequalities requires a deep, persistent and relentless focus on commissioning and funding services in a way which supports some areas of the primary care system more than others. Such an approach is espoused by the Deep End general practice movement, originating in Scotland but now spreading around the world [18].

Michael Marmot described the concept of proportionate universalism, in which there is recognition that the challenges of providing a universal system of care are greater in some areas, requiring extra focus and effort as needs increase [19]. For instance, in order to reverse the divergence in the

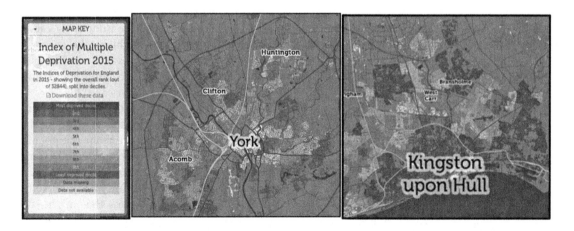

Figure 4.5 Illustration of deprivation in Hull and York.

Table 4.2 Change in Number of Patients per FTE GP in York and Hull 2005–2009 and 2009–2018

Region	Good times			Bad times		
	2005	2009	% change	2009	2018	% change
HULL	1838	1916	+4.0	1916	2556	+33
Ratio (Hull/York)	1.12	1.17		1.17	1.36	
YORK	1638	1624	−0.9	1624	1885	+16

number of patients per FTE, more than 50% of our newly qualified GPs would need to go to work in our more deprived areas.

But, as the saying goes, there is a 'well-known solution to every human problem – neat, plausible, and wrong' [20].

NO MAGIC BULLETS

There are no simple solutions or magic bullets to address the maldistribution of workforce capacity, capability and resilience. However, the literature describes three broad and overlapping strategies to improve the maldistribution of workforce [21] (Figure 4.6)

- Posting people to areas of deprivation might be described as *coercive.*
- Promising additional resources – a 'golden hello' or additional CPD opportunities might be *allocative/rational.*
- Setting minimum and maximum workforce thresholds might be a *normative* approach.

We must utilise ALL three strategies, adopting them and adapting them to local circumstances. Different strategies need to be used at different times and for different contexts. During times of relative growth, when the workforce is optimistic, incentive programmes may have more scope to nudge the natural system of allocation and

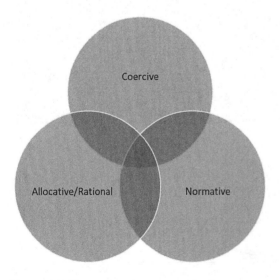

Figure 4.6 Illustrating the connection between the different approaches to workforce strategies.

encourage people to opt to work in more deprived areas. Almost all clinically trained staff want to make a difference to the world; where best to make that difference than where the needs are greatest? At other times, when workforce constraints are at their greatest, the system as a whole needs to provide greater direction, through strategic decisions on investment which recognise the dangers to the whole team of not supporting the players who are under greatest pressure.

Aligning lots of different actions across all three strategic areas is more likely to work than relying on a single intervention. How would this be achieved? Research suggests the resilience of GPs who work in such areas is maintained by the team and infrastructure they work with, not simply through some inner strength [22]. Encouraging GPs to work in deprived areas is therefore about much more than the 'golden handshakes' and financial incentives they receive, it's about co-creating the support and resources to allow whole primary care teams to flourish within these communities.

DEEP SOLUTIONS

We believe it is not enough to tackle variations in workforce resilience, capability and capacity, we must go deep to tackle the underlying causes of these variations. This might be the approach adopted by champions such as those in Bromley-by-Bow, London, who seek to build community capacity across the layers of our cake [23].

Another strategy might be to improve diversity and inclusion in our workforce. It is an admirable ambition to draw a workforce from the population it serves. This workforce could have a greater and more nuanced understanding of the context of healthcare for their community and could offer different insights into solutions that might succeed, including prevention and re-enablement solutions. But in order to draw a workforce from a population where educational attainment at school may be lower, you would need to improve education provision, recognise any equivalence of experience against academic attainment and perhaps select for academic potential rather than on past academic performance. This would require a radical rethink of selection to health and social care careers.

We need to look at where these doctors (along with other clinical staff) come from. Widening access to medicine to allow members of all communities to train and work as doctors is important. In a retrospective study of applications to UK medical schools from 2009–12, only 7.6% of accepted medical school places went to applicants residing in the two most deprived postcodes nationally [24]. Though the mobility of the workforce has increased dramatically, it is apparent that doctors trained from – and in – particular areas (e.g. rural and remote) are more likely to return to work in these areas [25, 26].

And let's be clear. It's not just about doctors. The data described earlier was used as a proxy measure for the wider team: healthcare assistants, nurses and advanced practitioners, receptionists, administrators and care navigators. The issue is about inequalities in access to good quality primary care, not simply to GPs. With the impending breakdown of services to some communities, the answer will also depend upon teams transforming into resilient multidisciplinary teams, working collaboratively with the communities they serve to work out ways of providing services that suit them as efficiently as possible. There will be many challenges, for example preserving continuity. Such a transformation increases the number of staff in face-to-face roles, building a team on the foundations of the most junior members of staff whilst providing a clear ethos, culture and understanding of the principles of generalist care within the team. We have previously described this transformation in the form of a Dalek [27] (Figure 4.7).

It may be necessary to differentially invest in career-long continuing professional development and support for the workforce serving a more deprived population, recognising the higher opportunity costs of supporting people working in challenging environments.

If a barrier to attracting and retaining a high-quality workforce to an area is a lack of spouse/partner employment opportunities, you might need to improve local employment opportunities outside healthcare.

A good transport infrastructure, cleaner air and access to good local amenities also play a role in recruitment and retention of workforce.

PERSISTENT SOLUTIONS

The effort required to sustain a capable, resilient workforce in sufficient numbers to meet a population's needs is not a one-off effort. It is not a see-saw of either (a) improved recruitment or (b) better retention but a climbing frame of both (a) and (b).

Individuals and providing organisations are not insulated from the system in which they work.

This aim must persist over time, across geographies and through organisational and sector boundaries (our cake again!). The purpose is to reduce inequalities by addressing the health and social care workforce despite changes in political administrations and the organisation of how that health and social care is delivered. How often have we seen the charade of good work having to

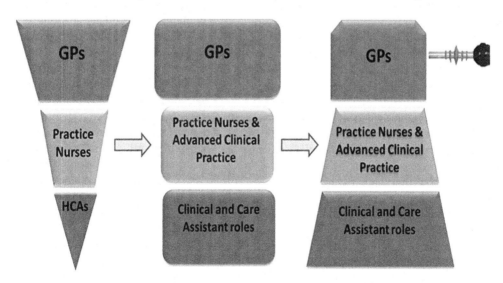

Figure 4.7 The 'Dalek' transformation in primary care workforce.

be retrofitted into the policy of the day: a Darzi review, a QIPP initiative, a vanguard, a sustainability and transformation plan, an integrated care system or a 'test bed' site [28–32].

Earlier we referenced the abolition of the medical practices committee as a factor contributing to workforce maldistribution. The underlying purpose of this committee – to manage the distribution of general practice services – was handed to the Family Health Services Authority (FHSA). The purpose was lost along with the skills and infrastructure. Successive re-organisations have diluted the mission to homoeopathic levels!

Change drivers may come and go, but purpose must persist.

RELENTLESS SOLUTIONS

It is not enough to go deeper and persist with our workforce efforts. A reduction of health inequalities must become our *meaning and mission*, it must be the very air that health and social care lives and breathes – no irony intended (as clean air is both a determinant of health and marker of workforce distribution) [13]. It must become meaning, mission and culture. Everything we do should be aligned to this. Everything should be tested against this.

We need to move from a state that is sometimes pathological – asking 'Why waste our time on workforce solutions to health inequalities' or reactive – solving workforce crises as and when they arise – towards a more proactive and generative stance. This will require new ways of measuring cultural change with respect to how programmes address inequalities.

What does this all mean? Imagine if these widening inequalities were allowed to accumulate over a further 10 years. Access to any primary care services would become a virtual impossibility for a growing proportion of people in our most deprived communities. Given the evidence for the effectiveness of primary care in supporting the health system, we can predict that our National Health Service would cease to exist for many.

We are aware that this chapter is light on solutions, certainly from the perspective of those working in our hardest pressed communities who need help now! We do not apologise for advocating co-production rather than prescription. However, we hope that our chapter will provoke the realisation that, if you have a strategy to address health inequalities and this strategy does not encompass workforce, you have no strategy!

REFERENCES

1. Wilkinson R, Pickett KE. *Spirit Level. Why Equality Is Better for Everyone.* London: Penguin; 2010.
2. House of Commons Health Committee. *Workforce Planning Fourth Report of Session 2006-07* [Internet]. London; 2007 [cited 2018 Jul 22]. Available from: https://publications.parliament.uk/pa/cm200607/cmselect/cmhealth/171/171i.pdf
3. Starfield B. State of the art in research on equity in health. *J Health Polit Policy Law.* 2006;31(1).
4. Starfield B. Primary care: An increasingly important contributor to effectiveness, equity, and efficiency of health services. SESPAS report 2012. *Gac Sanit.* 2012;26(Suppl. 1):20–6.
5. Payne RA, Abel GA, Guthrie B, Mercer SW. The effect of physical multimorbidity, mental health conditions and socioeconomic deprivation on unplanned admissions to hospital: A retrospective cohort study. *Can Med Assoc J* [Internet]. 2013 Mar 19 [cited 2016 Aug 30];185(5):E221–8. Available from: http://www.cmaj.ca/cgi/doi/10.1503/cmaj.121349
6. Walton E, Ahmed A, Mathers N. Influences of Socioeconomic Deprivation on GP's decisions to refer patients to cardiology: A qualitative study. *Br J Gen Pract.* 2018;1–9.
7. Barnett K, Mercer SWS, Norbury M, Watt GG, Wyke S, Guthrie B et al. Epidemiology of multimorbidity and implications for health care, research, and medical education: A cross-sectional study. *Lancet* (London, England) [Internet]. 2012 [cited 2017 Jan 2];380(9836):37–43. Available from: http://www.ncbi.nlm.nih.gov/pubmed/22579043
8. Rittel HWJ, Webber MM. Dilemmas in a general theory of planning. *Policy Sci.* 1973;4(2):155–69.
9. GP in-depth review. London; 2013.
10. Plint S. GP Taskforce. Securing the future GP workforce. Delivering the mandate on GP expansion. GP taskforce final report. 2014;(March):1–63. Available from: http://hee.nhs.uk/wp-content/uploads/sites/321/2014/07/GP-Taskforce-report.pdf
11. Charlesworth A, Firth Z, Gershlick B, Watt T, Johnson P, Kelly E et al. Securing the future: Funding health and social care to the 2030s.

The Health Foundation The Institute for Fiscal Studies [Internet]. 2018 [cited 2018 Sep 14]. Available from: http://www.ifs.org.uk

12. Mercer SW, Watt GCM. The inverse care law: Clinical primary care encounters in deprived and affluent areas of Scotland. *Ann Fam Med.* 2007;5(6):503–10.

13. Goddard M, Gravelle H, Hole A, Marini G. Where did all the GPs go? Increasing supply and geographical equity in England and Scotland. *J Health Serv Res Policy* [Internet]. 2010 [cited 2018 Sep 7];15(1):28–35. Available from: https://www.york.ac.uk/media/che/documents/papers/WheredidalltheGPsgo.pdf

14. Asaria M, Cookson R, Fleetcroft R, Ali S. Unequal socioeconomic distribution of the primary care workforce: Whole-population small area longitudinal study. *BMJ Open* [Internet]. 2016;6(1):e008783. Available from: http://www.pubmedcentral.nih.gov/articlerender.fcgi?artid=4735310&tool=pmcentrez&rendertype=abstract

15. Tudor Hart J. The Inverse Care Law. *Lancet.* 1971;(7696):405–12.

16. McLean G, Guthrie B, Mercer SW, Watt GCM. General practice funding underpins the persistence of the inverse care law: Cross-sectional study in Scotland. *Br J Gen Pract.* 2015;65(641):e799–805.

17. Levene LS, Baker R, Wilson A, Walker N, Boomla K, Bankart MJG. Population health needs as predictors of variations in NHS practice payments: A cross-sectional study of English general practices in 2013–2014 and 2014–2015. *Br J Gen Pract* [Internet]. 2016 Jan 1 [cited 2017 Jan 12];67(654):e10–9. Available from: http://www.ncbi.nlm.nih.gov/pubmed/27872085

18. Watt G. GPs at the deep end. *Br J Gen Pract* [Internet]. 2011;61(582):66–7. Available from: http://bjgp.org/lookup/doi/10.3399/bjgp11X549090

19. Marmot M. Fair society, Healthy Lives [Internet]. 2010. Available from: https://www.gov.uk/dfid-research-outputs/fair-society-healthy-lives-the-marmot-review-strategic-review-of-health-inequalities-in-england-post-2010

20. H.L. Menken. *Prejudices Second Series* [Internet]. New York: Borzoi; 1920 [cited 2018 Dec 2]. Available from: https://dspace.gipe.ac.in/xmlui/bitstream/handle/10973/22764/GIPE-002119.pdf?sequence=3&isAllowed=y

21. Sibbald B. Putting general practitioners where they are needed : An overview of strategies to correct maldistribution. National Primary Care Research and Development Centre October 2005.

22. Eley E, Jackson B, Burton C, Walton E. Professional resilience in GPs working in areas of socioeconomic deprivation: A qualitative study in primary care. *Br J Gen Pract* [Internet]. 2018 Oct 8 [cited 2018 Oct 19];bjgp18X699401. Available from: http://www.ncbi.nlm.nih.gov/pubmed/30297436

23. Catford J. Social entrepreneurs are vital for health promotion - but they need supportive environments too. *Health Promot Int* [Internet]. 1998;13(2):95–7. Available from: http://search.ebscohost.com/login.aspx?direct=true&db=cin20&AN=105931652&site=ehost-live

24. Steven K, Dowell J, Jackson C, Guthrie B. Fair access to medicine? Retrospective analysis of UK medical schools application data 2009–2012 using three measures of socioeconomic status. *BMC Med Educ* [Internet]. 2016 Dec 13 [cited 2018 Oct 12];16(1):11. Available from: http://bmcmededuc.biomedcentral.com/articles/10.1186/s12909-016-0536-1

25. Henry JA, Edwards BJ, Crotty B. Why do medical graduates choose rural careers? *Rural Remote Health.* 2009;9(1):1083.

26. Laven G, Wilkinson D. Rural doctors and rural backgrounds: How strong is the evidence? A systematic review. *Aust J Rural Health.* 2003;11(6):277–84.

27. Jackson B. General practice, the integrated care system and allied health professionals [Internet]. 2018 [cited 2018 Oct 23]. Available from: https://www.healthandcaretogether-syb.co.uk/application/files/8615/2507/7826/SYB_Primary_Care_Workforce_Group_from_Dr_Ben_Jackson.pdf

28. NHS England. Integrated care systems. [Internet]. NHS England website. 2018. Available from: https://www.england.nhs.uk/integratedcare/integrated-care-systems/

29. NHS England. Sustainability and transformation partnerships (STPs) [Internet]. NHS England website. 2017. Available from: https://www.england.nhs.uk/stps/

30. NHS England. NHS Test Beds programme [Internet]. NHS England website. 2018. Available from: https://www.england.nhs.uk/ourwork/innovation/test-beds/

31. NHS England. New Care Models: Vanguards – developing a blueprint for the future of the NHS and care services. 2016.

32. Darzi A. High quality care for all. High quality care for all NHS next stage review final report. 2008.

PART 2

Knowledge and Skills

5

Our Patients and the Benefit System

LISA CHATTINGTON

This process is traumatic for patients and difficult to navigate.

The UK benefit system can be complicated at the best of times and it has been constantly evolving in recent years as successive governments implement change. These issues should not detract from a simple fact: depending on personal circumstances, patients may be entitled to assistance. The benefit system exists to provide practical help and financial support for those who are unemployed or looking for work, have a low income, a disability, are bringing up children, are retired, care for someone or are ill themselves. Some of the most common benefits are discussed below.

UNIVERSAL CREDIT

Universal Credit (UC) is a fairly new benefit being rolled out across the country. In Greater Manchester it is almost fully active. The purpose of UC is to help with living costs and it is intended to eventually replace the following: Child Tax Credits, Housing Benefit, Income Support, income-based Job Seekers Allowance (JSA), income-related Employment and Support Allowance (ESA) and Working Tax Credit. [1]

Patients may be eligible to claim Universal Credit if they:

- Are on a low income or out of work.
- Are over 18 years of age.
- Are under state pension age or their partner is.
- Live in the UK.
- Between them (they or their partner) have less than £16,000 in savings. (A partner's income or savings will be taken into account even if they are not eligible for UC).

Universal Credit payments are made up of a standard allowance and any extra amounts which apply to individual patients, for example, if they have children, have a disability or health condition which prevents them from working, or need help to pay rent. Patients can use a benefits calculator on the gov.uk website to see how much money they could be eligible for.

Patients' circumstances are assessed every month and what they are paid may change. There is a benefit cap and this can limit the total amount of benefit received. If employed, the UC amount a patient gets depends on their earnings. A UC payment is reduced gradually the more a patient earns. For every £1 they earn, the payment is reduced by 63p. There is no limit to the hours a patient can work.

If a patient receives Universal Credit they may also be able to get other financial support.

Universal Credit is paid once a month, usually into a bank, building society or credit union account. Payments can include an amount for housing and patients are expected to pay their landlord. If a patient is unable to manage their money, a request can be made for rent to be paid directly to the landlord. This is known as an alternative payment arrangement (APA).

It will take approximately six weeks for patients to get their first Universal Credit payment. If they need help with living costs while they wait for this first payment, they can apply for an advance payment. Patients need to be made aware that by getting an advance payment they will immediately be in debt and a set amount will be deducted from their payments every month until this is paid back.

To apply for Universal Credit patients need to provide a significant amount of detail and evidence:

- Bank, building society or credit union account details.
- Email address.
- Telephone number.
- National insurance number.
- Proof of nationality.
- Information about their housing.
- Details of who lives in the property with the patient.
- Details of any earnings e.g. payslips, employer details.
- Details of any savings, investments or properties they own.
- Details of childcare costs.

If the correct information isn't provided at this stage, it will affect when a patient will get paid and how much they receive. The patient will also have to verify their identity online, to do this they will need a driving licence or passport and a debit or credit card.

This can be a very complicated process and doesn't always work. In this instance the patient will need to take three forms of identity proof to their first interview at their local Job Centre Plus.

If patients need help to apply for Universal Credit they need to ask straight away.

There are two ways to get help:

- Contact the Universal Credit helpline if they cannot use digital services at all, this might be due to disability or personal circumstances.
- Contact Citizens Advice.

The Help to Claim Department offer support in the early stages of a Universal Credit claim, from the online application through the stages until the patient receives their first full payment. This is a free, independent, confidential service provided by trained advisers. It is, however, a very busy service and patients may have to wait some time to get an appointment.

If a patient has a disability or illness affecting their ability to work they may need a Work Capability Assessment. A booklet will have to be completed which covers aspects of physical and mental health. Patients will then have to attend a health assessment. Their GP will also be contacted so they can give medical evidence about the patient's condition. Attending the health assessment can be very traumatic for patients. Some of the assessors are lacking in compassion and have little or no experience of the conditions affecting patients. The reports the assessors write are sent to a case manager at the Department for Work and Pensions (DWP) who will then look at all the evidence provided (booklet, notes from the GP practice and assessor's report) to make a decision as to whether the patient is entitled to additional money because of their condition. The same process will apply if a patient has a terminal illness. This should be declared at the very beginning of the application. A patient with a terminal illness may not have to go for a health assessment. Home assessments are also made available at the discretion of the assessment centre or DWP. They are, however quite rare.

If a patient is claiming Universal Credit they may be entitled to other financial support:

- Cold Weather Payment.
- Disabled Facilities Grant.
- Energy Company Obligation (ECO), Affordable Warmth Scheme Programme (Really good!).
- Free early education for 2-year-olds.
- Free school meals.
- Funeral Expenses Payment.
- Healthy Start vouchers.
- Help with some health costs, including prescriptions and dental treatment.
- Help with prison visiting costs.
- Sure Start Maternity Grant.

When patients have submitted a claim for Universal Credit, they then have to manage their

UNIVERSAL CREDIT AND FOODBANK USE

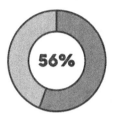
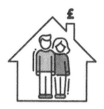
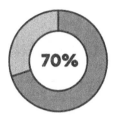

56% had experienced issues with housing

8% of respondents said their full Universal Credit payment covered their cost of living

70% had experienced debt during the wait

Figure 5.1 Universal credit and food bank use.

claim online and make contact with their work coach via their portal. Patients will need to report any changes to their circumstances so that they keep getting the right amount of money each month. A claim will be stopped or reduced if a change of circumstance isn't reported promptly. Patients will be asked to complete other activities depending on their circumstances. These could include going to the job centre and speaking to their work coach via telephone or online. Again, if these activities aren't completed on time, patients will have their benefit reduced or sanctioned. If a patient doesn't have access to the internet they can use the facilities at their local library or at the job centre.

Claiming Universal Credit is never straightforward. It is a difficult, lengthy process. Patients are not treated as individuals. For many patients, going through the process of claiming Universal Credit can negatively impact their health further. There has been a rise in food bank usage with the implementation of UC and the Trussell Trust, together with Mind, provided evidence of the negative impact UC is having [2].

> Under Universal Credit, even those who are severely unwell and at crisis point are still being required to look for work or risk losing their benefits. We've also seen a real lack of support for people who aren't well enough to manage an online claim or monthly payments. While some people with mental health problems are able to manage their money well, for others receiving one payment

and being responsible for ensuring rent and bills are paid can be problematic. Taken together these problems are driving too many people into a cycle of debt, housing problems, and deteriorating mental health.

Figure 5.1 highlights issues food bank users identified as a result of UC [2].

JOB SEEKERS ALLOWANCE

Job Seekers Allowance (JSA) is a benefit for people who are actively seeking employment and are capable of work. Patients must be under state pension age and over the age of 18 and not in full-time employment or working more than 16 hours a week.

EMPLOYMENT AND SUPPORT ALLOWANCE (ESA)

Employment and Support Allowance (ESA) is a benefit for patients who have a limited capability for work due to illness or disability and are not receiving Statutory Sick pay. Patients must be over 16 years old and under state pension age to claim. A form will be completed over the phone and a copy sent to the patient. They will then have to attend a health assessment, similar to the one for Universal Credit.

INCOME SUPPORT

Income Support is a means-tested income replacement benefit and is available to patients who are either pregnant, a carer or a lone parent of a child under 5 years of age. Patients need to apply for this benefit by telephone.

PERSONAL INDEPENDENCE PAYMENT

Personal Independence Payment (PIP) is a benefit for patients between the ages of 16 and 64 years old who, due to illness or disability, have additional care needs. It is not means-tested and any savings or capital are ignored.

There are two parts to the benefit: the daily living component and the mobility component. The application process is very similar to the one described for UC but looks more closely at the areas of daily living and mobility. Again, this process is traumatic for patients and difficult to navigate.

Additional evidence from GPs, consultants and other health professionals is always useful. Claiming this benefit can lead to entitlement to other means-tested benefits. This benefit will eventually replace Disability Living Allowance (DLA) for patients over the age of 16 years.

DISABILITY LIVING ALLOWANCE

Disability Living Allowance (DLA) is a benefit for children who have additional care or mobility needs. DLA is not means-tested. To apply, patients need to go online to the gov.uk website and search for 'DLA for children'.

ATTENDANCE ALLOWANCE

Attendance Allowance is for patients aged over 65 years who are either physically or mentally disabled and require assistance or supervision with their personal care needs to ensure they are safe. It is available to patients who live on their own or with others. It is not means-tested.

CARERS ALLOWANCE

Carers Allowance is available for patients who provide care for more than 35 hours a week to someone who has an illness or disability. The person being cared for must be in receipt of Attendance Allowance, the daily living component of PIP benefit or, if a child, the middle or higher rate of DLA of the care component.

PENSION CREDIT

This is a means-tested benefit for pensioners who are on a low income. Checking eligibility and form completion must be done over the phone.

TAX CREDITS

There are two types of tax credits, Working Tax Credits and Child Tax Credits:

Working Tax Credit – is a benefit that is available to people who work and are on a low income. Eligibility takes into consideration how many hours of paid work a patient does, if they have a disability, children or any childcare costs (that must be provided by an approved childcare service).

Child Tax Credit – is a benefit to assist with the costs of bringing up a child. Patients do **not** need to be working to be eligible. Eligibility takes into consideration if patients work, how many children they have, when they were born and if they have a disability.

HOUSING BENEFIT

This is available to assist patients with rental costs if they are on a low income. Patients can be employed or unemployed, it is a means-tested benefit and takes into consideration income and capital. If Universal Credit is live in the patient's area then this benefit will be paid via UC. If it is not live, then it will be paid via the local council and patients should apply directly to their council.

COUNCIL TAX SUPPORT OR REDUCTION

This is administered by the local council and designed to assist patients with their council tax bill if they are on a low income. Patients can be employed or unemployed and the amount paid depends on where they live. It is a means-tested benefit and takes into account income and capital. It is available to patients who live in rental properties and to homeowners. Patients need to contact their local council directly to apply.[1]

CASE STUDY

Tom

Tom is 54 and has worked for most of his life in a local bakery, moving pallets of products around the warehouse. When the bakery experiences financial issues, a number of staff are laid off – Tom is one of them.

Tom has always worked, with little time off sick, and is proud to be considered a hard worker. Initially he thinks he will find a job quickly as he is open to almost any kind of employment that will pay his bills. Tom applies for several positions but is told that he lacks the necessary skills or qualifications, even for entry-level work. He soon exhausts the job opportunities available locally and looks further afield but finds nothing that will meet his outgoing costs once the cost of travel is taken into account.

Tom keeps looking but soon his very limited savings run out. His pride and optimism had, thus far, kept him from applying for benefits but now he realises that this is a necessity. Tom is not tech-savvy but manages to access the internet at his local library to try to claim online. He accesses information about the range of benefits available in baffling detail and makes several attempts to apply but is unable to supply all the required evidence and successfully navigate the system. Eventually Tom gives up.

Unable to pay the rent, he borrows money from friends and other lenders but is unable to repay them. Fearing he will be evicted, he stops leaving the house, remaining quietly hidden when anyone comes to the door. He begins to spend what money he has on cheap alcohol and borrows cigarettes whenever he can. When he develops a chest infection, he reluctantly attends the GP who spots his dishevelled state and recognises his low mood. As part of a holistic consultation, she asks him about his financial situation and the full picture quickly becomes clear.

The GP introduces Tom to a Focused Care practitioner who quickly takes account of his circumstances, recognising that his physical and mental health are suffering due to his financial issues. She sets up appointments at the job centre and initially accompanies Tom to them, ensuring he brings the correct documents with him. It is a laborious process establishing Tom on Universal Credit but they manage to secure him an advance payment and negotiate staged repayments with his landlord so he doesn't become homeless. With some reluctance Tom starts to use the food bank.

A few months later Tom is healthier and much less stressed. He has stopped smoking and takes daily walks around the local area. He takes opportunities in conversation to ask about any jobs going and, eventually, finds a position in a small hardware business run by someone around his age.

THE DEEP END ADVICE WORKER PROJECT

In 2017, GPs at the Deep End in Scotland published details of their Deep End Advice Worker Project in which a financial advice worker was embedded in GP practices in areas of deprivation for half a day a week. Working in six practices from December 2015 to May 2017, the project received 276 referrals, the large majority of whom hadn't accessed services before. Overall, 65% engaged with the project and gained £848,001 – a median of £6,967 per annum each – through helping people access benefits to which they were entitled; £155,766 of debt was also identified and then managed. The return on investment was 39:1. [3]

SUGGESTIONS FOR PRACTICE

- If you are asked to supply a supporting letter or information, please do so as this could be the information needed to ensure your patient has a successful claim. The mental and physical health benefits of reducing poverty will be manifest.
- There may be regional variation in processes in different parts of the UK and wherever you are is likely subject to frequent change. All up to date information should be available at www.gov.uk.

REFERENCES

1. GOV.UK. 2019. Benefits. Available from: https://www.gov.uk/browse/benefits [Accessed 10th June 2019].
2. Trussell Trust & MIND. *Mind and The Trussell Trust evidence problems with Universal Credit*. July 2018. Available from:

https://www.trusselltrust.org/2018/07/10/
mind-trussell-trust-evidence-problems-
universal-credit/ [Accessed 10th June 2019].

3. Sinclair J. The Deep End Advice
    Worker Project: embedding an advice
    worker in general practice settings.
    Glasgow Centre for Population Health.
    September 2017. Available from: https://
    www.gcph.co.uk/assets/0000/6242/
    Deep_End_FINAL_WEB.pdf [Accessed 9th
    June 2019].

6

Fuel Poverty and Cold-Related Ill Health

JAMIE-LEIGH RUSE

Estimates suggest 20% of excess winter deaths can be attributed to cold homes.

WHAT IS FUEL POVERTY?

Fuel poverty occurs when a household is unable to afford their required energy costs for adequate health and well-being. The term normally refers to a household's inability to heat their home, though it can include other uses of energy such as hot water and lighting. Fuel poverty occurs through the interplay of poor, energy inefficient housing, high energy prices and low incomes.

In England, 11.1% of households (equating to 2.55 million) are in fuel poverty. Across the UK, that figure reaches to over 4 million households. The official definition of fuel poverty in England is based on a Low-Income High Costs (LIHC) calculation, whereby a household is considered to be in fuel poverty if its required fuel costs are higher than the national median and if the inhabitants should spend that amount, their income would fall below the official poverty line. In the rest of the UK, a household is considered to be fuel poor if its required energy costs are more than 10% of its income.

The reality of fuel poverty means [1]:

- Living in a home which is insufferably cold.
- Not turning the heating on for fear of the cost.

- Heating only one or two rooms in a house.
- Spending the day in places that are warm, such as a library or A&E.
- Resorting to barbeques or portable stoves for cooking. In some cases, eating only cold meals.
- Boiling a kettle to wash, rather than heating a water tank.
- Sleeping in damp bedrooms with walls covered in mould.
- Going without food or other essential items to meet the cost of energy bills. This might mean having to rely on food banks.
- Going to bed early to stay warm and/or to forget about the hunger.
- Living in the dark because you don't want to use electricity by turning on the lights. Candles become a main source of light.
- Leaving curtains closed all day or putting newspaper over windows to keep the heat in.
- Using inappropriate appliances, like ovens or unsafe, old and un-serviced secondary heaters to stay warm (increasing the risk of burns and carbon monoxide poisoning).
- Being isolated because you're too embarrassed to invite friends and families into a cold and damp home.

- Informal borrowing from friends and family, or formal borrowing from elsewhere, to meet basic living costs.

Such experiences have consequences for physical and mental health and well-being, as well as a patient's ability to cope with existing illness.

IDENTIFYING WHETHER A HOUSEHOLD IS IN FUEL POVERTY

In England assessing whether a household can be classed as fuel poor under the official, LIHC definition requires a complex calculation that considers household income, occupancy and property characteristics. As it is not always feasible or practical for practitioners and support agencies to gather the information needed for such a calculation, proxy fuel poverty risk indicators can be used.

A patient is likely to be in fuel poverty if:

- They live in a property which is energy inefficient.
- They live in a home which is older, has solid walls and can be considered hard-to-treat with mainstream energy efficiency measures.
- Their home is not connected to the mains gas grid.
- They pay for their energy using a prepayment metre (PPM) or standard credit.
- They have limited or no access to the internet (are at risk of digital exclusion).
- They are living on a low-income.
- They live in private rented accommodation.
- Someone in the household has a long-term illness or disability.
- They are a single-parent family with young children or a multi-adult household with children.
- Have limited English language and/or literacy skills.

SUGGESTIONS FOR PRACTICE

Be aware that patients are unlikely to state that they are in fuel poverty. Common complaints in a consultation may be:

- *Struggling to pay for gas or electricity.*
- *At point of being disconnected.*
- *Can't afford to have the heating on.*

- *House is cold.*
- *House is damp.*
- *Repeated illness, especially respiratory ill health.*
- *Falls at home.*
- *Experiencing other forms of crisis (in debt, struggling to meet food needs).*

CLINICAL CONCERNS ASSOCIATED WITH FUEL POVERTY

The World Health Organisation (WHO) recommends that indoor temperatures be kept at 21°C in living rooms and 18°C in bedrooms for at least 9 hours a day, in order to prevent ill health from cold temperatures [2]. According to Public Health England (PHE), groups who may be particularly vulnerable to ill health from cold homes include those with sensitive or immature thermoregulatory systems (the elderly and young children), as well as those who spend more time at home or who have underlying and chronic illnesses (especially cardiorespiratory disease) [3].

EXCESS WINTER MORTALITY AND MORBIDITY

- Thermally inefficient housing stock in the UK has been linked with higher rates of excess winter deaths (EWDs) than in countries that experience harsher and colder winters [4, 5].
- Studies have associated higher rates of excess winter deaths with older properties (28.2% winter excess deaths occurred in properties built before 1850, compared with 15% in properties built after 1980) [6] and in areas with low central heating coverage [7].
- People living with cold-related health conditions have been shown to be more likely to be limiting their fuel use and living in a home which is cold and mouldy [8].
- For those living in the coldest 10% of homes mortality increases by 2.8% for every 1°C drop in outdoor temperature below 19°C. It increases by only 0.9% for those in the warmest 10% of homes. Overall, those living in coldest 25% of homes have a 20% higher risk of dying during the winter than those living in the warmest 25% of homes.
- Estimates suggest 20% of excess winter deaths can be attributed to cold homes, with 10% of those being directly attributable to fuel poverty [9].

Temperatures below 16°C	Impaired respiratory function.
Temperatures below 12°C	Strain placed on the cardiovascular system.
Temperatures between 5-8°C	Increased risk of death at population level.
3 days after a cold spell	Deaths from coronary thrombosis peak.
12 days after a cold spell	Deaths from respiratory conditions peak.

Figure 6.1 Temperature thresholds.

Around half of UK excess winter deaths are caused by cardiovascular disease [10], and a third by respiratory disease. According to Public Health England different temperature thresholds have varying clinical impacts (Figure 6.1).

Evaluation of the Warm Front Scheme (a national energy efficiency scheme) found that the risk of mortality during winter did not increase for the 70% of scheme beneficiaries that increased indoor temperatures to WHO recommended levels after receiving energy efficiency improvements. For those who did not increase indoor temperatures post intervention, mortality risk increased by 2.2% with every 1°C fall in outdoor temperatures. The programme evaluation estimated that providing energy efficiency measures to households could increase the life expectancy of men by 10 days and women by 7 days. If replicated at a population level, winter deaths would be reduced annually by 0.4 per 1000 occupants [11–13].

RESPIRATORY DISEASE

Breathing in cold air can cause airways to constrict, which stimulates the production of mucus. The risk of bronchitis and pneumonia increases, as does the risk of broncho-constriction in patients with asthma and COPD. By overcoming the heat exchange ability of the upper respiratory tract, cold air is inhaled directly into the lower respiratory tract, potentially leading to inflammation and infection. Inflammatory responses can result in increased fibrinogen production and therefore the risk of arterial thrombosis. Further evidence shows:

- GP consultations for respiratory conditions in older people increase by 19% each time there is a 1°C drop in temperature below 5°C [15].
- Chronic obstructive pulmonary disease (COPD) sufferers are four times more likely to be admitted to hospital over winter for respiratory complications.
- Studies have found that the fuel poverty index can act as a predictor for respiratory-related hospital admissions for people who are aged over 65.
- Unlike other forms of debt, fuel debt has been independently associated with respiratory illness.
- A study of COPD patients in Scotland found that respiratory health was significantly worse for those who spent fewer days with the living room heated to 21°C for 9 hours [16].

Inflammatory responses during respiratory infections are furthermore related to the incidence of ischaemic heart disease as a result of the increased production of fibrinogen. Short-term exposure to the cold has been associated with mild inflammatory reactions and tendencies towards hypercoagulability [17].

People that live in a home that is damp and mouldy are 30–50% more likely to have respiratory problems, and patients with asthma are 2–3 times more likely to live in a damp home [18]. Asthma, allergy symptoms and upper respiratory tract infections in children are particularly associated with living in a damp and mouldy home. A significant correlation between the severity of airflow obstruction and the level of damp within a home has been identified, indicating a dose-response relationship [19–21].

CASE STUDY

Cornwall

A pilot scheme to install energy efficiency measures saw incidents of nocturnal coughing in children from 'most nights' to only 'one or several nights' in the previous months. Before central heating measures were installed, children lost 9.3 school days per 100 to asthma, this dropped to 2.1 days afterwards [22–26].

CARDIOVASCULAR DISEASE

Increased plasma fibrinogen levels and factor VII clotting during winter account for a 15% and 9% rise in coronary heart disease respectively [27]. Research has estimated that 9% of hypertension in people in Scotland could be prevented if indoor temperatures were maintained above 18°C [28].

Systolic and diastolic blood pressure have both been shown to increase as an effect of cold temperatures and poor housing. Prolonged haemoconcentration starts to occur almost immediately following a decrease in temperature, lasting for up to 2 days [29, 30]. In older people, this starts when they are exposed to temperatures below 12°C for more than 2 hours, [31, 32] although other studies suggest that the association actually begins with exposure to indoor temperatures below 18°C.

MENTAL HEALTH AND WELL-BEING

Evidence shows:

- Patients such as those with Alzheimer's Disease or related dementias (ADRD) tend to see competence worsen around independently managing the basic needs of shelter and food, as well as experiencing disturbances in thermoregulation. This can make managing heating and energy routines at home difficult to maintain [33, 34].
- People experiencing difficulties in paying their fuel bills are four times more likely to suffer from mental ill health, including common mental disorders (CMD).

- Children in poor housing have less task persistence and suffer from more psychological symptoms than those in adequate housing [35, 36]. Energy insecurity at home can increase the likelihood of a child experiencing food insecurity, hospitalisation, developmental delay and poor health more generally [37].
- Homes which are inadequately heated have been independently shown to be the only housing quality indicator associated with four or more negative mental health outcomes in young people [38].
- Being cold at home can affect the educational attainment of children, and often means that they cannot find an appropriate and comfortable space to study.
- Living in a cold home can result in social isolation, with subsequent implications for mental health and well-being.
- Being unable to meet the cost of energy, or a home which is damp and mouldy, can cause significant stress, worry and embarrassment. Dampness is associated with mental ill health even after other confounding variables have been controlled for [40].

Energy efficiency interventions can improve mental health and well-being by:

- Improving thermal comfort.
- Alleviating financial strain.
- Providing greater control over heating management.
- Improving social and familial relationships.
- Improving quality of life [41–43].

Evaluation of the national Warm Front Scheme and Scottish Central Heating Programme found that post intervention, recipients who maintained bedroom temperatures of 21°C were 50% less likely to suffer from depression and anxiety than those who maintained bedrooms at 15°C. Two-thirds of participants felt more comfortable at home, and a quarter felt more relaxed and content. A third used more space within the house and had more confidence in their new heating system. People were almost 40% less likely to report high levels of psychological distress following the receipt of central heating and insulation measures than they did before. The incidence of CMDs also fell from 300 to 150 per 1000 residents [14].

The National Energy Action's Health and Innovation Programme (HIP) was a £26.2 million programme which provided fuel poverty and affordable warmth support to vulnerable households. It did so by working with local authority and housing association partners, who coordinated with local front-line health and social care professionals to both identify and target households. Over half of households who received larger energy efficiency measures and just under half of those who received smaller measures associated changes in their pre-existing health conditions to the receipt of their HIP interventions. Over a third of households who received larger measures reported improvements to general mental health, and almost half (43.7%) reported improvements to pre-existing health conditions or disabilities [44, 45].

OTHER HEALTH CONDITIONS AFFECTED BY COLD TEMPERATURES

Sickle Cell Disease (SCD)

- A crisis can be triggered by being cold.
- Comfortable temperature range is 20–30°C.
- Patients living with the condition are likely to have elevated heating needs, with higher energy costs (difficult if on a low-income).
- Cost of SCD-related hospital admissions ranges from £637 to £11,367 a time. Some researchers have argued that part or fully subsidising the heating bills of SCD sufferers (with an average fuel bill of £1,200 per year) would be a cost-effective means of avoiding cold-related SCD admissions [46–49].

Musculoskeletal

- Arthritic and rheumatic pain can worsen in cold and damp housing and have been shown to improve after the installation of central heating [50].
- Experiencing cold at home can affect strength and dexterity, increasing the risk of falls and accidents amongst the elderly.

Nutrition

Paying for energy may mean that families spend less on food, choosing between heating or eating. This increases the risk of malnutrition and can be detrimental to infant weight gain, as well as impacting upon other illnesses that require dietary content or calorific intake to be managed [51].

A study conducted amongst low-income families in the US found that, in families who spent less on food in order to pay for their energy, single adults consumed 47 fewer calories, adults with children consumed 241 fewer calories, and children consumed 197 fewer calories per day over the winter [52]. Another US study found that, in families who received the winter fuel subsidy, infants were 30% more likely to be admitted to hospital or primary care clinics in their first 3 years of life. They were also 20% more likely to be underweight than in families not in receipt of the subsidy [53].

THE COST OF COLD HOMES

The Building Research Establishment (BRE) has calculated that poor housing containing category 1 hazards (as per the housing health and safety rating system [HHSRS]), including excess cold, costs the NHS £1.4bn, with wider societal costs of £18.6bn [54].

Others have calculated cold homes cost the NHS £3,124 per case of cardiovascular disease; £4,359 per case of respiratory illness; and £2,453 per case of injury through falls. Cold homes cost £1,543 per case of CMD [55].

SUPPORT FOR PATIENTS

Patients who are in or at risk of fuel poverty may need multiple forms of support, including:

- Energy efficiency improvements to their home.
- Energy efficiency advice.
- Support to switch energy supplier or access services such as the priority services and register for the warm home discount scheme.
- Income maximisation advice.
- Debt and fuel debt support.
- Onward referrals for falls prevention (including handyman services), social isolation, food poverty (amongst others).

SUGGESTIONS FOR PRACTICE

- *Raise awareness and understanding of the health risks associated with fuel poverty and living in a cold home (and be able to identify signs of energy vulnerability) by attending training courses or facilitating the provision of training to relevant staff members.*

- *Proactively identify patients who may be in fuel poverty using available data and where appropriate, signposting or referring them to local support services.*
- *Develop or participate in local referral pathways so that patients that present at health services displaying signs of cold-related ill health can be linked with appropriate support services.*
- *Embed fuel poverty and cold homes into winter resilience plans (including messaging, referral mechanisms and discharge support).*

In 2018, the public health team at Cornwall Council, together with Citizens Advice, produced a 'cold homes toolkit' [56] aimed at health professionals looking to support patients in or at risk of fuel poverty.

Each year, the National Energy Action publishes a Fuel Poverty Action Guide. It considers the most common areas of concern for domestic energy consumers and describes their rights and entitlements, and the agencies available to assist them. The action guide also provides contact details for agencies able to deliver support around paying for energy, financial help and warmer homes [57–59].

REFERENCES

1. NEA. 2018. *Warm and Safe Homes Campaign: Dangerous Strategies People in Fuel Poverty Adopt to Cope.* Newcastle-upon-Tyne: NEA.
2. Friends of the Earth and Marmot Review Team. 2011. The health impacts of cold homes and fuel poverty. Available at: http://www.foe.co.uk/sites/default/files/downloads/cold_homes_health.pdf [Accessed 03/06/2017]
3. Public Health England. 2014. *Cold weather Plan for England.* Making the case: *Why long-term strategic planning for cold weather is essential to health and wellbeing.* Crown Copyright.
4. Friends of the Earth. 2015. Briefing: Cold homes and respiratory ill-health in England and Sweden. A comparison of health service statistics.
5. Department of Health. 2001. *Health Effects of Climate Change in the UK: An Expert Review.*
6. Healy JD. 2003. Excess winter mortality in Europe: A cross country analysis identifying key risk factors. *Journal of Epidemiology and Community Health,* 57(10), pp.784–789.
7. Isaacs N and Donn M. 1993. Health and Housing - Seasonality in New-Zealand Mortality. *Australian Journal of Public Health,* 17(1), pp.68–70.
8. Rudge J and Gilchrist R. 2007. Measuring the health impacts of temperatures in dwellings: Investigating excess winter morbidity and cold homes in the London borough of Newham. *Energy and Buildings,* 39, pp. 847–858.
9. Wilkinson P, Landon M, Armstrong, B, Stevenson S, Pattenden S, McKee M and Fletcher T. 2001. *Cold Comfort: The Social and Environmental Determinants of Excess Winter Deaths in England,* 1986–96. Bristol: The Policy Press
10. Khaw K-T. 1995. Temperature and cardiovascular mortality. *The Lancet,* 345, pp.337–338.
11. Harris J, Hall J, Meltzer H, Jenkins R, Oreszczyn T and McManus S. 2010. *Health, Mental Health and Housing Conditions in England.* London: National Centre for Social Research.
12. Hills J. 2012. Getting the measure of fuel poverty: Final report of the fuel poverty review. Centre for Analysis of Social Exclusion: Case Report 72.
13. Rudge J. 2011. Indoor cold and mortality. In: Braubach M, Jacobs DE, Ormandy D (Eds) WHO Europe. *Environmental Burden of Disease Associated with Inadequate Housing. Methods for Quantifying Health Impacts of Selected Housing Risks in the WHO European Region.* Available at: http://www.euro.who.int/__data/assets/pdf_file/0003/142077/e95004.pdf [Accessed 06/03/2017].
14. Green G and Gilbertson J. 2008. Warm Front: Better Health: Health Impact Evaluation of the Warm Front Scheme. Sheffield: Sheffield Hallam University, Centre for Regional Social and Economic Research. (page 18).

15. Mason V and Roys M. 2011. *The Health Costs of Cold Dwellings*. Watford: Building Research Establishment.

16. Public Health England, Sept 2014, Local action on health inequalities: Fuel poverty and cold home-related health problems. *Health Equity Evidence Review 7.*

17. Collins K. 2000. Cold, cold housing and respiratory illness. In: Rudge J, Nicol F (Eds) *Cutting the Cost of Cold: Affordable Warmth for Healthier Homes*. London: Taylor & Francis.

18. Hajat S, Kovats RS and Lachowycz K. 2007. Heat-related and cold-related deaths in England and Wales: Who is at risk? *Occupational and Environmental Medicine*, 64(2), pp.93–100.

19. Osman LM, Ayres JG, Garden C, Reglitz K, Lyon J and Douglas JG. 2008 Home warmth and health status of COPD patients. *European Journal of Public Health*, 18(4), pp.399–405.

20. Fisk W, Lei-Gomez Q and Mendell M. 2007. Meta-analyses of the associations of respiratory health effects with dampness and mould in homes. *Indoor Air*, 17(4), pp.284–296.

21. Press V. 2003. *Fuel Poverty + Health: A Guide for Primary Care Organisations, and Public Health and Primary Care Professionals*. London: National heart Forum.

22. Williamson I, Martin C, Mcgill G, Monie R and Fennerty A. 1997. Damp housing and asthma: A case-control study. *Thorax*, 52, pp.229–234.

23. Bornehag CG, Sundell J, Hagerhed-Engman L, Sigsggard T, Janson S, Aberg N and the DBH Study Group. 2005. Dampness at home and its association with airway, nose and skin symptoms among 10,851 pre-school children in Sweden: A cross-sectional study. *Indoor Air*, 15(S 10), pp.48–55.

24. Andriessen JW, Brunekreef B and Roemer W. 1998. Home dampness and respiratory health status in European children. *Clinical and Experimental Allergy*, 28(10), pp.1191–1200.

25. Koskinen O, Husman T, Meklin T and Nevalainen A. 1999. Adverse health effects in children associated with moisture and mould observations in houses. *International Journal of Environmental Health Research*, 9(2), pp.143–156.

26. Somerville M et al. 2000. Housing and health: Does installing heating in their homes improve the health of children with asthma? *Public Health*, 114, pp.434–439.

27. Woodhouse PR et al. 1994. Seasonal variations of plasma fibrinogen and factor VII in the elderly: Winter infection sand death from cardiovascular disease. *The Lancet*, 343, pp.435–439.

28. Shiue I and Shiue M. 2014. Indoor temperature below 18°C accounts for 9% population attributable risk for high blood pressure in Scotland. *International Journal of Cardiology*, 171(1), pp.e1–2.

29. Collins KJ et al. 1985. Effects of age on body temperature and blood pressure in cold environments. *Clinical Science*, 69, pp.465–470.

30. Keatinge WR et al. 1984. Increase in platelet and red cell counts, blood viscosity and arterial pressure during mild surface cooling: Factors in mortality from coronary and cerebral thrombosis in winter. *British Medical Journal*, 289, pp.1405–1408.

31. Neild PJ, Syndercombe-Court D, Keatinge WR, Donaldson GC, Mattock M and Caunce M. 1994. Cold induced increases in erythrocyte count, plasma cholesterol and plasma fibrinogen of elderly people without a comparable rise in Protein C or Factor X. *Clinical Science*, 86(1), pp.43–48.

32. Woodhouse PR, Khaw K-T and Plummer M. 1993. Seasonal variation of blood pressure and its relationship to ambient temperature in an elderly population. *Journal of Hypertension*, 11(11), pp.1267–1274.

33. Saeki K, Obayashi K, Iwamoto J, Tanaka Y, Tanaka N, Takata S, Kubo H, Kamoto N, Tomioka K, Nezu S and Kurumatani N. 2013. Influence of room heating on ambulatory pressure in winter: A randomised controlled study. *Journal of Epidemiology and Community Health*, 67(6), pp. 484–490.

34. Goodwin J. 2000. Cold stress, circulatory illness and the elderly. In: Rudge J, Nicol F (Eds) *Cutting the Cost of Cold*. London, Taylor & Francis.

35. Collins KJ. 1986. Low indoor temperatures and morbidity in the elderly. *Age and Ageing*, 15, pp.212–220.

36. Chesshire Lehmann Fund: Understanding Fuel Poverty, June 2016. Gray B, Allison S, Thomas B, Morris C and Liddell C. Univeristy of Ulster. Excess winter deaths among people living with Alzheimer's Disease or related dementias (ADRD [page 27]).

37. Gilbertson J, Grimsley M and Green G, for the Warm Front Study Group. 2012. Psychosocial routes from housing investment to health gain. Evidence from England's home energy efficiency scheme. *Energy Policy*, 49, pp.122–133.

38. Evans G, Saltzman H and Cooperman J. 2001. Housing quality and children's socio-emotional health. *Environmental Behaviour*, 33(3), pp.389–399.

39. Harker L. 2006. *Chance of a Lifetime: The Impact of Housing on Children's Lives*. London: Shelter.

40. Cook JT et al. 2008. A brief indicator of household energy security: Associations with food security, child health, and child development in US infants and toddlers. *Pediatrics*, 122, pp.e867–e875.

41. Barnes M et al. 2008. *The Dynamics of Bad Housing: The Impacts of Bad Housing on the Living Standards of Children*. London: National Centre for Social Research.

42. NEA and The Children's Society (for National Grid Affordable Warmth Solutions). 2015. Making a house a home: Providing affordable warmth solutions for children and families living in fuel poverty. Available at: http://www.nea.org.uk/wp-content/uploads/2016/01/Making-a-House-a-Home.pdf [Accessed 06/03/2017]

43. Hopton JL and Hunt SM. 1996. Housing condition and mental health in a disadvantaged area in Scotland. *Journal of Epidemiology and Community Health*, 50, pp.56–61.

44. Shortt N and Rugkåsa J. 2007. "The walls were so damp and cold" fuel poverty and ill health in Northern Ireland: Results from a housing intervention. *Health and Place*, 13(1), pp.99–110.

45. Liddell C and Morris C. 2010. Fuel poverty and human health: A review of the recent evidence. *Energy Policy*, 38, pp.2987–2997.

46. Thomson H, Thomas S, Sellstrom E and Petticrew M. 2013. Housing improvements for health and associated socio-economic outcomes (Review) The Cochrane Collaboration. Available at: http://www.thecochranelibrary.com/details/file/4426391/CD008657.html [Accessed 06/03/2017]

47. Gilbertson J, Stevens M, Stiell B and Thorogood N. (For the Warm Front Study Group). 2006. Home is where the hearth is. Grant recipients views of the Warm Front Scheme. *Social Science and Medicine*, 63, pp.946–956.

48. Chesshire Lehmann Fund: Understanding Fuel Poverty, June 2016. Cronin de Chavez, Centre for Health and Social Care Research, Sheffield Hallam University. Keeping Warm with Sickle Cell Disease.

49. Cronin de Chavez. 2015. Keeping Warm with Sickle Cell Disease Research Project: Report for the Chesshire Lehmann Fund, Sheffield Hallam University: Centre for Health and Social Care Research

50. Anderson W, White V and Finney A. 2010. "You just have to get by" Coping with low incomes and cold homes. Centre for Sustainable Energy. Available at: https://www.cse.org.uk/downloads/reports-and-publications/fuel-poverty/you_just_have_to_get_by.pdf [Accessed 06/03/2017].

51. Beatty T, Blow L and Crossley T. 2011. *Is There a Heat or Eat Trade Off in the UK?* London: Institute of Fiscal Studies.

52. Cooper N, Purcell S and Jackson R. 2014. *Below the Breadline: The Relentless Rise of Food Poverty in Britain*. Church Action on Poverty, Oxfam, The Trussell Trust.

53. Grey C, Jiang S and Poortinga W. 2015. Arbed recipient's views and experiences of living in hard-to-heat, hard-to-treat houses in Wales: Results from three focus groups conducted in South Wales, Welsh school of Architecture, Cardiff University: Cardiff WSA Working Paper Series ISSN 2050–8522.

54. Bhattacharya J, DeLeire T, Haider S and Currie J. 2003. Heat or eat? Cold weather shock and nutrition in poor American families. *American Journal of Public Health*, 93(7), pp.1149–1154.

55. Liddell C. 2008. *Policy Briefing – The Impact of Fuel Poverty on Children*. Belfast: Ulster University & Save the Children. http://tinyurl.com/STC-Policy-Briefing-FP

56. Roys M, Nicol S, Garrett H and Margoles S. 2016. *The Full Cost of Poor Housing*. Berkshire, United Kingdom, BRE Press,.

57. Stafford B. 2014. The social cost of cold homes in an English city: Developing a transferable policy tool. *Journal of Public Health*, 37(2), pp.251–257.

58. Cornwall Council and Citizens Advice. 2018. Building cold homes referrals within the health sector. Available: https://www.citizensadvice.org.uk/Global/CitizensAdvice/Health%20professionals%20cold%20homes%20toolkit.pdf [Accessed 2nd May 2019].

59. NEA. 2017. Fuel poverty action guide. Available: http://www.nea.org.uk/wp-content/uploads/2018/10/Fuel-Poverty-Action-Guide-2018-15th-Edition-for-print-reviewed-Mar-2018.pdf

7

Child Safeguarding and Social Care

PAUL BYWATERS

The new LA decided they would not be eligible for any ongoing support "because they did not meet the thresholds".

'Child maltreatment is a leading cause of health inequality, with the socioeconomically disadvantaged more at risk. It worsens inequity and perpetuates social injustice because of its far-reaching health and development consequences'. [1]

The scale of child maltreatment is uncertain but large [2]. Retrospective studies of adults suggest that at least one in ten report childhood maltreatment [3]. The long-term effects on children's health and development can be severe, affecting their educational progress and subsequent employment, material well-being, physical and psychological development and capacity to make strong, secure relationships [4]. Consequences in young adults include low educational attainment, high levels of early pregnancy and parenthood, homelessness, unemployment and imprisonment.

Recent research in the UK has reinforced longstanding evidence that the chances of a child being on a child protection plan or being 'looked after' in out-of-home care are strongly related to the same social determinants that contribute to inequalities in health [5]. The most significant single contributory factor is the socio-economic conditions affecting adults' capacity to parent, often reflecting longstanding disadvantage, and hence children's

physical and emotional development. But inequalities in children's involvement with child protection services are also influenced by other factors in parents' lives and by differential access to services which may be more or less well aligned to families' needs. Children's age and ethnicity are also influential in the rates of involvement of children's services in complex ways.

Each of the four UK countries has a different legal policy framework which determines local responses to child protection concerns, which are the responsibility of local authorities in all countries except in Northern Ireland, where joint Health and Social Care Trusts manage services. However, a similar overall approach has dominated social care practice in all four countries in recent years with a tendency to prioritise the investigation of child protection concerns and the separation of children from their parents over family support and prevention. This has been exacerbated since 2010, especially in England where children's services have faced unprecedented cuts in expenditure, with more disadvantaged areas facing larger reductions.

Partly in response to the ensuing crisis in children's services, new approaches are now under consideration in the UK and internationally. The most important developments are a move towards public health [6] or social models [7] for protecting children and the poverty-aware paradigm [8]. These approaches espouse working closely in partnership with families and communities to build protective models from the ground up, rather than emphasising legalistic and investigatory approaches.

Health practitioners can contribute to children's safety and development by being alert to the widespread experience of disadvantage in childhood, particular stress points and the consequences for children of pressures on parents. Maximising parents' capacities and resources, engaging families and communities in responding to children's needs and building alliances across organisations and services are key factors in good practice.

KEY TERMS

Child in need: A child in need is defined under the Children Act 1989 as a child who is unlikely to reach or maintain a satisfactory level of health or development, or their health or development will be significantly impaired without the provision of services, or the child is disabled.

Child on a child protection plan: A child protection conference is held when, following a section 47 enquiry, a child is deemed to be at continued risk of significant harm. The conference will lead to a decision whether or not to make a child subject to a child protection plan. In April 2008 plans replaced the child protection register in England. Wherever possible, plans should be agreed by parents and professionals and state what the intended short- and long-term outcomes are for the child, how social services will monitor the child's welfare, what changes are needed to reduce the risk to the child and what support will be offered to the family. Local authority children's services departments oversee children in their area subject to child protection plans.

A looked-after child: The term 'looked after' has a specific, legal meaning, based on the Children Act 1989. A child is looked after by a local authority if they are provided with accommodation for a continuous period of more than 24 hours; are subject to a care order or are subject to a placement order. Children are most commonly placed in foster care but may be in residential care, or placed with relatives or family friends.

DEFINITIONS

Concepts of child maltreatment have widened greatly in the 50 years since Kempe and colleagues first identified the battered-child syndrome [9]. The World Health Organisation report on violence and health [10] defined child maltreatment as 'all forms of physical and/or emotional or sexual abuse, deprivation and neglect of children, or commercial or other exploitation resulting in harm to the child's health, survival, development or dignity in the context of a relationship of responsibility, trust or power.' In the UK, child protection concerns are usually defined as either physical, sexual or emotional abuse or neglect. In recent years, sexual exploitation, particularly affecting adolescents, and the trafficking of children have emerged as new concerns.

DEFINITIONS OF ABUSE AND NEGLECT

Neglect: Neglect is the persistent failure to meet a child's basic physical and/or psychological needs, which is likely to result in the serious impairment of the child's health or development. For instance, a parent or carer may fail to provide adequate food, shelter, or clothing (including exclusion from home or abandonment); protect a child from physical harm, emotional harm, or danger; ensure adequate supervision (including the use of inadequate caregivers); ensure access to appropriate medical care or treatment. It may also include neglect of, or unresponsiveness to, a child's basic emotional needs.

Sexual abuse: Sexual abuse involves forcing or enticing a child to take part in sexual activities, including prostitution, regardless of whether or not the child is aware of what is happening. Such activities may involve physical contact, including non-penetrative and penetrative acts (for example rape, buggery, or oral sex) or non-penetrative acts such as masturbation, kissing, rubbing and touching outside of clothing. They may also include non-contact activities, such as involving children in looking at, or in the production of, sexual images, watching sexual activities, encouraging children to behave in sexually inappropriate ways or grooming a child in preparation for abuse (including via the internet).

Physical abuse: Physical abuse may involve hitting, shaking, throwing, poisoning, burning or scalding, drowning, suffocating or otherwise causing physical harm to a child. Physical harm may also be caused when a parent or carer deliberately fabricates symptoms or induces illness in a child. The fabrication and deliberate inducement of symptoms relate to conditions such as Munchausen syndrome by proxy.

Emotional abuse: Emotional abuse is the persistent ill-treatment of a child that causes severe and continual adverse effects on the child's emotional development. It may involve conveying to the child that they are inadequate, worthless or unloved, or valued only as far as they meet the needs of another person. It may include not giving the child opportunities to express their views, deliberately silencing them or making fun of what they say or how they communicate. It may feature the imposing of age or developmentally inappropriate expectations on the child. Such expectations may include interactions that are beyond the child's developmental capability. It includes overprotection and limitation of exploration and learning, or preventing the child from participating in normal social interactions. It may involve the child seeing or hearing the ill-treatment of another. It may also involve serious bullying (including cyberbullying), causing children frequently to feel frightened or in danger, or the exploitation or corruption of children.

SCALE AND DISTRIBUTION

Recent evidence shows that by the age of five, 20% of all children will have been referred to children's services in England, rising to over 50% of all children in the most deprived 10% of neighbourhoods [11]. On average two children in every school class of 30 were assessed as a 'child in need' at some time during the year 2017–2018 in England [12], more than half said to be primarily because of abuse or neglect. One child in every 70 was investigated by children's services over a child protection concern during the year.

The past ten years have seen an acceleration in the upward trend in reported cases of child abuse and neglect in the UK. However, it is less clear whether this represents a real rise in maltreatment rather than a growing investigation culture and widening definitions of maltreatment. In 2009–2010 in England there were 87,700 Section 47 (child protection) investigations with some 33,000 not leading to child protection plans. In 2017–2018 there were almost 200,000 investigations but 120,000 resulted in no confirmed maltreatment requiring a plan [12]. Critics [13] have argued that, following high profile cases such as Baby P. and Daniel Pelka, the current focus in children's services on identifying risk rather than prevention and support is profoundly damaging for relationships between social care services and families and has drawn attention and services away from prevention and support.

In England and internationally, neglect and emotional abuse have become by far the most common forms of maltreatment as recorded in child protection plans (Table 7.1). Because there are no reliable data for the total numbers maltreated in the child population, the rate of children on protection plans i.e. with substantiated maltreatment concerns, is the best available proxy. The rise in the proportion of neglect and emotional abuse cases reflects heightened concern about the consequences for children of living in households where they are exposed to parents' domestic abuse, substance use or mental ill health, rather than directly experiencing physical or sexual abuse themselves.

The proportion of children on child protection plans is heavily patterned by age with younger children more likely to be investigated and placed on plans (Table 7.2). By contrast older children

Table 7.1 Percentage of Child Protection Plans Starting during the Year 2017–18

Category of Abuse	% of plans
Neglect	49
Physical Abuse	8
Sexual Abuse	4
Emotional Abuse	39
Total	100

and young people are more likely to be in care (a looked-after child), the majority because of concerns about maltreatment.

There are also very large differences in the proportions of children on child protection plans by ethnic categories [14]. Children identified as being of Asian heritage are half as likely to be on a child protection plan as white children, while children of mixed heritage are over-represented. If you control for family socio-economic circumstances, black children are also significantly **less** likely to be on child protection plans than white children (Table 7.3).

Limited evidence suggests that children with disabilites are more likely than others to be maltreated but the data collected by UK national governments does not include reliable and valid data on child disability [15].

Despite the understandable public concern which occurs when a child dies as a result of maltreatment, the death rate from abuse and neglect is and has long remained low in the UK [16]. In the five years leading up to 2018 there were an average of 68 deaths due to assault or undetermined intent a year in the UK, around six per million children. The influence that child deaths have on policy and

Table 7.2 Rate of Children on Child Protection Plans at 31st March 2015 per 10,000 Children

Age Group	Rate per 10,000 children
0–4	61
5–9	48
10–15	36
16–17	12

Table 7.3 Rate of Children on Child Protection Plans at 31st March 2015 per 10,000 Children by Broad Ethnic Category

Ethnic Category	Rate per 10,000 children
White	45
Mixed	76
Asian	21
Black	43
Other	43

practice is arguably out of proportion to the numbers, albeit that any death is a tragedy for those involved.

CAUSES OF AND INEQUALITIES IN MALTREATMENT

A child's chance of being maltreated is profoundly unequal as a result of their family circumstances, aspects of their identity and where they live. Research on inequalities in child maltreatment is at a very early stage compared to work on inequalities in health but recent UK studies have found a steep social gradient in the proportion of children on child protection plans or registers in every UK country and in all of the 55 local authorities studied [5]. No systematic demographic or socio-economic data is collected on the parents of children on child protection plans, so the best available evidence to date uses index of multiple deprivation scores for small neighbourhoods (Lower Layer Super Output Areas) as a proxy for families' material circumstances. A child in the most deprived 10% of neighbourhoods is more than ten times more likely to be on a child protection plan than a child on the least deprived 10% (Figure 7.1).

Just as Blackpool had the lowest male life expectancy at birth and Kensington and Chelsea the highest (in 2015–2017), so Blackpool had the highest rate of children on child protection plans or in care (looked after) in 2017–2018, nearly five times the rate for Kensington and Chelsea. There is a very high correlation between local authorities with low life expectancy at birth and those with high rates of child protection interventions.

While poverty does not cause maltreatment and the vast majority of parents, whatever their circumstances, want the best for their children, families' financial resources are the most significant single contributory factor in maltreatment. This works in two main ways evidenced by the social gradient [17, 18].

Each step reduction in family resources increases financial stress, a common cause of relationship problems in families, and at low levels of income families can be forced to go without essentials such as food, heating or clothing. The majority (70%) of families in poverty now have a family member who is working but most working and non-working households in poverty share common experiences of insecure and often inconsistent patterns of

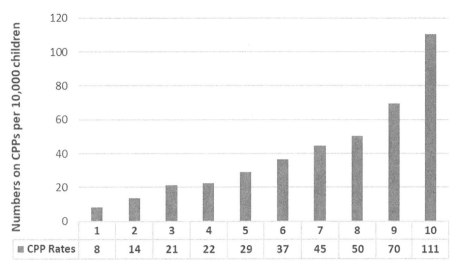

Figure 7.1 Child protection plan (CPP) rates per 10,000 children by Deprivation Decile.

income. Welfare reforms have made financial management more difficult with frequent use of sanctions, erroneous assessments, and the withdrawal of direct payments for rent and utilities exacerbating the effects of substantial cuts in headline benefit rates. Zero-hours contracts reflect the wider issue of the limited bargaining power of workers in lowest-wage jobs. The practical difficulties in making ends meet, the processes of negotiating benefit claims or applying for food bank help and the public discourse about 'scroungers' exacerbate feelings of shame and worthlessness. Children can feel particularly acutely their disadvantaged status compared to their peers, especially when, for example, reinforced by visible markers of free school meals or the inability to afford fashionable clothing. Poverty can impact considerably on educational opportunities if families cannot afford IT equipment which is increasingly essential to school performance.

Each increase in family resources increases the range of solutions that families can command to care well for their children. Better resources enable parents to secure the essentials, purchase occasional treats to ease relationships or as rewards, to buy replacement or additional support with childcare or education and to exercise greater control over the housing and neighbourhood in which they live.

Four separate quasi-experimental studies in the United States have compared populations matched in all respects except the levels of income available

to families and all found that even small increases in income are associated with lower rates of child maltreatment [20–23]. No equivalent studies have been carried out in the UK but all available evidence, as well as common sense, points to the relevance of socio-economic resources as a key factor in family pressures.

In the UK in recent years there has been a dominant focus in child protection practice on domestic violence, mental health difficulties and substance use as the three key factors in maltreatment, but the close connections of these factors with poverty has been largely ignored. In all three cases, low and insecure incomes are commonly both causal and consequential factors. For example, poverty makes poor mental health more likely and poor mental health increases the chances that parents and children will be living in poverty. Once again, having more money gives parents more options in managing difficult circumstances and protecting children's well-being and development. Another concern has been that these problems have sometimes been treated by service providers just as risk factors for children rather than as difficulties with which parents need help. So parents experiencing, for example, domestic violence are sometimes warned that unless they can protect their children from exposure they will be taken into care, although the parent may have no means of securing safe accommodation and are offered no help by children's services.

POLICY CONTEXT AND DEVELOPMENTS

Central government cuts in funding for local authorities since 2010 have radically changed children's services in England [24–26]. Almost all the cuts in funding per child have been managed by reducing prevention and family support services, especially early years services, such as Sure Start children's centres, and youth services. These reductions in children's services have been exacerbated by budget cuts or constraints for allied services – such as health, domestic violence, money advice, drug and addiction services. As far as children's services in England are concerned, more deprived local authorities have faced much larger cuts. This has created a vicious circle of rising demand and reduced provision. Children's services have had to increase the rationing of services and most have done so by raising the thresholds at which children and families are considered eligible for particular kinds of intervention [27]. Families with disabled children, for example, complain that unless they present their children as being at risk of maltreatment, it can be impossible to secure support, while other families are refused support until relatively minor problems become much more serious and difficult to resolve [7].

However, despite the growing evidence, the Department for Education in England [28], sometimes backed by reports from the National Audit Office [29] and Ofsted [30], has argued that the quality of a particular local authority's children's services is not related to levels of funding or to the levels of deprivation in the child population served but reflects the quality of leadership and the particular models of practice followed. Because of the financial pressures facing local authorities, some see the solution in the search for data analysis tools to predict which children are at risk, despite the paucity of evidence about the circumstances which lead to maltreatment or clear evidence about the outcomes of risk-focused intervention.

PRACTICE PATTERNS AND LIMITATIONS

This risk-based approach to policy and practice has come under increased attack in recent times as the Association of Directors of Children's Services, researchers, parents' groups and independent sector organisations have argued that there is a growing gap between the focus and availability of services and what families require to help them keep their children safe [31]. Internationally there are three key emerging models of interest:

1. A public health model of policy and practice incorporating a population focused rather than individualising approach [6].
2. A social model of child protection [7].
3. A 'poverty-aware paradigm' for practice [8].

These approaches, which share many significant features, are based on similar criticisms of current practice internationally. These can be illustrated in two examples. Emerging concerns in English towns and cities about the sexual exploitation of so-called 'vulnerable' teenagers were initially responded to as individual cases. They were identified either as promiscuous behaviour by the young people concerned or parental failure to protect their daughters (and sometimes their sons). These victim-blaming service responses meant that too often agencies ignored what was happening or focused on removing the children into care. Two key shifts changed this individualising focus on behaviour and parenting. Firstly, the scale and systematic patterns of exploitation had to be recognised in a switch from an individual to a population focus. Secondly, the behaviours had to be reframed as criminal abuse by perpetrators rather than individual failures on the part of victims and their parents.

CASE STUDY

Charlotte

A family of four came to the attention of children's services after A&E alerted them that an eight-year-old girl, Charlotte, had been left in charge of her three-year-old sibling while her father took his wife – her mother – to hospital at night. The family were recent migrants to the UK. The wife suffered from a pre-existing serious brain injury, requiring almost full-time care. The family had no recourse to public funds and only a very limited support network. A financial assessment of the family's circumstances revealed that, although the father was doing everything within his power to keep the family afloat, there was no leeway within the household budget whatsoever and all wages were being used to meet the family's most basic needs. This left Charlotte with a number of caring responsibilities, both for her mother and younger sibling. Children's services responded with a support plan including funded child minding for the three-year-old, relieving pressure on the father, and twice weekly 'out of the house' activities for Charlotte, giving her some time to pursue her own interests and to interact with peers. The family were connected with a local community association for refugees and gifts provided at Christmas. A few months later the family moved to another local authority for work. The new LA decided they would not be eligible for any ongoing support 'because they did not meet the thresholds'. The family were warned that if Charlotte and her younger sibling were left alone again, they would be subject to a child protection investigation and possible removal into care.

In this case, two profoundly different approaches are demonstrated. The first sees the role of the state as supporting parents in difficult circumstances in the care of their children. Despite the complex legal and ethical situation, putting the children's welfare first meant supporting the family in material and practical ways. Following the move, the family were seen as solely responsible for their children's care with the state's role as being to enforce that responsibility even if the financial costs to the state – never mind the human costs to the family - were much greater.

These examples illustrate how models of child protection which focus on behaviours and individual responsibility without consideration of the social, economic and environmental context of children's and parents' lives can lead to counterproductive and expensive outcomes, and damage what should be a relationship of trust between state services and citizens.

The social model of Featherstone et al. argues for at least three key changes in practice and policy.

A SHIFT OF ATTENTION

Attention has shifted from identifying individual risk to understanding and responding to root causes. For services, this means thinking strategically about what and where to focus resources. For example, given that domestic violence is a contributory factor in over half of all cases of children in need and a key child protection concern, a

strategic investment in services which support parents to keep children safe where violence is occurring would seem obvious [7]. This means investing in a nexus of financial, housing, policing, child care and other provision to enable parents and children to be safe. Similar arguments could be made about, for example, addiction and mental health services where the connections with financial and other material resources are equally important for keeping children safe.

A CHANGE OF THINKING ABOUT THE ROLE OF THE STATE

There has been a change of thinking about the role of the state from investigative, legalistic and controlling to being responsible for creating the conditions in which children can flourish, preferably in their birth families. These conditions, Morris suggests [7], include provision which enhances participation, reduces inequalities and responds to children's and parents' immediate needs. For example, Sure Start children's centres, at their best, provided universal services to support parents and young children thereby building social solidarity, equalised children's chances by prioritising the allocation of resources to disadvantaged families including through outreach, and offered rights and advocacy services to maximise the take up of entitlements and parents' capacity to deal with a range of external organisations. This is the opposite of a state that accuses 200,000 families a year of failing to protect their children with a 60% rate of false positives.

PRACTICE BASED ON BUILDING RELATIONSHIPS BETWEEN PROVIDER ORGANISATIONS, FAMILIES AND COMMUNITIES

Practice is now based on building partnerships between families, communities and provider organsiations with services being co-produced, emphasising partnerships which respect the strengths of those involved. The chief social worker of Northern Ireland has argued that 99% of parents want the best for their children and services should be built on recognition of common ground *with* parents rather than seeing parents as the problem. The poverty-aware paradigm (PAP) developed by Michal Krumer-Nevo [8] exemplifies that this approach and has much to offer. The PAP views families' socio-economic circumstances not just as a distant structural issue but as vital to relationships between family members and professionals. Poverty is not just a matter of material and social capital (although these are real and important) but also of symbolic capital resulting in stigma, shame and a lack of recognition of the voice and knowledge of people living with poverty. PAP approaches depend on workers' entering into close relationships with families and the communities in which they live in order to understand what it means to live with both the practical constraints and the emotional microaggressions of poverty. In recent years government attitudes and policies, reinforced in media presentations, have exacerbated a longstanding hostile environment for parents and children in poverty. This creates daily shaming experiences in negotiating for basic needs in the absence of an adequate or secure income.

> For example, our project observed one father who had just attended a meeting which decided to take his child into care (at an average cost of £50,000 per year) in tears when he was refused money for the bus fare home. If professionals communicate their understanding of these undermining experiences, this can provide the basis for jointly developed problem solving with children's safety and development in mind, including through workers using their social capital as advocates.

Recent research in Northern Ireland [32] has found features of practice which reflect these ideas, albeit that much more could be done within an inequalities framework. Northern Ireland has – surprisingly, given its higher levels of deprivation – the lowest rates of looked-after children in any of the four UK countries. The research has shown:

- There is evidence of a higher routine awareness of poverty and deprivation in social workers' general practice. Poverty, and its consequences, is more of a foreground factor in social workers' consideration of family needs. Similarly, holding families individually responsible for their poverty in risk assessments is certainly less evident than in the other comparable UK sites.

- Care and protection plans reveal some evidence of the children's and families' socio-economic circumstances being addressed. This includes examples such as provision of direct financial support, income maximisation services and support plans to address the consequences of economic hardship.
- There is significant recognition of the capacity of extended family and community members to care for children, and this is played out in the higher kinship care rates evident in Northern Ireland.
- There is evidence of a greater awareness of, and access to, community support services.
- Use of early help services, and engagement of social workers in providing early help is more evident in NI sites, with some areas having access to a varied and much valued range of family support services.

Safeguarding children is health work. Good and safe development in childhood protects children from immediate harm and ill health, builds the economic and social capital for a healthy life and prevents ill health and shortened lives in adulthood.

State responses to child and family difficulties have become dominated by a focus on identifying individual children at risk, with UK government policies emphasising austerity in public finances and ideological commitments, to reducing the state's role while also increasing individual and parental responsibility; a wide range of relevant services and welfare benefits that supported families have experienced unprecedented cuts. The largest proportionate cuts have affected children in early years (Sure Start) and adolescence (youth services). But it is not only the amount spent on services but the focus of services on individualised risk which is currently problematic. This is leading to increasing numbers of child protection investigations coupled with growing numbers of children in care: a response which is both expensive, destructive of trust between the state and families and is supported by little evidence of benefit to children overall.

In this crisis new practice models are emerging which emphasise:

- The significance of families' and communities' material, social and environmental resources.

- The value of mutually respectful relationships which recognise strengths, knowledge and the right to a voice.
- Populatio-based, strategic as well as personal and human responses.
- A policy goal of reducing inequalities in children's lives, including in rates of abuse and neglect.

Those working with families can usefully test their practice against these emerging models.

REFERENCES

1. Sethi, D., Bellis, M., Hughes, K., Gilbert, R., Mitis, F. and Galea G. European report on preventing child maltreatment European report on preventing child maltreatment [Internet]. WHO; 2013. Available from: http://www.euro.who.int/__data/assets/pdf_file/0019/217018/European-Report-on-Preventing-Child-Maltreatment.pdf?ua=1

2. Gilbert, R., Widom, C.S., Browne, K., Fergusson, D., Webb, E. and Janson, S. Burden and consequences of child maltreatment in high-income countries. *Lancet* [Internet]. 2009 Jan 3 [cited 2014 Jul 10];373(9657):68–81. Available from: http://www.ncbi.nlm.nih.gov/pubmed/19056114

3. Radford, L., Corral, S., Bradley, C. and Fisher, H.L. The prevalence and impact of child maltreatment and other types of victimization in the UK: Findings from a population survey of caregivers, children and young people and young adults. *Child Abuse and Neglect* [Internet]. Elsevier Ltd;2013;37(10):801–813. Available from: http://www.ncbi.nlm.nih.gov/pubmed/23522961

4. Bunting, L., Davidson, G., McCartan, C., Hanratty, J., Bywaters, P., Mason, W. and Steils, N. The association between child maltreatment and adult poverty – a systematic review of longitudinal research. *Child Abuse and Neglect*. 2018;77:121–133. https://doi.org/10.1016/j.chiabu.2017.12.022

5. Bywaters, P., Brady, G., Bunting, L., Daniel, B., Featherstone, B., Jones, C., Morris, K, Scourfield, J., Sparks, T. and Webb, C. Inequalities in English child protection practice under austerity: A universal challenge? *Child Fam Soc Work*. 2018;23:53–61. doi:10.1111/cfs.12383

6. Bywaters, P. Understanding the Neighbourhood and Community Factors Associated With Child Maltreatment in Lonne, B., Scott, D., Higgins, D. &Herrenkohl, T. (eds.) *Re-Visioning Public Health Approaches for Protecting Children*. 2019. New York: Springer Press.

7. Featherstone , B., Gupta, A., Morris, K. and White, S. *Protecting Children: A Social Model*. 2018. Bristol: Policy Press.

8. Krumer-Nevo, M. Poverty-aware social work: A paradigm for social work practice with people in poverty. *Br J Soc Work*. 46:1793–1808.

9. Kempe, C.H. and Helfer, R. (eds) *The Battered Child*. 1st edition. 1968. Chicago: Chicago University Press.

10. Krug, E.G., Dahlberg, L.L., Mercy, J.A., Zwi, A. and Lozano, R. *World Report on Violence and Health*. 2002. Geneva: World Health Organization.

11. Bilson, A., Martin, K.E.C. Referrals and child protection in England: One in five children referred to children's services and one in nineteen investigated before the age of five. *Br J Soc Work*. 2016. doi:10.1093/bjsw/bcw054

12. Department for Education. Characteristics of children in need: 2017 to 2018. 2018. https://www.gov.uk/government/statistics/characteristics-of-children-in-need-2017-to-2018

13. Featherstone, B., Morris, K. and White, S. A marriage made in hell: Early intervention meets child protection. *Br J Soc Work*. 2013:1–15.

14. Bywaters, P., Scourfield, J., Webb, C., Morris, K., Featherstone, B., Brady, G., Jones, C. and Sparks, T. Paradoxical evidence on ethnic inequities in child welfare: Towards a research agenda. *Child Youth Serv Rev* [Internet]. 2019;96(November 2018):145–154. Available from: https://linkinghub.elsevier.com/retrieve/pii/S019074091830728X

15. Taylor, J., Stalker, K., Fry, D. and Stewart, A. Disabled Children and Child Protection in Scotland: An investigation into the

relationship between professional practice, child protection and disability. Scottish Government Social Research. 2014. https://www.pkc.gov.uk/media/39936/Research-Paper-Disabled-Children-and-Child-Protection-in-Scotland/pdf/Research_Paper_-_Disabled_Children_and_Child_Protection_in_Scotland

16. Pritchard, C. and Steven, K. Child mortality and child-abuse-related deaths in Albania, Bulgaria, Croatia, Cuba, Czech Republic, Estonia, FRY Macedonia, Hungary, Latvia, Lithuania, Moldova, Poland, Romania, Russia, Serbia, Slovakia and Slovenia compared to western comparators the USA and the UK (1988–90 to 2012–14). *Br J Soc Work*. 2018;48:236–253. http://doi.org/10.1093/bjsw/bcw179

17. Graham, H., (ed.) *Understanding Health Inequalities*. 2000. Buckingham: Open University Press.

18. Bywaters, P., Bunting, L., Davidson, G., Hanratty, J., Mason, W., McCartan, C. and Steils, N. *The relationship between poverty, child abuse and neglect: An evidence review.* 2016. York: Joseph Rowntree Foundation.

19. Bywaters, P., Scourfield, J., Jones, C., Sparks, T., Elliott, M., Hooper, J., McCarten, C., Shapira, M., Bunting, L. and Daniel, B. Child welfare inequalities in the four nations of the UK. *J Soc Work*. 2018. http://journals.sagepub.com/doi/10.1177/1468017318793479

20. Cancian, M., Yang, M.-Y. and Slack, K.S. The effect of additional child support income on the risk of child maltreatment. *Soc Serv Rev*. 2013;87(3):417–437.

21. Slack, K.S., Font, S., Maguire-Jack, K. and Berger, L.M. Predicting child protective services (CPS) involvement among low-income U.S. families with young children receiving nutritional assistance. *Int J Environ Res Public Health*. 2017;14(10). doi:10.3390/ijerph14101197

22. Maguire-Jack, K., Purtell, K.M., Showalter, K. and Barnhart, S. Preventive benefits of US childcare subsidies in supervisory child neglect. *Children & Society*. 2018. doi:10.1111/chso.12307

23. Brown, D. and De Cao, E. The Impact of Unemployment on Child Maltreatment in the United States∗. Department of Economics Discussion Paper Series, Oxford University. 2017. Number 837.

24. National Audit Office. Pressures on children's social care. 2019. HC 1868 Session 2017–2019 January.

25. Kelly, A.E., Lee, T., Sibieta, L. and Waters, T. *Public Spending on Children in England: 2000 to 2020*. 2018. Insititute of Fiscal Studies report for the Children's Commissioner's Office.

26. Webb, C.J.R. and Bywaters, P. Austerity, rationing and inequity: Trends in children's and young peoples' services expenditure in England between 2010 and 2015. Local Gov Stud. 2018:1–25. Available from: https://doi.org/10.1080/03003930.2018.1430028

27. Devaney, J. The trouble with thresholds: Rationing as a rational choice in child and family social work. *Child Fam Soc Work*. 1–9. doi:10.1111/cfs.12625

28. Department for Education. Children's services: Spending and delivery. 2016. https://www.gov.uk/government/publications/childrens-services-spending-and-delivery

29. National Audit Office. Children in need of help or protection. 2016. HC 723 Session 17 12 October.

30. Ofsted. Ofsted Annual Report 2016. https://www.gov.uk/government/collections/ofsted-annual-report-201516

31. The Association of Directors of Children's Services. Research Report: Safeguarding pressures phase 6. 2018 (November). Available from: http://adcs.org.uk/safeguarding/article/safeguarding-pressures-phase-6

32. Mason, W., Morris, K., Bunting, L., Bywaters, P., Davidson, G., Featherstone, B. and McCartain, C. (forthcoming) *Poverty, family and community: Exploring child welfare inequalities in Northern Ireland.*

8

Domestic Violence and Abuse

CATHERINE CUTT AND CLARE RONALDS

Power and control is at the core.

Domestic violence and abuse (DVA) are a breach of human rights and a public health problem which have a significant, long-lasting impact on physical and mental health [2, 3]. Studies report that 21–55% of women will suffer DVA in their lifetime [3, 4], however its prevalence is difficult to measure as it remains predominantly hidden.

DEFINITIONS

Domestic violence

'Any incident or pattern of incidents of controlling, coercive or threatening behaviour, violence or abuse between those aged 16 or over who are or have been intimate partners or family members regardless of gender or sexuality. This can encompass but is not limited to the following types of abuse: psychological, physical, sexual, financial, emotional.'

Controlling Behaviour

A range of acts designed to make a person subordinate and/or dependent by isolating them from sources of support, exploiting their resources and capacities for personal gain, depriving them of the means needed for independence, resistance and escape and regulating their everyday behaviour.

Coercive Behaviour

An act or a pattern of acts of assault, threat, humiliation and intimidation or other abuse that is used to harm, punish, or frighten their victim.

This definition, which is not a legal definition, includes so called honour-based violence, female genital mutilation (FGM) and forced marriage, and is clear that victims are not confined to one gender or ethnic group' [1].

Despite individual preconceptions, DVA occurs across all socioeconomic groups, sexualities, cultures and ethnicities. Socially disadvantaged individuals may be more vulnerable to DVA, however robust research into this area is lacking. Deprivation, particularly when coupled with gender, can place women at greater risk of DVA due to financial hardship/dependency, lack of affordable childcare, shared benefits claims, withholding of child support and an assumption that the lead carer will be the woman. Both men and women suffer DVA, however, it remains a gendered crime with women suffering more frequent and more severe attacks [4, 5]. They are more likely to be sexually assaulted, be killed by a partner or ex-partner and to fear for their lives [4, 6]. Women in same-sex relationships suffer the same level of abuse as those in heterosexual relationships but up to 50% of gay and bisexual men may suffer DVA [7].

Women who suffer DVA experience poorer health, with increased use of both primary and secondary care services [5]. It is estimated to cost the UK £16bn per annum, with at least £1.7bn being attributable to the NHS [8, 9], however, as much DVA is hidden these figures are likely to be an underestimate of its true cost. The impact on children living in households where DVA occurs is significant and enduring [10].

Power and control are at the core of DVA. The Duluth power and control wheel (Figure 8.1) illustrates some of the behaviours that perpetrators use to keep control over their partners. This can be a useful tool in consultations to help a patient recognise what is happening to them. It is used by DVA professionals in their work to help explain the behaviours of perpetrators and highlight the breadth of actions perpetrators may use to maintain power and control in the relationship.

In order to improve the health inequalities of those suffering DVA, clinicians need to work closely with specialist DVA agencies who can support their patients to address the abuse and improve their quality of life [12].

LEARNING EXERCISE

- *Find your local DVA provider and their referral criteria for patients affected by DVA.*

HEALTH IMPACTS AND PRESENTATIONS

The health impacts of DVA are significant (Table 8.1). Epidemiological studies demonstrate the wide and long-lasting disease burden from DVA-related illness, disability and premature death [13, 14]. The consequences of abuse can be immediate and acute, long-lasting and chronic, can persist long after the abuse has stopped and can be fatal [13, 15].

Women who suffer DVA are more likely to be frequent health service attenders, be issued more prescriptions, have more visits to pharmacies, be admitted to hospital more often and undergo more operations. They are more likely to suffer gynaecological problems (3 times more likely than women who don't suffer DVA)), depression (2.8 times more likely), suicidal ideation (3.6 times more likely), alcohol problems (5.6 times more likely) and post-traumatic stress disorder (PTSD) (7.3 times more

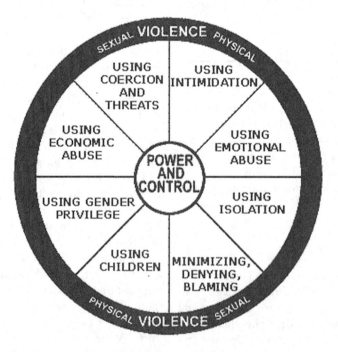

Figure 8.1 The Duluth power and control wheel [11].

Table 8.1 Health Presentations of DVA, IRISi

Physical	Gynaecological/ Reproductive	Psychosocial	Situational
• Chronic gastrointestinal symptoms. • Chronic abdominal pain. • Chronic back pain. • Chronic headaches • Other chronic pain (especially where unexplained). • Unexplained hearing loss. • Injuries, especially to head/neck or multiple regions. • Bruises in various states of healing. • Lethargy. • Cardiovascular disease. • Hypertension.	• Chronic pelvic pain. • Sexual dysfunction. • Vaginal bleeding (especially repeated cases). • Sexually transmitted infections. • Multiple unintended pregnancies/ terminations. • Miscarriages. • Delayed antenatal care. • Low infant birth weight.	• Anxiety. • Depression. • Eating disorders. • Panic disorders. • Post-traumatic stress disorder. • Sleep disorders. • Somatoform disorders. • Alcohol abuse (OR 5.6, 3-9). • Substance use. • Suicide ideation or attempts. • Self-harm.	• Frequent healthcare service use and/or hospital admissions. • Frequent/high level medication use. • Abuse of a child in the family. • Delays in seeking treatment. • Not following through with treatment and/or appointments. • Inconsistent, implausible or vague explanation of injuries. • Partner who is intrusive or over attentive in consultations. • Social isolation. • Recent separation or divorce.

likely). Women who have depression, PTSD or are suicidal as a result of DVA have approximately twice the level of usage of general medical services and between 3 and 8 times the level of usage of mental health services [6]. An Australian study showed DVA to be responsible for more ill-health and premature deaths in women aged 15–45 than any other of the well-known risk factors: high blood pressure, obesity, smoking, drugs, alcohol or physical inactivity [18]. Yet DVA as a health issue is not taught routinely in medical school curricula.

WHY ASK ABOUT DVA?

DVA prevalence is high in our practice populations with evidence from general practice waiting rooms showing that 41% of women have experienced physical violence from a partner or former partner, 74% have experienced some form of controlling behaviour and 46% have been threatened [18]. These figures are significantly higher than those reported by the Crime Survey of England and Wales. As many as 80% of women in a violent relationship seek help

from health services [16], who may be their first or only point of contact. Referral to, and engagement with specialist DVA services improves outcomes for patients in practical terms, such as safe accommodation and civil/criminal justice support in addition to improvements in their health and well-being [12, 17].

Research concludes that routine screening of all patients for DVA in general practice does not meet established criteria [18], however routine enquiry should be incorporated as good practice in maternity, sexual health [19] and A&E settings. NICE guidance is that all health professionals are able to ask, respond and refer patients experiencing DVA [20, 21]. Clinicians must recognise how domestic abuse may present in healthcare settings and how living with trauma translates into health problems [15].

People affected by DVA present to healthcare settings and regard health professionals as a source of help, however, they rarely disclose being affected by DVA unless asked directly and safely.

COMMUNICATION SKILLS – HOW TO ASK AND RESPOND

Asking

Asking about domestic abuse can be incorporated into everyday consultations. There is insufficient evidence for routine screening [18] but clinicians should have a low threshold for asking.

- Ask when patients present with certain problems or conditions, see Table 8.1.
- In particular, always ask pregnant patients as abuse often starts or escalates in pregnancy.
- Do not assume someone else has asked; disclosure is a process.
- Only ask the patient when they are on their own and it is safe to do so.
- The patient must be seen on their own, with no children or accompanying adults.
- Do not use a family member or friend to translate.
- You may have to organise to see the patient on her own to make safe enquiry.

After asking an open-ended question, be ready to pick up on cues (e.g. 'you mentioned stress at home…')

SUGGESTIONS FOR PRACTICE

- *Ask a specific question about domestic abuse, for example*:
  - *Is anyone harming you or intimidating you?*
  - *Does anyone control what you do or who you see?*
  - *Do you feel safe at home?*
- *Try linking the presenting problem to the possibility of DVA, for example: 'Sometimes when someone is suffering from [insert their reason for attending] there may be someone harming or intimidating them.'*

LEARNING EXERCISE

- Discuss with at least one patient each surgery the above suggestions.

RESPONDING

It is really important that your patient feels believed. This might be the first time they have disclosed the abuse.

SUGGESTIONS FOR PRACTICE

- *Respond positively to the disclosure, for example*:
  - *It's not your fault.*
  - *You are not alone.*
  - *I am pleased you felt able to tell me.*
  - *I know someone/an organisation you can talk to*
- *Offer a referral to your local DVA specialist service. The patient may not remember the exact question asked but will welcome the positive response.*
- *'It was the doctor's reaction when I spoke. If she hadn't believed me or showed some empathy I wouldn't have bothered' [17].*
- *'She was just different, really friendly, acted as though she really cared, listened and helped me talk about it' [17].*

GP REGISTRARS

GP registrars can practise asking about DVA during video surgeries and discuss with their GP trainers. DVA scenarios are included in the Membership of the Royal College of General Practitioners (MRCGP) clinical skills assessment examination.

Ensure there are clear referral pathways available from your local DVA specialist providers and safeguarding board. This may include provision by the community and voluntary sector as well as statutory provision for high-risk patients – such provision may need to come from an IDVA (Independent Domestic Violence Adviser) and/or MARAC (Multi Agency Risk Assessment Conference).

Ensure there are DVA posters up in every clinical consulting room, patient waiting areas and all staff and patient toilets. This can act as a prompt to remind clinicians to ask about DVA and to encourage patients to make disclosures. Remember that staff may also be suffering DVA too and may need help to access specialist DVA services.

RISK ASSESSMENT

If a patient discloses DVA it is vital that the health professional is able to gauge an accurate picture of the **current** risk that the individual is experiencing. There are various tools available to help with this assessment and it is essential that healthcare professionals (HCP) know the expectations in their local area. This may be different in areas that commission specialist programmes such as hospital IDVAs and IRIS (Identification and Referral to Improve Safety).

LEARNING EXERCISE

- Check your practice/organisation has the relevant risk assessments and referral guidance for your area available.
- Resources are available from SafeLives (www. safelives.org.uk) [29] and from your local safeguarding board.

A brief initial risk assessment should always be carried out following a disclosure of DVA:

- Are you safe to go home today?
- What threats have been made?
- What about the children?

If the patient says they are not safe to go home then the patient should be encouraged to contact the police immediately who can complete a detailed risk assessment and if necessary, remove the perpetrator from the property or take the patient to a place of safety, such as specialist refuge accommodation or temporary housing. Risk is dynamic and can fluctuate on a daily basis so needs regular reassessing.

There are also a number of triggers that can indicate or increase risk:

- Separation.
- Pregnancy/postnatal period.
- Escalation of severity of DVA or frequency, particularly threats to kill.
- Cultural considerations such as honour-based violence and forced marriages.
- Stalking/harassment.
- Sexual violence.

If any of the above have occurred recently (last 3 months) and there is no specialist DVA provider arrangement, the HCP should complete a risk assessment using the local risk-assessment tool and follow local referral pathways/guidance; these are usually based on the SafeLives

risk indicator checklist (RIC). Specialist training is available and should be undertaken by professionals in order to ensure that the risk assessment is completed in a meaningful way. All high-risk cases should be referred to MARAC where they will automatically be offered specialist support from an IDVA. In some areas this high-risk intervention is the only specialist DVA local support available.

At the MARAC a number of agencies meet to share confidential information known about the victim, the perpetrator and any children in the household to ascertain the level of risk involved. With a clear, multi-agency picture the agencies work together to try to mitigate as much of the risk as possible.

The longest and most enduring effect of DVA is on women's mental health. If the abuse is historic, although it presents no immediate risk to their safety, it is important to acknowledge the significant effects of experiencing this trauma. Talking to a DVA specialist and having their experiences validated can prove significant in helping patients come to terms with their experiences and moving forward in their lives. Not all specialist DVA providers work with survivors of historic abuse, so it is important to check what provision is available locally.

People are at most risk at the point of separation from their partner or shortly afterwards, because this is the point at which the perpetrator is about to lose/has lost the power and control over the relationship. Never advise a patient to leave; refer them for specialist DVA support where they can explore their options whilst ensuring their safety. If they are at immediate risk encourage them to report to the police and seek advice from your local high-risk provider. If a high-risk patient declines a referral to police, the IDVA service or MARAC, seek advice from the practice safeguarding lead and local safeguarding team. There are legal criteria for GPs to breach medical confidentiality, details of these are available from SafeLives [22].

SAFEGUARDING

Safeguarding is everyone's responsibility. If a patient discloses DVA a safeguarding assessment must be carried out. If there are children in the household, they will be affected by the abusive behaviours. Research is clear about the significant and long-lasting effects on children [10]. High-risk cases should be referred to children's social care. For lower risk families, the HCP should refer them within the local pathways, such as early help hubs or similar types of multi-agency provision. If the patient is vulnerable with multiple needs, including disabilities or learning disabilities, a referral to adult services for support should be considered.

RECORDING DVA SAFELY

In 2017 RCGP/IRISi issued new national guidance on recording disclosures of DVA from the victim, child, or perpetrator, using an agreed national code 'History of domestic abuse 14XD'. This guidance is summarised in Figure 8.2.

SUGGESTIONS FOR PRACTICE

- *Disclosures should be recorded using the patient's own words. Note symptoms and observed injuries, frequency, type (emotional, psychological, financial, physical and sexual) and severity of abuse.*
- *Describe the facts, don't judge or assume, and record your action e.g. referral and safety advice given. It is also important to record if a patient does not consent to referral or to a record being made.*
- *Make it clear in the consultation text if the disclosure is made by a perpetrator and add code 'Alleged perpetrator of domestic violence 14XC'.*
- *Consider computer screen safety; ensure notes are not visible to accompanying third parties.*
- *From April 2015 patients have right of access to medical records online, however this may leave them at risk of the perpetrator obtaining access and reading their records. Use the EMIS online visibility button, or equivalent, to hide consultations from patient online access. Review your practice protocol regarding patients' online access to records and redaction policy.*
- *A GP medical record of DVA (or an IRIS referral form – see next section) can be evidence to support a patient's application for Legal Aid.*

Domestic abuse is under-recorded in GP medical records [3]. It requires due consideration of safety issues and a robust redaction practice policy if records are shared with third parties.

LEARNING EXERCISE

- Audit your practice or clinic's methods of recording instances of DVA.
- Consider how it can be improved?

IRIS is an evidence-based training, referral and support programme for general practice. It is a collaboration between primary care and a local DVA specialist organisation, usually from the voluntary and community sector. IRIS DVA training is usually jointly delivered by a GP and the IRIS specialist domestic abuse worker, the Advocate Educator (AE) to the whole GP practice. The training includes the evidence base for the health impacts of DVA, learning how to ask, respond, risk assess, refer and record DVA safely. Consenting patients are referred to the IRIS AE who sees the patient in their own practice, enhancing safety and confidentiality.

Following its successful MRC clinical trial [12], the IRIS model was developed as a commissionable model for implementation nationally. It has been commissioned in over 34 sites in England and Wales and is available in over 800 general practices.

The success of the IRIS model is reflected in the NICE guidance (recommendations 15 and 16) on effective primary care responses to DVA and the recent standards that have been published to support these [20, 23]. The chief medical officer's annual report (2014) references this guidance and the importance of developing integrated commissioning of gender-based violence (GBV) services and supported referral pathways between health services and the GBV sector [24].

The difference that a successful and committed IRIS programme can make is significant. In Manchester, over the past 7 years, IRIS has been commissioned and supported to grow from providing IRIS training and service in 16 practices to having trained all practices. This has seen DVA referrals from general practice increase to 826 in 2018–19. Before IRIS, DVA referrals from all Manchester GPs were less than 10 per annum (Figure 8.3).

Victim discloses DVA to clinician in the practice

Victim's EMR
- Record the disclosure under 'History of domestic abuse' (14XD)
- Nature of abuse can be coded through the HARK template and/or free text
- Use the online visibility function to hide this consultation from online access

Children's (or vulnerable adult's) EMR
- If you are confident of your practice's redaction protocol, record the under 14XD code
- Use the online visibility function to hide this consultation from online access
- Ensure that any reference to DVA is redacted from children's records if provided to the perpetrator or provided to children who are deemed to have capacity to request their information

Perpetrator's EMR
- Do not record

Child discloses DVA to clinician in the practice

Children's (or vulnerable adult's) EMR
- Record the disclosure under 'History of domestic abuse' (14XD)
- Use the *online visibility function* to hide this consultation from online records

Perpetrator's EMR
- Do not record

Non-abusing parent and sibling's EMR
- Record the disclosure under the 14XD code
- Use the *online visibility function* to hide this consultation from online records
- Ensure any reference to DVA is redacted from children's records if provided to the perpetrator or provided to children who are deemed to have capacity to request their information

Perpetrator discloses DVA to clinician in the practice

Perpetrator's EMR
- Record the disclosure under 'History of domestic abuse' (14XD)
- Nature of abuse and perpetrator status should be recorded as free text

Children's (or vulnerable adult's) EMR
- Record the disclosure under the 14XD code
- Use the *online visibility function* to hide this consultation from online access

Victim's EMR
- Record the disclosure under the 14XD code
- Use the *online visibility function* to hide this consultation from online records

Figure 8.2 IRISi/RCGP DVA recording flow charts.

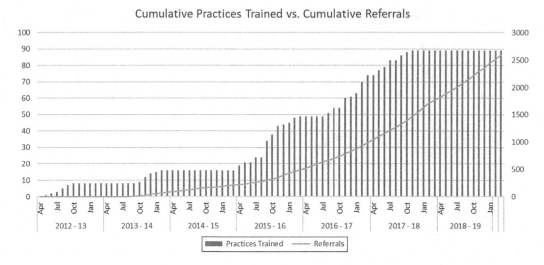

Figure 8.3 Cumulative practices trained in IRIS vs. cumulative DVA referrals.

FORCED MARRIAGE (FM), HONOUR-BASED VIOLENCE (HBV) AND FEMALE GENITAL MUTILATION (FGM)

Forced marriage, where victims are coerced into marrying against their will, is different from a mutually agreed arranged marriage. Pressure may be applied in subtle ways over an extended period of time with threats that may include physical violence, financial and emotional control. Forced marriage has been a crime in the UK since June 2014 and can result in up to 7 years in prison. In an arranged marriage, families may take an active role in choosing a spouse, however the prospective participants are involved in the process and have the final say.

Individuals may incur, or may be told they are incurring shame and dishonour by behaving in ways that may be viewed as inappropriate in their culture e.g. wearing make-up, wearing inappropriate clothes, having boy/girlfriends outside their approved group, running away and refusing an arranged marriage. There are differences in the dynamics of FM/HBV and DVA in that the breach of the family's honour code may be very slight e.g. being out later than the curfew, but the punishment can be severe, long-lasting and involve multiple perpetrators [25, 26]. A community may be involved in the abuse, informing on and punishing the individual. Forced marriage and HBV are not confined to a single ethnic group. In 2018, of the 1,764 cases the Forced Marriage Unit dealt with 17% involved

males, with 74 countries involved, 7% of them taking place entirely within the UK [27].

Female genital mutilation (FGM) is also included in the definition of DVA. It is thought to affect 140 million women in 29 countries and it is estimated that 66,000 women in the UK are affected. It has been illegal in the UK since 1985, and in 2003 the law was amended to make it illegal to take girls abroad for FGM. Mandatory reporting is required in some areas of health, including in general practice, and safeguarding should be considered for female children in families with known instances of FGM (the GP can record the patient to be at risk) with the NHS FGM information sharing system now flagging all girls born to mothers who have experienced FGM. GPs are uniquely placed to help combat FGM, although the RCGP have acknowledged that clear guidelines on how to support successful prosecutions remain inadequate. When considering FGM in a patient population it is important to know that although FGM is usually performed on pre-pubertal girls, infants and adult women are also targeted. The most important role of the GP remains identification and where it is suspected that FGM has taken place or that it is about to occur, a GP should refer the case to social services under their Local Safeguarding Children Board (LSCB) procedures. Significant factors to consider are if the girl/woman originates from a community known to practice FGM and whether her mother or sister have been affected. Girls are more at risk during school summer holidays when there is time for them to be taken out of the country to have FGM performed, followed by time to recover before any external adults (such as school teachers or nurses) may raise any concerns. This is often referred to as the 'cutting season' and there may be initiatives at airports in an attempt to raise awareness and intercept those at risk.

DOMESTIC HOMICIDE REVIEWS

In 2011 Domestic Homicide Reviews (DHRs) were setup to enable agencies to learn and improve their responses to DVA. These reviews occur when a patient dies from suspected domestic abuse. DHRs have shown that most victims have had contact with at least one health professional. In most cases the victim presented to their GP and in a number of cases the perpetrators presented to their GP too. Health professionals were well placed to identify both victims and perpetrators but missed multiple opportunities to ask about DVA.

PERPETRATORS

Perpetrators are patients too! They may have health problems, present with anger issues or disclose losing their temper; however, they should not be referred for anger management. Perpetrators are able to manage their anger and in fact use it as means to exercise control over their victim. If a patient presents with suicidal ideation, always ask if they have thoughts about harming others as well as themselves. Sources of help vary locally; some probation services have a perpetrator programme and there may be local perpetrator-specific programmes which also support the victims of abuse such as Manchester's TLC (Talk, Listen, Change) Bridging to Change programme. A national helpline is available via the charity Respect.

Domestic abuse causes significant health impacts and results in a burden of illness for patients, children, their families and society. The health inequality of domestic abuse is threefold: patients living with abuse, current or historic, have poorer health than those not suffering abuse; it is a gendered issue – overall women suffer worse and more severe DVA, and there are significant inequalities in the provision of specialist domestic abuse provision nationally.

GPs are well placed to recognise domestic abuse and need to recognise the expertise of specialist DVA services and work closely with them.

There is robust evidence to show that models such as IRIS training combined with a specialist DVA service delivered safely to patients in their own practice dramatically improve responses to DVA with health benefits to the patients and cost benefit to the NHS and society [4].

LEARNING EXERCISE

- Look at commissioning specialist DVA provision such as IRIS for general practice or hospital IDVAs

PATIENT QUOTES FROM MANCHESTER IRIS: HEARING THE VOICES OF THE IRIS SERVICE USERS [17]

A woman who was suffering from family abuse was surprised at being referred to Advocate Education (AE):

'She told me about (AE) who could help with DV issues. I was surprised, as I had not thought of this as DV as I thought that was only with partners. I did not know anything about DV services' (Woman J).

'I have more confidence now. I talk to people and have lots of friends. Before I had none. I am happy now, doing a range of courses to lead to a job' (Woman I).

'Before I felt bad about myself and depressed but now I think about a good future. I am starting a college course and want to look for a job' (Woman G).

'I now have less contact with the GP. I am not so scared because there is someone there (AE)' (Woman M).

'(AE) has been brilliant, I wouldn't be where I am now without her support' (Woman K).

ACKNOWLEDGEMENTS

Clare and Catherine would like to thank the IRISi team for their continuing endeavours to provide evidence-based interventions in healthcare to support and improve the lives of women and their children in the UK and beyond. Further information is available at www.irisi.org. A special thanks goes to the commissioners of IRIS in Manchester, jointly commissioned between health and social care and delivered by a superb team at The Pankhurst Trust (incorporating Manchester Women's Aid).

REFERENCES

1. Cross Government definition of DVA available at www.gov.uk/government/news/new-definition-of-domestic-violence [accessed 28/05/2019].

2. World Health Organization. (2005). WHO multi-country study on women's health and domestic violence against women: Initial results on prevalence, health outcomes and women's responses / authors: Claudia Garcia-Moreno... [et al.]. World Health Organization. http://www.who.int/iris/handle/10665/43309 [accessed 28/05/2019].

3. Feder G, Responding to interpersonal violence: What role for general practice? *British Journal of General Practice* 2006; 56 (525): 243–244.

4. Office for National Statistics (ONS). (2017). Domestic abuse in England and Wales: Year ending March 2017 available at www.ons.gov.uk/peoplepopulationandcommunity/crimeandjustice/bulletins/domesticabuseinenglandandwales/yearendingmarch2017 [accessed 28/05/2019].

5. Ulrich Y et al. Medical care utilization patterns in women with diagnosed domestic violence. *American Journal of Preventive Medicine* 2003; 24(1): 9–15.

6. Walby S, Allen J. (2004). Home Office Research Study 276. *Domestic Violence, Sexual Assault and Stalking: Findings from the British Crime Survey*. London, Home Office, Research, Development and Statistics Directorate.

7. Domestic Abuse Stonewall Health Briefing, 2012 available at www.healthylives.stonewall.org.uk [accessed 28/05/2019].

8. National Institute for Health Care and Excellence (NICE) 2014 Costing statement: Domestic violence and abuse Implementing the NICE guidance on Domestic violence and abuse – how services can respond effectively (PH50) available at www.nice.org.uk/guidance/ph50/resources/costing-statement-pdf-69194701 [accessed 28/05/2019].

9. Walby S. (2009). The Cost of Domestic Violence Up-date 2009. Lancaster University, available at www.lancs.ac.uk/fass/doc_library/sociology/Cost_of_domestic_violence_update.doc

10. Bellisi MA et al. (2015). *Adverse Childhood Experiences and their impact on health-harming behaviours in the Welsh adult population* available at http://www2.nphs.wales.nhs.uk:8080/PRIDDocs.nsf/7c21215d6d0c613e80256f490030c05a/d488a3852491bc1d80257f370038919e/$FILE/ACE%20Report%20FINAL%20(E).pdf

11. Domestic Abuse Intervention Project Duluth Power and Control Wheel available at www.duluthmodel.org/wheels

12. Feder, G et al., Identification and Referral to Improve Safety (IRIS) of women experiencing domestic violence with a primary care training and support programme: A cluster randomised controlled trial. *The Lancet* 2011;378(9805): 1788–1795.

13. World Health Organisation (WHO). 2012 *Understanding and addressing violence against women Intimate partner violence* available at www.apps.who.int/iris/bitstream/handle/10665/77432/WHO_RHR_12.36_eng.pdf?sequence=1 [accessed 28/05/2019].

14. Vic Health. (2004). *The Health Costs of Violence: Measuring the Burden of Disease Caused by Intimate Partner Violence*. State Government Victoria, Australia, Department of Human Services.

15. Bessel A. Van der Kolk. *The Body Keeps the Score: Mind, Brain and Body in the Transformation of Trauma*. Penguin Books Ltd. 2015.

16. Richardson J et al., Identifying domestic violence: Cross sectional study in primary care. *BMJ* 2002; 324(7332): 274–278.

17. Gillian Granville. *Identification and Referral to Improve Safety (IRIS). Hearing the voices of the IRIS service users Study Report* 2014 available at www.gilliangranville.com/wp-content/uploads/IRIS-service-users-study-April-2014-Report2.pdf [accessed 28/05/2019].

18. Feder G, Ramsay J, Dunne D, Rose M, Arsene C, Norman R et al. How far does screening women for domestic (partner) violence in different health-care settings meet the UK National Screening Committee criteria for a screening programme? Systematic reviews of nine UK National Screening Committee criteria. *Health Technol Assess* 2009; 13(16).

19. Sacks et al. (2016). *Responding to Domestic Abuse in Sexual Health Settings* BASHH Sexual Violence Group available at www.bashh.org/documents/Responding%20to%20Domestic%20Abuse%20in%20Sexual%20Health%20Settings%20Feb%202016%20Final.pdf [accessed 28/05/2019].

20. National Institute for Health Care and Excellence (NICE). (2016). Domestic violence and abuse: Multiagency working (PH50) available at www.nice.org.uk/guidance/ph50/resources/domestic-violence-and-abuse-multiagency-working-pdf-1996411687621 [accessed 28/05/2019].

21. National Institute for Health Care and Excellence (NICE). (2016). Quality statement 1: Asking about domestic violence and abuse.

22. SafeLives available at www.safelives.org.uk/practice-support/resources-identifying-risk-victims-face [accessed 28/05/2019].

23. SafeLives available at http://www.safelives.org.uk/sites/default/files/resources/SafeLives_GP_guidance_manual_STG1_editable_0.pdf [accessed 28/05/2019].

24. Home Office Domestic Homicide Reviews Common Themes Identifed as Lessons to be Learned available at http://data.parliament.uk/DepositedPapers/Files/DEP2013-1881/Domestic_Homicide_Review:-_Common_themes_v2__2_.pdf [accessed 28/05/2019].

25. Department of Health Commissioning services for women and children who experience violence or abuse – a guide for health commissioners available at https://assets.publishing.service.gov.uk/government/uploads/system/uploads/attachment_data/file/215635/dh_125938.pdf [accessed 28/05/2019].

26. HM Government Violence against Women and Girls Strategy 2016–2020 available at https://assets.publishing.service.gov.uk/government/uploads/system/uploads/attachment_data/file/522166/VAWG_Strategy_FINAL_PUBLICATION_MASTER_vRB.PDF [accessed 28/05/2019].

27. Home Office 2019 Forced Marriage Unit Statistics 2018 available at https://assets.publishing.service.gov.uk/government/uploads/system/uploads/attachment_data/file/804044/Forced_Marriage_Unit_Statistics_2018_FINAL.pdf [accessed 28/05/2019].

9

Substance Use: Our Patients, Drugs and Alcohol

JAMES MATHESON*

Once you've been starving, you never forget that feeling.

In 2017 the Office for National Statistics (ONS) reported 3,756 deaths from drug poisoning in England and Wales [1] – two thirds related to drug misuse. Whilst male deaths had reduced, drug deaths in women had increased for the eigth year running. It is difficult to prove a death is drug-related and gather specific data on the circumstances, so most believe the true figure is much higher. In 2018 the ONS conducted a 'deep dive' into coroners' reports concerning drug-related deaths. They found;

'...a vulnerable, at-risk population engaging in unsafe drug-taking practices such as taking drugs alone and consuming multiple different types of drug alongside alcohol' [2].

CASE STUDY

Ashley

Ashley is late for her appointment but not by long. She missed the last one and Neil, her support worker from the drug and alcohol service,

had worked hard to track her down and persuade her to come in today for a methadone restart. When Ashley is on a binge she is high on the list of people I worry about adding to the drug-related deaths that bring our practice's age-at-death list to well below the national average.

These 'deaths of despair' [3] amongst our patient population at the harsh end of growing national inequalities are recorded in the mounting number of entries in our coroner's case file and in our memories, for these are often the patients we see the most and invest the most in trying to heal.

When I last saw Ashley she had been almost unbearably sad. It was nearly a year since her husband, John, had died. In anticipation of the anniversary she had returned her three children to their grandmother's care. We both knew what would happen next, though we discussed ways to avoid it. After that we talked about harm reduction.

WHAT IS 'SUBSTANCE ABUSE'?

The World Health Organisation (WHO) describes substance abuse as referring to:

* With thanks to Graham Parsons, Graham Shiels and Martyn Hull.

'…the harmful or hazardous use of psychoactive substances, including alcohol and illicit drugs…', adding that use can lead to a dependence syndrome in which users have, '…difficulties in controlling its use, persisting in its use despite harmful consequences, a higher priority given to drug use than to other activities and obligations, increased tolerance, and sometimes a physical withdrawal state' [4].

In the UK it is more commonly called substance misuse.

Ashley has heard this term used many times and it makes her smile. 'What else are you going to use heroin for?' she asks. Ashley defines her addiction differently. 'It's a hunger', she says, 'an all-consuming hunger like you haven't eaten for days and all you can think about is food. But, once you've been starving, you never forget that feeling so, as soon as you've eaten, the first thing you're thinking about is doing it again'.

THE COMPLEXITIES OF SUBSTANCE MISUSE

Headlines from NHS Digital's substance misuse statistics 2017–2018 include, in England alone, 2,503 deaths and 17,031 hospital admissions due to drug poisoning and 7,258 hospital admissions due to the mental health effects of drugs [5]. 9% of people aged 16–54 and 19.8% of people aged 16–24 had used illicit drugs in the preceding year [5]. Again, with the difficulties in gathering reliable data, the true figure is likely to be much higher.

In Scotland, there were 934 drug-related deaths in 2017, more than double the figure for 2007 [6] and a rate higher than any other EU country. On the same webpage as National Records of Scotland reported that Jack and Olivia were Scotland's most popular baby names, it also recorded that the country's previous increases in life expectancy had stalled, that deaths outstripped births by 5,000 and that life expectancy varied by council area by up to 7.2 years [6].

Wales also reported higher rates of drug-related death than England in 2017 at 185, a rate of 64.5 deaths per million population compared with England's rate of 42.7 per million [7]. Northern Ireland recorded 136 deaths from drug use, a figure 68% higher than a decade ago [8]. The cost of dealing with drug-related harm, including its health effects, are estimated at £780 million (for Class A drugs) in Wales, £3.5 billion in Scotland and £10.7 billion in England [9].

For those working in deprivation it can seem like the figures should be much higher because drug-related harm is concentrated in more socio-economically disadvantaged areas. Areas with the most neighbourhood deprivation bear the highest number of drug-related deaths [9]. Drug use is higher in groups who experience marked social exclusion. Aldridge et al. found that people in the most deprived parts of England and Wales had an all-cause standardised mortality rate (SMR) for women 2.1 times higher than more affluent areas and 2.8 times higher for men. In marginalised and excluded populations including homeless people, those in contact with the criminal justice system, people involved in sex work and those with substance use issues, the SMRs were 7.9 for men and 11.9 for women [10]. It has been suggested that substance use is a bigger driver of health inequalities than even socio-economic inequalities [9].

Whilst illicit drug use is a huge problem, problem drinking is even more so. Hospital admissions linked to alcohol have increased by 17% over the last 10 years and alcohol-related harm is estimated to cost the NHS around £3.5 billion each year in England alone [11]. In 2017, in England, 5,843 deaths were directly attributed to alcohol with a further 1,659 partially attributed [12]. Again, in reality the figures should be much higher.

In Wales between 2015–2017 1,170 deaths were attributed to alcohol – mostly from alcoholic liver disease but also including cancers, poisoning and mental/behavioural problems. Summarising alcohol-related statistics in 2017, the Public Health Observatory Wales stated that, 'the consumption of alcohol is deeply ingrained in the culture of Wales' with almost a fifth of Welsh drinkers reporting very heavy drinking within the last week [13].

In 2017, in Scotland, 1,235 alcohol-attributable deaths were recorded – a reduction on the previous year but more than double the rates in the

1980s. Alcohol was implicated in many more [14]. In Scotland, adult drinkers consume a fifth more alcohol than in England and Wales. The Scottish Government has described the nation's relationship with alcohol as 'unbalanced', with the amount of alcohol sold each year enough for every adult in Scotland to be drinking 20 units per week. The impact of this is costing Scotland £3.6 billion a year, around £900 for each adult in the country [15].

> Ashley has never been a big drinker. She says the memories of her father keep her away from alcohol. As a child, Ashley lived in a household fraught with domestic violence. When her father drank she feared even more for her safety and the safety of her mother who she felt took more of the violence to protect her daughter.

The consumption and harm of alcohol in the UK can appear paradoxical. Figures illustrate that, whilst alcohol consumption is markedly higher in affluent areas than more deprived locations, levels of harm are much higher in deprivation. Wales' most deprived quintile had double the rates of hospital admission due to alcohol than its least deprived quintile, and double the rates of mortality from alcohol [13]. Katikireddi et al. examined socio-economic status and risk of alcohol-related admission or death in a paper published in *The Lancet Public Health*. They found that, controlling for smoking and obesity and removing known problem drinkers, even light drinkers in deprived areas faced disproportionate risks of harm: Hazard Ratio (HR) 6.12 in advantaged areas compared with 10.22 in disadvantaged areas [16].

Nor are the drinkers the only ones to come to harm. The Scottish Government reported that in 2017 40% of people in prison, including 60% of young offenders, were drunk at the time of their offence [15]. In more than half of violent crimes in England and Wales over the last decade the victim has reported that their assailant was drunk. Alcohol was also involved in a third of reported domestic violence incidents [13].

> Ashley has frequently been in contact with the criminal justice system. Her notes contain many entries detailing injuries she has sustained from various assailants. Prior to meeting her husband she engaged in sex work to fund her drug addiction. She has come today to ask to restart antidepressants. Her mood has worsened, she says, at the prospect of returning to jail. She says she has been shoplifting, amongst other forms of theft, to feed the children. Jane, her Focused Care worker, had helped her claim benefits after her husband died but that money goes on rent and drugs – she is in debt to more than one dealer and worries for her and her family's safety.

Women make up only 5% of the prison population at any one time [17] but, because these are usually short sentences (half less than 6 months), around 12,000 women are imprisoned each year through the UK [18]. Ashley's children will be amongst the estimated 17,240 children separated from their mothers each year in the UK due to imprisonment [18]. It is estimated around 80% of women in prison have a diagnosable mental disorder and, despite their small numbers in prison, they carry out 47% of prisoner self-harm episodes and have a higher rate of suicide than men in prison or women outside [17]. One survey found more than half of women in prison had used heroin, cocaine or crack in the month before being imprisoned and funding their or a partner's drug addiction was a common reason for offending [17].

The relationship between drugs, alcohol and mental health is complex. Early alcohol use has long been acknowledged as predictive of later alcohol addiction, substance misuse and major depression [19]. To what extent reverse causation, i.e. early depression leading to substance use, is present in the UK may be less clear. In America, the National Bureau for Economic Research suggested that 69% of that country's alcohol and 84% of its cocaine were consumed by people with mental illness [20].

In reality it is rare for human behaviour to be solely attributable to one factor. In *Youthoria*, Harris examines risk factors for substance use problems including, amongst many others:

Societal: socio-economic status especially extreme deprivation, education and availability of substances.

- Interpersonal: family substance use, family conflict and instability, permissive parenting and drug-using peers.
- Psycho-behavioural: problematic behaviour, low academic achievement and alienation.
- Biogenetic: susceptibility to substance use and its effects, sensation-seeking, and poor impulse control [21].

Lankelly Chase's 2015 publication, *Hard Edges*, looked at those living with severe and multiple disadvantages (SMD) – those with combinations of contact with the criminal justice system, homelessness and substance use problems – a population totalling 586,000 people in England; 58,000 had all three. As children, large numbers of these people had experience, amongst other traumas, of family breakdown, abuse and neglect. As adults they reported high levels of poverty, isolation and loneliness. Across the categories around 40%· reported a mental health problem, but poor mental health was reported by 58% of those with substance use issues. Areas of high SMD prevalence mapped similarly to deprivation [22].

BASIC PRINCIPLES OF HARM REDUCTION

An important theme running through substance use interventions is the principle of harm reduction. The UK Harm Reduction Alliance has defined harm reduction principles [23]as:

- Pragmatic – in accepting that substance use is common and that reducing harm may be more feasible than complete elimination of substance use behaviours.
- Prioritising goals – the first of which may be engaging the individual.
- Non-judgemental.
- Focusing on risks so harms can be reduced or avoided, rather than on abstinence.
- Maximising use of available interventions.

Harm reduction advice will vary according to the substance and the way it is used. The ability to deliver pragmatic harm reduction interventions is often defined by how far a society will tolerate such interventions when the substance in use is illegal. An example of pragmatism successfully applied is the increasing presence of drug-testing facilities at clubs and festivals. The Loop (www.weretheloop.org) is a group who provide on-the-spot drug testing so potential users can know exactly what they have bought prior to taking it and receive harm reduction advice at the same time. This also provides information on what is being sold, allowing for warnings to be delivered when required.

In 2013 GPs at the Deep End Project discussed the role of primary care in alcohol addiction in deprived areas as assessing risk, providing brief interventions, minimising harm, managing physical and mental co-morbidities and signposting to other agencies [24]. The same could be said for drug problems. At first contact, many substance users will not yet be ready to engage with other services or be considering abstinence. America's Harm Reduction Coalition (www.harmreduction.org) provides detailed harm reduction advice.

Ashley was given harm reduction advice by Neil, who later became her addiction service keyworker. 'He even told me the safest way to draw up water from a public loo', she recalls, smiling. She also received informal support from Erin, our practice nurse. 'Erin was someone I could talk to, who I felt I could trust. She got me thinking how life could be different if I had more control of the drugs rather than the drugs controlling me'.

SUGGESTIONS FOR PRACTICE

- *Harm reduction advice can be a life-saving intervention. Consider finding out more about harm reduction for the different substances your patients may use.*
- *Identify substance users and use motivational interviewing techniques and apply a non-judgemental strength-based approach to encourage patients towards addressing their addictions.*
- *Questions to ask could include, 'Have you considered how the amount you're drinking may be affecting your health?' or 'What benefits do you think controlling your drug use might have for you?'*
- *Targeted brief interventions are effective in reducing consumption and harm [25]. It is estimated that if drinkers consuming more than 14 units per week were given brief advice, the number of high-risk drinkers would fall by 18% [26].*

OPIOID SUBSTITUTION THERAPY (OST)

For heroin users, OST forms a large part of harm reduction and the pathway back to well-being. Early mortality is up to 20 times higher than in non-users, with the main cause of premature death being overdose, alongside other causes including violence, accidents and suicide, as well as the medical consequences of injecting [27].

Full details of OST and other interventions to help substance users are beyond the scope of this short chapter but can be found in *Drug Misuse and Dependence: UK Guidelines on Clinical Management,* known as 'The Orange Book' [28].

Receiving OST leads to a marked decrease in mortality from overdose [27]. Both methadone and buprenorphine are effective in reducing all-cause mortality and drug-related poisoning. There is a high-risk period in the first 4 weeks of starting methadone treatment, but it has better long-term adherence than buprenorphine. Buprenorphine has better figures for reducing all-cause mortality, especially in the first 4 weeks of treatment, possibly due to a ceiling effect on respiratory depression [29]. Buprenorphine may also be the medication of choice in certain populations due to being available in oral lyophilizate form, reducing the risk of diversion.

Initiation of OST can be a difficult and potentially risky time for patients, so frequent contact and supervised consumption are usually called for. Overdose awareness and training are important, especially at this time. Once started on a medication, dose optimisation is crucial. At times there has been a focus on establishing people on the minimum dose to control withdrawal symptoms, often with a plan to progressively reduce the OST dose with the aim of coming off it and remaining abstinent. This aim will not be appropriate for all patients and a more suitable initial aim may be for dose optimisation at a sufficiently high dose to control drug cravings and reduce or eliminate heroin use on top [27].

When she was first established on methadone Ashley used heroin once or twice a week. She had initially been reluctant to increase her methadone dose as she assumed she would be made to come off it eventually and feared this would make the process harder. She found, as her methadone wore off around three in the morning, however, that she couldn't always resist calling her dealer. After discussions with Ashley and Neil we increased her methadone and Ashley reported injecting much less frequently.

The length of treatment should be determined by the patient and, with the knowledge that relapse is common, treatment should be reviewed and adjusted regularly. OST is only one part of the intervention to support people moving away from addiction. Psychosocial interventions, relapse prevention counselling and support are all beneficial to success [30]. Contingency management – incentivising achieving agreed goals with, for example, shopping vouchers – has been shown to be effective in promoting abstinence in drug, alcohol and smoking cessation [31].

Interventions to support patients with alcohol are also multi-faceted. Opinion and evidence are mixed as to the roles of inpatient and outpatient detoxes. Whilst some may benefit from an environment away from the stressors which trigger their drinking and be more likely to complete a detox in an inpatient setting, the risk remains that returning them to the same stressors will likely trigger relapse. Benzodiazepine reducing regimes are effective in reducing withdrawal symptoms from alcohol dependence and in reducing seizures and life-threatening complications. Amongst benzodiazepines, chlordiazepoxide performed best (though differences did not reach statistical significance) and is widely used [32].

A Cochrane systematic review found Acamprosate to be an effective and safe treatment to help former drinkers stay off alcohol, preventing relapse and no more side effects than the placebo [31].

Ashley's brother Chris never took drugs but he drank, increasingly, from an early age. 'I was an alcoholic', he now recognises, 'for a long time before I realised it. Because I could hold down a job and because my family put up with it, I thought I had it under control. Then my wife said she was leaving and taking the kids. It was a big wake up call'. Chris paid for his first detox – it cost him

£1,600 he couldn't really afford, and he started drinking the day after he finished it. He attended the surgery the next day, inebriated and begging for a Librium (chlordiazepoxide) prescription so he could try again. I noted he had been prescribed disulfiram in the past but, having experienced its very unpleasant effects when taken with alcohol, he had stopped the disulfiram rather than the alcohol.

Alcohol withdrawal syndrome is associated with a 5–15% risk of death [32]. Alcohol withdrawal may precipitate delirium tremens, seizures may follow and death may occur from cardiac arrhythmias and respiratory failure [33]. These risks can be reduced through pharmacologically supported detox [33], but risks increase with multiple attempts to detox especially when in close succession, in a process called 'kindling' [34].

Chris didn't get a Librium prescription that day or for some time later. After several detoxes when he had presented with withdrawal symptoms at A&E, Chris eventually followed up on our referral to local services and engaged with counselling and a support group. He had a supervised detox in the community, seeing a support worker on alternate days. A year on from this he still hasn't had a drink. 'At first I didn't want to stop drinking', says Chris. 'I was only doing it because other people said I had to. Once I realised I needed to do it for me, I found the motivation to push through it and I feel so much better now. My life is coming back together'. Chris is now off his thiamine but stays on Acamprosate and attends regular meeting of Alcoholics Anonymous. 'I still think about booze a lot and the idea of never drinking again is still terrifying. That's why I've promised myself a drink on my 80th birthday', he says laughing.

NICE have produced guidance on the diagnosis and management of alcohol-use disorders [35] and on their complications [36–37]. In years past, it was not uncommon for GPs to prescribe detox regimes for their patients. Best practice in terms of risk reduction and likelihood of success is for specialist services to support patient detoxes as part of a package of pre-and post-detox interventions.

People may struggle to engage with drug and alcohol services which are at a distance or used by people they are trying to avoid. There may also be perceived stigma attached to attending these locations.

SUGGESTIONS FOR PRACTICE

- *Consider offering a shared care OST clinic at your surgery or offering space at the practice for addiction services to see local patients.*

GPs at the Deep End in Scotland trialled embedding nurse alcohol workers in primary care and found it an effective way of reaching patients who had had difficulty engaging with services.

OPIOIDS

Alcohol and heroin are not the only drugs that will cause issues for your patients but they are big issues. Of opioid drug users entering treatment across Europe, 78% cited heroin as their primary drug, 9% cited methadone, 5% buprenorphine, 0.5% fentanyl (small numbers but with high risk due to the strength of fentanyl and its more potent variant carfentanyl) and 7% opioids [38]. The UK tops the list for high-risk opioid use in this year's *European Drug Report* with an estimated 341,576 users [38]. Risk is increased by combining opioids with other medications including sedating antidepressants, antipsychotics, gabapentinoids, benzodiazepines and other hypnotics, or with alcohol.

COCAINE

The UK also tops the European list for cocaine use prevalence [38]. The quantities of cocaine seized in the UK were surpassed only by the amounts of cannabis seized [38]. Cocaine is a psychostimulant which produces euphoric effects in the user. In its different forms it can be snorted, smoked or injected. Cocaine can dangerously affect many organs but is particularly associated with increased risk of cardiac arrhythmia, myocardial infarction and stroke [39]. Chronic use can lead to neurobiological changes in the brain and cognitive impairment. Previously regarded as a party drug for the wealthy, its increased availability, purity and reduced cost have made it increasingly prevalent amongst drug users. There is no specific medication treatment for those wanting to stop using cocaine – psychosocial interventions form the mainstay of treatment [28]. Using cocaine alongside other substances is common, with powder cocaine users often having drinking problems and heroin users commonly also injecting cocaine [28].

> Ashley's husband John died unexpectedly aged 40. The coroner's enquiry concluded the cause of death was likely to be cardiac following many years of cocaine use. Ashley continued to use cocaine after his death though recognising the risk.

Deaths caused by cocaine and fentanyl continue to rise based on 2017 figures [1].

CRACK COCAINE

Since 2013 there has been a marked rise in crack use in England. Whilst use in London has dropped, other parts of the country, especially the south east and east of England have seen large increases. A number of reasons have been put forward to explain the increases including better purity, crack being cheaper to buy (due to being sold in smaller quantities rather than the price per rock coming down) and the reduction of stigma previously associated with its use. County lines activity has also been blamed. The increased use is seen across most age groups, reversing the previous downward trend in use by younger people [40]. Anecdotal evidence has crack use being much more socially acceptable with rooms dedicated to crack-smoking at parties and builders smoking crack on building sites prior to starting work [41] whilst dealers, aware that people on crack and heroin spend more than users of either drug alone, are selling bundles of two bags of one drug with one of another thrown in cheaper on top.

ECSTASY

Ecstasy or 'MDMA' after its chemical name, 3,4-Methylenedioxymethamphetamine is a psychedelic stimulant, known for making people affectionate and adding a vivid quality to colours and other sensory experiences [42]. Drug dealers, users and the press will often use a multitude of names for substances which can lead to a confused history – a list of common names can be found at https://www.talktofrank.com/drugs-a-z[43] but beware of the potential for misidentification. Chronic use can cause cognitive impairments and acute use has shown effects on the body's homeostatic mechanisms resulting in deaths from dehydration [42]. One of the principal risks is the variability of the drug – in terms of strength of dose and other psychoactive substances in the tablet. Slower or lower effects may result in the user re-dosing i.e. taking another tablet which can result in overdose or much more prolonged symptoms [44]. Again, there is no specific medication to assist in stopping MDMA use and psychosocial interventions are employed.

These can include: cognitive behavioural therapy, behavioural approaches, family or social network interventions, social skills training, vocational training, engaging in other activities, assistance with housing services and income support [28]. Where users will persist in taking ecstasy, harm reduction advice and directing them towards onsite drug-testing services are pragmatic interventions.

AMPHETAMINES

Amphetamines, commonly known as 'speed', are stimulants which can be snorted, swallowed, injected or dabbed onto gums [42]. Its impurity leads to a high risk of overdose and it is particularly dangerous when injected [42]. Long-term use can result in cardiovascular and neurological toxicity [45]. Users exposed to high doses can become agitated or aggressive and risk seizures in these situations benzodiazepines are sometimes used for sedation and seizure prevention [45].

NOVEL PSYCHOACTIVE SUBSTANCES (NPS)

NPS started out with the trend of 'legal highs' where new psychoactive substances could be bought legally, often in 'head shops'. These were widely available, cheap and popular among young people. The first generation of NPS were generally stimulants such as mephedrone which could be snorted, smoked, swallowed or injected [46]. Gradually these new substances were made illegal but were quickly replaced by new chemical variants increasing in potency. The next generation of substances were synthetic cannabinoid receptor agonists (SCRAs), often referred to (though with much crossover with other NPS) as 'spice'. These seemed particularly prevalent among vulnerable populations such as the homeless [46]. Use was increasingly seen in prisons where complications included cardiac arrhythmias, dangerous hypertension and seizures [47]. Some variants triggered the bizarre behaviours for which they became known in the populist media. As more NPS were outlawed, other variants proliferated with as many as 620 substances being monitored and deaths from NPS increasing [46]. In 2016 the UK's Psychoactive Substances Act provided a blanket ban on NPS after which numbers dropped. In 2017 deaths related to NPS halved [1]. NPS now include stimulants, sedatives and hallucinogens – their use remains highly prevalent and very risky among vulnerable groups, especially those in prison.

SUGGESTIONS FOR PRACTICE

- *Neptune, the novel psychoactive treatment: the UK network provide detailed clinical guidance and free e-learning modules on their website neptune-clinical-guidance.co.uk.*

CANNABIS

The majority of young people in treatment in the UK cite cannabis as their main drug problem, often in combination with alcohol [28]. Its psychoactive potency depends on the percentage of tetrahydrocannabinol (THC). Heavy use can result in lethargy, depression, cognitive impairment, paranoia and drug-induced psychosis [28]. Cost varies according to form – herbal or resin – and strength. More than half of UK drug offences in which the drug was specified are attributed to cannabis [28]. Its use in areas of deprivation is high and can be related to contact with the criminal justice system through use, cultivation and dealing. There is no medication to assist withdrawal but there is a strong evidence base for behavioural change interventions [28].

There are many, many drugs in use amongst our practice populations with diverse effects and harms beyond the scope of this chapter. Where specific drugs are locally prevalent, further reading or discussion with a drug service is recommended. As well as physical and mental health risks, drug users may come to harm through contact with the criminal justice system and interactions with dealers when debt is incurred. Vulnerable people or those in debt to dealers may find themselves holding stock, hosting deals or even coerced into the cultivation of drugs. Relationship breakdown, job loss and social isolation can compound the problems of people using drugs.

> Ashley is imprisoned for a short sentence. Whilst in prison she reduces her methadone dose gradually and eventually comes off OST. She engages with psychological services at the prison and makes significant progress in moving on from her childhood experiences. She declines the offer of a 'retox', restarting her methadone in anticipation of the increased risk of overdose on release. She does, however accept the take-home prescription of naloxone.

CHANGING THE TRAJECTORY: CARE FOR THE WHOLE PERSON

In his insightful book *In the Realm of Hungry Ghosts: Close Encounters with Addiction* Maté describes how his patients' drug use often follows severe and repeated trauma in childhood and through life, with patients describing how they attempt to fill emotional voids in their past or present with the sensations or the release from sensation offered by intoxication [48].

It is rare that people with serious substance dependency have only that one problem in their lives. It will remain unlikely that the problem will be overcome without addressing the things which drove them to substance use originally and the stressors which maintain their use. A holistic assessment of a patient's medical, psychiatric and emotional needs is recommended, alongside assessment of their accommodation, financial situation and food security. Discussion about the use of other substances is also important.

Drug use and mental health problems are frequently seen in conjunction. In order to treat one issue successfully, the other also needs to be addressed. Sometimes specialist 'dual diagnosis' services are available but at others dual diagnosis can be a reason patients are excluded from one service or the other.

SUGGESTIONS FOR PRACTICE

- *Consider targeting high-risk patients such as people with mental health problems, homeless people and those with other vulnerabilities for assessment and extra support.*
- *Patients can be at an increased risk of overdose after a period of abstinence when their tolerance levels have dropped, for example on leaving prison. Consider targeting people for extra care at such times.*

Ashley is released from prison and, according to local hearsay, is planning a fresh new start. Her listed phone number no longer works so we sent her a letter asking her to book an appointment for review. Two weeks later Erin comes in with sad news – Ashley has been admitted to hospital following an overdose of mixed substances including heroin. Fortunately, her friend had received training on administering naloxone whilst staying at a hostel. It sounds like this saved her life. After discharge, her first call is to Neil, to restart her methadone.

For infrequent attenders, the most should be made of any contact with the practice. Things to consider when opportunity arises would include screening tests such as smears, vaccinations and blood tests including for blood-borne viruses, especially in at-risk groups such as injecting drug users.

Of people who inject drugs around 1 in 100 are estimated to have HIV and, with increased awareness and testing, it is thought that most are in treatment [49]. It remains a risk, however, that HIV may be detected late in intravenous drug users, worsening outcomes and increasing the risk of the disease spreading.

It is estimated that around 1 in 200 people who inject drugs are living with hepatitis B (HBV), half the number of a decade ago [49]. Infection can be passed by needle sharing, sexual intercourse and other means. If chronic infection ensues, carriers may be asymptomatic and risk spreading the disease or being unwell with symptoms of fatigue or

malaise. Chronic HBV infection can lead to liver cirrhosis and hepatocellular carcinoma [50]. Infection risk can be reduced by vaccination and around 75% of intravenous drug users are now vaccinated [49].

SUGGESTIONS FOR PRACTICE

- *Take the opportunity to protect any unvaccinated IV drug users as they present.*

An estimated 200,000 people in the UK have chronic hepatitis C (HCV) with around 2,000 developing end-stage liver failure or cancer each year [51]. HCV is particularly prevalent in vulnerable groups including people who inject drugs, and as many as 50% of people carrying the disease are unaware of their status [52]. Hepatitis C is curable, therefore elimination of the disease is possible. New oral medications with few or no side effects make treatment a more appealing prospect, but stigma still remains around the disease and people may be deterred by fears of the side effects of older treatment regimes. The World Health Organisation has set a target to reduce HCV-related mortality by 10% by 2020, and by 65% by 2030 [51]. NHS England has set a target to eliminate HCV by 2025 at the latest [52]. Testing and referring patients when opportunities present will play a large part in achieving these goals.

Local infections and abscesses in injecting drug users are common causes of hospital admissions, but can be treated more easily when caught early. It can be worth advising patients to seek help promptly when they see the signs.

IT'S NOT JUST ABOUT HEROIN

OST will only be of use to those people with opioid problems but it is a powerful incentive for people who might not usually be effective users of healthcare to regularly attend the surgery and much else can be positively achieved whilst they are there. Withholding scripts, however, should not be used as a threat as dealers will make it very easy to obtain the drug the doctor withholds.

Of patients receiving OST, 80–98%. also smoke. Up to 50% will die of tobacco-related causes, but 75% are open to the idea of receiving a smoking cessation intervention [53]. Smoking cessation pharmacotherapies may be less effective in OST but chances of successful quitting are increased once patients are on a stable OST dose and abstinent from other drug use. Smoking cessation does not worsen outcomes for OST [53].

Estimates of alcohol-use disorders in patients on OST range from 17–50% and are associated with worse outcomes and increased mortality [53]. Usual interventions for alcohol dependence apply to those on OST though use of nalmefene and naltrexone, as opioid antagonists, would be precluded [53].

Concurrent use of cocaine in heroin users is common and associated with lower levels of treatment retention and poorer outcomes [53]. Optimisation of OST dose may bring about reduction or cessation of cocaine use [53].

Prevalence of benzodiazepine use in patients receiving OST is estimated at 50–75% and increases the risk of overdose, with benzodiazepines implicated in up to 80% of heroin-related deaths [53]. Long-term benzodiazepine use is associated with poorer outcomes so a switch to diazepam with gradually reducing doses is an approach once a stable OST dose is achieved – concurrent detox from opioids and benzodiazepines in the community is not recommended [53, 54].

SUGGESTIONS FOR PRACTICE

- *The market in illicit drugs can change rapidly causing variations in drug use and the risks associated with them. Consider joining the email mailing list for your local drugs bulletin to keep you abreast of drug news. Your local drug and alcohol service can put you in touch.*

For most, addiction is a cycle of use, treatment and relapse until, one day, they break the cycle and real-life change is achieved. There is much we can do to help people achieve this end and to support them on the journey towards it.

Ashley recognises the effect her traumatic childhood had on her and is determined to break the cycle before she sees the same effects in her children. She attends the surgery with both her children, looking startlingly well and happy. She has decided to stay on a maintenance dose of methadone believing it to be the best way to protect her from relapse for the foreseeable future.

Since we last saw her she has moved from being a service user with her local drug service to volunteering to support other patients in their journey away from addiction. She is studying online and hopes to become a key worker in the future. Her daughters are home and her mother has moved in with them. More than anything else now, she says, she is just enjoying time with her family.

For healthcare professionals, working with or as part of drug and alcohol services can be interesting, challenging but highly rewarding as well as a positive way to improve outcomes for our patients.

REFERENCES

1. Office for National Statistics. Deaths related to drug poisoning in England and Wales: 2017 Registrations. 2018. Available from: https://www.ons.gov.uk/peoplepopulation-andcommunity/birthsdeathsandmarriages/deaths/bulletins/deathsrelatedtodrugpoisoninginenglandandwales/2017registrations [Accessed 28 April 2019].
2. Office for National Statistics. Drug-related deaths "deep dive" into coroner's records. 2018. Available from: https://www.ons.gov.uk/peoplepopulationandcommunity/birthsdeathsandmarriages/deaths/articles/drugrelateddeathsdeepdiveintocoronersrecords/2018-08-06 [Accessed 25 April 2019].
3. Press release: *Are the inequalities seen today a sign of a broken system? Launch of the IFS Deaton Review of inequalities.* Institute for Fiscal Studies. Available from: https://www.ifs.org.uk/inequality/press-release/are-the-inequalities-seen-today-a-sign-of-a-broken-system-launch-of-the-ifs-deaton-review-of-inequalities/ [Accessed 8th June 2019].
4. World Health Organisation. Health topics: Substance abuse. Available from: https://www.who.int/topics/substance_abuse/en/ [Accessed 18th May 2019].
5. NHS Digital. Statistics on drug misuse, England, 2018. (November 2018 update). Available from: https://www.who.int/topics/substance_abuse/en/ [Accessed 18th May 2019].

6. National records Scotland. 134 drug-related deaths in Scotland in 2017. Available from: https://www.nrscotland.gov.uk/news/2018/934-drug-related-deaths-in-scotland-in-2017 [Accessed 18th May 2019].

7. Turner D, Smith J. *Drug Deaths in Wales 2017*. Cardiff: Public Health Wales; 2018.

8. Northern Ireland Statistics and Research Agency. Drug-related and drug-misuse deaths registered in Northern Ireland (2007–2017). Available at: https://www.nisra.gov.uk/sites/nisra.gov.uk/files/publications/Drug%20Related%20Deaths%20Press%20Release%202017.pdf [Accessed 18th May 2019].

9. Advisory Council on the Misuse of Drugs. *What Are the Factors Which Make People Susceptible to the Substance Misuse Problems and Harms?* London: Advisory Council on the Misuse of Drugs; 2018.

10. Aldridge RW et al. Morbidity and mortality in homeless individuals, prisoners, sex workers, and individuals with substance use disorders in high-income countries: A systematic review and meta-analysis. *The Lancet*. 2018; 391: 241–250.

11. NHS England. NHS Long Term Plan will help problem drinkers and smokers. Available online from: https://www.england.nhs.uk/2019/01/nhs-long-term-plan-will-help-problem-drinkers-and-smokers/ [Accessed 25th May 2019].

12. NHS Digital. Statistics on alcohol, England 2019. Available from: https://digital.nhs.uk/data-and-information/publications/statistical/statistics-on-alcohol/2019/part-2 [Accessed 25th May 2019].

13. Public Health Observatory Wales. Alcohol in Wales. Available from: https://publichealthwales.shinyapps.io/AlcoholinWales/#section overview page export [Accessed 25th May 2019].

14. National Records of Scotland. (Alcohol-related Deaths (old National Statistics definition. Available from: https://www.nrscotland.gov.uk/statistics-and-data/statistics/statistics-by-theme/vital-events/deaths/alcohol-related-deaths/main-points [Accessed 25th May 2019].

15. Scottish Government. Alcohol. Available from: https://www2.gov.scot/Topics/Health/Services/Alcohol [Accessed 25th May 2019].

16. Katikireddi SV, Whitley E, Lewsey J, Gray L, Leyland AH. Socioeconomic status as an effect modifier of alcohol consumption and harm: analysis of linked cohort data. *The Lancet Public Health*. 2017; 2(6): 267–276.

17. Ginn S. Women prisoners. *British Medical Journal*. 2013; 346: e8318.

18. Prison Reform Trust. Welcome to the women's programme. Available from: http://www.prisonreformtrust.org.uk/WhatWeDo/Projectsresearch/Women [Accessed 25th May 2019].

19. Brook DW, Brook JS, Zhang C, Cohen P, Whiteman M. Drug use and the risk of major depressive disorder, and substance use disorders. *Archives of General Psychiatry*. 2002; 59(11): 1039–1044.

20. Smith K. Substance abuse and depression. *Psycom*. Available from: https://www.psycom.net/depression-substance-abuse [Accessed 25th May 2019].

21. Harris P. *Youthoria. Adolescent Substance Misuse – Problems, Prevention and Treatment*. Lyme Regis: Russell House Publishing; 2013.

22. Bramley G, Fitzpatrick S, Edwards J, Ford D, Johnsen S, Sosenko F, Watkins D. *Hard Edges: Mapping Severe and Multiple Disadvantage in England*. London: Lankelly Chase; 2015.

23. UK Harm Reduction Alliance. Definition of harm reduction. Available from: http://www.ukhra.org/harm_reduction_definition.html [Accessed 27th May 2018].

24. GPs at the Deep End. Deep End Summary 11: Alcohol problems in under 40s. Available from: https://www.gla.ac.uk/media/media_277943_en.pdf [Accessed 27th May 2019].

25. Public Health England. *The Public Health Burden of Alcohol and the Effectiveness and Cost-Effectiveness of Alcohol Control Policies: An Evidence Review*. London: Public Health England; 2016.

26. Angus C, Willott S, Harris L. *Baby Boomers vs Millennials: How our drinking patterns are changing and what we can do about it*. Presentation at Royal College of General Practitioners SMMGP Annual Conference. 29th November 2018.

27. Brinksman S. OST – *why treatment optimisation matters*. Presentation at Royal College of General Practitioners SMMGP Annual Conference. 29th November 2018.

28. Clinical Guidelines on Drug Misuse and Dependence Update 2017 Independent Expert Working Group. *Drug Misuse and Dependence: UK Guidelines on Clinical Management*. London: Department of Health; 2017.

29. Hickman M, Steer C, Tilling K, Lim AG, Marsden J, Millar T, Strang J, Telfer M, Vickerman P, MacLeod J. The impact of buprenorphine and methadone on mortality: A primary care cohort study in the United Kingdom. *Addiction*. 2018; 113(8): 1461–1476.

30. Amato L, Minozzi S, Davoli M, Vechhi S. Psychosocial and pharmacological treatments versus pharmacological treatments for opioid detoxification. *Cochrane Database of Systematic Reviews*. 2011. Available from: https://www.cochrane.org/CD005031/ADDICTN_psychosocial-and-pharmacological-treatments-versus-pharmacological-treatments-for-opioid-detoxification [Accessed 29th May 2019].

31. Prendergast M, Podus D, Finney J, Greenwell L, Roll J. Contingency management for treatment of substance use disorders: A meta-analysis. *Database of Abstracts of Reviews of Effects: Quality-assessed Reviews*. Available from: https://www.ncbi.nlm.nih.gov/books/NBK72392/ [Accessed 29th May 2019].

32. Amato L, Minozzi S, Hackl-Herrwerth A, Leucht S, Lehert P, Vecchi S, Soyka M. Benzodiazepines for alcohol withdrawal. *Cochrane Database of Systematic Reviews*. 2010. Available from: https://www.cochrane.org/CD005063/ADDICTN_benzodiazepines-for-alcohol-withdrawal [Accessed 29th May 2019].

33. Rosner S, Hackl-Herrwerth A, Leucht S, Lehert P, Vecchi S, Soyka M. Acamprosate for alcohol dependence. *Cochrane Database of Systematic Reviews*. 2010. Available from: https://www.cochrane.org/CD004332/ADDICTN_acamprosate-for-alcohol-dependent-patients [Accessed 29th May 2019].

34. Band RM, Meena MC, Kandpal A, Mittal S. Rapid death due to alcohol withdrawal syndrome: Case report and review of literature. *Asia Pacific Journal of Medical Toxicology*. 2015; 4: 51–55.

35. National Clinical Guideline Centre (UK). *Alcohol Use Disorders: Diagnosis and Clinical Management of Alcohol-Related Physical Complications*. London: Royal College of Physicians (UK); 2010.

36. Becker HC. Kindling in alcohol withdrawal. *Alcohol Health and Research World*. 1998; 22(1): 25–33.

37. *Alcohol-Use Disorders: Diagnosis, Assessment and Management of Harmful Drinking and Alcohol Dependence*. Clinical guideline 115. London: National Institute for Health and Care Excellence; 2011. Available from: www.nice.org.uk/guidance/cg115 [Accessed 8th June 2018].

38. *Alcohol-Use Disorders: Diagnosis and Management of Physical Complications*. Clinical guideline 100. London: National Institute for Health and Care Excellence; 2010 (updated April 2017). Available from: www.nice.org.uk/guidance/cg100 [Accessed 8th June 2019].

39. Doonan L, Daly E, Smith M, Cribbin L, Dargan S, Martin A, Robinson M, Craig M, Williamson A. *Deep End Report 31. Attached Alcohol Nurse Deep End Pilot (July 2015–2016): Final Report*. Glasgow: GPs at the Deep End; 2016.

40. *European Drugs Bulletin 2019: Trends and Developments*. Lisbon: European Monitoring Centre for Drugs and Addictions; 2019.

41. Gray JD. Medical consequences of cocaine. *Canadian Family Physician*. 1993; 39: 1975–1981.

42. O'Conner R. What the latest estimates on opiate and crack use tell us. *Public Health Matters Blog*. Public Health England. 2018. Available from: https://publichealthmatters.blog.gov.uk/2019/03/25/what-the-latest-estimates-on-opiate-and-crack-use-tell-us/ [Accessed 25th April 2019].

43. Flemen K. Cracks in the mirror. *Drink and Drugs News*. June 2018: 6–7.

44. *The Effects of Drugs*. National Health Service. Available online from: https://www.nhs.uk/live-well/healthy-body/the-effects-of-drugs/#ecstasy-mdma-pills-crystal-e [Accessed 8th June 2019].

45. *Drugs A-Z*. Talk to Frank. Available from: https://www.talktofrank.com/drugs-a-z [Accessed 8th June 2019].

46. Couchman L, Frinculescu A, Sobreira C, Shine T, Ramsey J, Hecht M, Kipper K, Holt D, Johnston A. Variability in content and dissolution profiles of MDMA tablets collected in the UK between 2001 and 2018 – A potential risk to users? *Drug Testing and Analysis*. 2019; doi: 10.1002/dta.2605.

47. Vasan S, Olango GJ. Amphetamine toxicity. *StatPearls*; 2018. Available from: https://www.ncbi.nlm.nih.gov/books/NBK470276/ [Accessed 8th June 2019].

48. Bowden-Jones O. *Novel psychoactive substances*. Presentation at Royal College of General Practitioners SMMGP Annual Conference. 29th November 2018.

49. Brew I. Novel psychoactive substances. *British Journal of General Practice*. 2016; 66 (644): 125.

50. Gabor Maté. *In the Realm of Hungry Ghosts: Close Encounters with Addiction*. London: Vermilion; 2018.

51. *Shooting Up: Infections among people who inject drugs in the UK, 2016. An update, November 2017*. London: Public Health England; 2017.

52. Henderson R. *Hepatitis B*. Patient.co.uk. Available from: https://patient.info/doctor/hepatitis-b-pro [Accessed 8th June 2019].

53. *Hepatitis C in the UK 2018 Report: Working to Eliminate Hepatitis C as a Major Public Health Threat*. London: Public Health England; 2018.

54. *Eliminating Hepatitis C in England*. London: All-Party Parliamentary Group on Liver Health; 2018.

55. Hull M. *It's not just about heroin: The management of other substance use for those on OST*. Presentation at Royal College of General Practitioners SMMGP Annual Conference. 29th November 2018.

56. Hughes K, Bellis MA, Sethi D, Andrew R, Wood YY, Ford K, Baban A, Boderscova L, Kachaeva M, Makaruk K, Markovic M, Wlodarczyk J, Zakhozha V. Adverse childhood experiences, childhood relationships and associated substance use and mental health in young Europeans. *European Journal of Public Health*. 2019: ckz037. Available from: https://doi.org/10.1093/eurpub/ckz037 [Accessed 26th May 2019].

10

How to Address Smoking Cessation in Areas of Deprivation

CAMRAN MIAH

If services can help reduce the stress it will reduce the emotional triggers and tackling the biochemical addiction is more likely to be successful.

Smoking tobacco is a negative health behaviour and has been much examined in association with health inequalities [1, 2]. Smoking initiation and continuation is partly influenced by nicotine activating the brain's reward pathway [3], but is also heavily influenced by factors such as socio-economic status (SES), academic background and parental support [4]. Long-term smoking has a strong association with Chronic obstructive pulmonary disease (COPD) and many cancers [5]. The World Health Organisation (WHO) states that smoking is the world's leading cause of preventable illness, impoverishment and death [6] and in the UK smoking-related deaths accounted for 19% of all deaths in 2009. Studies suggest members of deprived populations are less likely to access smoking cessation services, less likely to quit smoking and suffer higher levels of harm [7]. The Office for National Statistics (ONS) has shown that smoking is more common in individuals who earn less than £10,000 per year [8].

It is estimated the NHS spent £2.6 billion treating smoking and smoking-related diseases in 2015 [9]. An estimated £905.7 million was spent in primary care through GP and practice nurse visits and an estimated £851.6 million through hospital admissions [9].

SMOKING IN AREAS OF DEPRIVATION

Smokers may be identified at registration through questionnaires or simply by asking [10]. Although primary care is incentivised to identify smokers through the Quality and Outcomes Framework (QOF), many practices are failing to reach the required 90% [10, 11]. In a study of 415 practices, 26% of adults registering did not have their smoking status checked, suggesting opportunities may be missed for discussing smoking cessation in consultations [10].

COPD, if adequately diagnosed, can be seen as a proxy measure for smoking prevalence [5]. A case-control study of 38,597 pairs demonstrated 2.9 times greater prevalence of COPD in the most deprived compared with the least deprived areas based on the Index of Multiple Deprivation (IMD) [12]. In a national study of 51,804 patients, Simpson et al. observed epidemiological trends of COPD identifying that the rise in prevalence of lifelong COPD was significantly higher in more deprived areas with 10.2 per 1,000 people in the most affluent areas and 31.1 per 1000 people in the most deprived [13]. This three-fold increase between areas represents a serious inequality in health. The same study observed changes in reported smokers between 2001 and 2005. Though both areas showed decreases, the more affluent areas showed greater reductions (6.5%) than the deprived areas (1.5%) [13]. Gershon et al.'s systematic review in 2012 concluded that there was an inverse relationship between SES and COPD [14]. Those of the lowest SES were shown to be at a higher risk of developing COPD, consistent with controlling for factors such as age, gender and population [14]. It was also observed that there were worse outcomes for these individuals, seen especially in COPD progression. Ultimately, the smoking status of individuals change many times throughout the year as smoking addiction is a cycle of smoking and smoking cessation [15].

CASE STUDY

Arthur

Arthur is 69 years old and has COPD. He began smoking aged 14 and continued throughout his life when socialising with family and friends, but also as a way of coping with stress. He doesn't see smoking as a big health issue as his COPD symptoms are reasonably well controlled with medication. He is concerned however, about the increasingly frequent chest infections he has been suffering. He feels smoking affects his life very little compared to other things that are going on in his life. Arthur is struggling to take care of his sick wife who has dementia and whose care needs are increasing. He is also having difficulties keeping up with his rent and bill payments. He sees smoking as his only form of stress relief and is reluctant to give up something which both relieves his stress and gives him a little joy in life.

Health Impact

Tobacco smoke contains harmful substances including tar, carbon monoxide and arsenic, which have been implicated in conditions including coronary artery disease, peripheral arterial disease, COPD and cancer [16, 17]. A population-based study in Spain suggested increased risk of later diagnosis in areas of lower SES; reducing opportunities to manage the condition [18]. Under-diagnosis is widespread; NICE have estimated that a further, under-diagnosed 2 million people in the UK are living with the condition [19]. Miravitlles et al. assessed how socioeconomic status affected quality of life (QoL) for COPD patients, with those from a lower SES group reporting poorer QoL, and associations with substandard housing, dangerous jobs, worse diets and increased prevalence of smoking [20, 21]. Those individuals of a low SES had more severe COPD based on their COPD severity scale (COPDSS) questionnaire with additional evidence also suggesting worsening lung function in these groups [20]. COPD's effect was worse on people of low SES and is associated with a greater prevalence of multiple morbidity and mental health issues in this population [22].

Smoking cessation should still be prioritised for those with conditions such as COPD. Though COPD is irreversible, progression can be reduced through smoking cessation [23]. The US Lung Health Study recorded changes in 5,887 smokers over 5 years, demonstrating that smoking cessation reduced deterioration in lung function to 34ml/year loss of FEV1 compared to 63 ml/year in continued smokers [24]. Importantly, there was also a 32% reduction in all-cause mortality in those who stopped smoking over the 5 years. Furthermore, studies have shown the link between the risk of lung cancer and lung function, especially when FEV1 is below 80% [25]. Those who stop smoking reduce mortality from lung cancer by 50% [24]. Stopping smoking has also shown benefit to people with asthma, leading to reduced medication use and improving lung function better than high dose steroids [24] (Figure 10.1).

Smoking and Pregnancy

Studies have shown a higher prevalence of smoking in pregnancy in lower SES groups, affecting the child beyond pregnancy and contributing to an increased risk of the child smoking. This continues the cycle of addiction affecting deprived areas more. A retrospective cohort study in Scotland showed

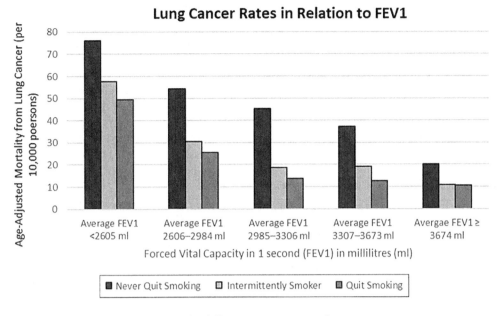

Figure 10.1 Decline in lung cancer deaths following quitting smoking.

smoking in pregnancy led to increased lower and upper respiratory tract infections within the first year of life and suggested 20% of postneonatal mortality was preventable if the mother stopped smoking [26]. In an Australian study, Mohsin et al. looked at changes in smoking rates of pregnant women between 1995–1997 and 2005–2007, showing declines in smoking prevalence but greater reductions in affluent populations compared to deprived. It was calculated that low SES pregnant women were more likely to smoke (2.7 times more) with a greater likelihood in 2005–2007 than 1995–1997 [27]. This may be due to health literacy issues and ineffective smoking cessation services targeting this group [27, 28]. The infant feeding survey carried out in 2010 showed professionals were less likely to smoke while pregnant (14%) compared to manual workers (40%) [29]. A Finnish study concluded that there is an increased risk of adolescents smoking if their mothers smoked after the first trimester [30]. One study showed that they were 5.5 times more likely if the mother smoked more than 10 cigarettes per day [31] and another concluded that in these groups there would be lower chances of quitting smoking, possibly due to the early stimulation of nicotine during foetal development [32]. It appears that women of low SES are smoking more,

are less successful in smoking cessation and their smoking may contribute to the continuing cycle of smoking addiction in their offspring.

CASE STUDY

Anna

Anna is 24 years old and is having her first child. She has smoked since her teens as it was a popular thing to do during school and has now become a regular smoker of half a pack a day. Though she knows smoking is bad for her she doesn't think it is likely to cause serious risks to her baby as many of her friends smoked during their pregnancies and their babies were fine. She has had thoughts of quitting but doesn't think she can, especially with the stresses of raising a child on her own.

Smoking Cessation in Areas of Deprivation

A systematic review of 27 trials including 11,000 participants displayed consistent evidence that tailored behavioural support services increased smoking cessation, with results showing a rise from 40% to 80% within a minimum 6 month period [33]. Stead et al. showed increases when behavioural therapy was paired with nicotine replacement therapy (NRT) [34]. Text messaging is a non-traditional approach to smoking cessation which showed cessation rates of 9.2% compared to the control of 4.3% where abstinence was checked via carbon monoxide testing [35]. Another systematic review of the effectiveness of internet interventions for smoking cessation saw greater quit attempts compared to control groups [36]. Most studies demonstrate the benefit of behavioural therapy alone and in conjunction with NRT.

Varenicline (Champix) is a smoking cessation pharmacotherapy which works by partially agonising nicotine acetylcholine receptors [37]. Its effectiveness has been analysed, with most studies supporting its benefits. A systematic review by Cahill et al. demonstrated the effectiveness of varenicline with a two- to three-fold increase in successful smoking cessation compared to placebo. The review also showed that it had more benefit than bupropion and nicotine patches [38]. In the past, varenicline use has been linked to neuropsychiatric adverse events such as suicidal ideation and psychosis, however, the EAGLES study, the largest of its kind researching varenicline, showed no statistical difference in neuropsychiatric events when compared to placebo [39]. Varenicline has been shown to have side effects such as insomnia, headaches and nausea but is generally well tolerated [38].

An Australian qualitative study by Bryant et al. examined smoking cessation interventions for disadvantaged people [40]. The results suggested better success for patients in communities and relationships where smoking was a social norm, if a personalised approach was adopted [40]. Systematic reviews looked at the effectiveness of NHS smoking cessation services and observed that smokers from deprived areas had good access to services but still had lower quit rates. Barriers to clinic attendance included perceived effectiveness, lack of childcare and shortage of time [41]. It was postulated that people in deprived areas were less successful in quitting smoking due to higher nicotine dependence and more difficult life circumstances [42]. Evidence associates lower SES groups with greater nicotine dependence due to earlier onset of smoking and increased consumption [41].

Vangeli et al. found that age, gender and levels of education had no association with successful quit attempts. They did, however, find a quit attempt in one year doubles the likelihood of another attempt the year after [42]. Further studies suggested a strong correlation between achieving long-term abstinence (more than 6 months) and increasing quit attempts [43]. One study suggested self-motivation predicted a successful quit attempt, supporting the longitudinal cohort study by Chaiton et al. that found that up to 30 attempts may be needed for successful cessation [44, 45]. A person's motivation to persevere increases likelihood of success.

Tackling Smoking Cessation in the Consultation

Brief interventions involve opportunistic advice given to patients who smoke, with cessation promoted by the 4 As: ask, advise, assist, arrange [46, 47]. Assess the patient's desire to stop smoking and offer further support such as behavioural therapy, NRT and more intensive support from the NHS stop smoking service. These interventions primarily help with inducing a quit attempt [47]. A study of 2,138 cigarette smokers based in London practices showed brief interventions could yield 25 long-term quit successes each year and potentially even greater numbers in larger surgeries [48]. A Cochrane review of 17 trials by Stead et al. showed statistically significantly higher quit rates when brief intervention was compared to control. Brief advice was considered less than 20 minutes (generally less than 5 minutes) with no follow-up [49], demonstrating the possible benefit clinicians can produce from minimal interventions with their patient population.

Motivational interviewing (MI) techniques may be used to introduce the idea of smoking cessation in consultations. In a randomised trial of 255 daily smokers, MI was shown to be more beneficial than brief advice and this related to patients having greater motivation to quit [50, 51]. MI encourages 'change talk' among patients using phrases such as, 'How important is it for you to change?' and 'How confident do you feel about changing?' [52]. The effectiveness of MI has been shown in studies across many health domains but particularly in smoking cessation – in a randomised control trial, Butler et al. concluded that MI produced better outcomes than brief interventions especially in those who were 'not ready to change' [53].

CASE STUDY

Arthur

To help Arthur address his smoking habit, we might begin by reducing stressors in his circumstances. This could be done by assessing and facilitating more care for his wife and introducing him to people who can help him manage his finances. If we can help him see the benefits in stopping smoking and reduce his need for stress relief, then we might proceed with NRT and behavioural therapies to support him towards a successful quit attempt.

Anna

Anna would be a priority for smoking cessation services especially with the potential for harm to her child. There may be a need to improve health literacy among pregnant women in areas of deprivation and, through reinforcing the message of smoking-related harm in pregnancy, we might improve uptake of cessation services. The same conversations might also be had, in a nonconfrontational and supportive manner, with her GP. NRT in pregnancy is considered less risky than smoking. Belfast Health and Social Care Trust information for pregnant smokers includes advice on licensed NRT available from GPs, joining a support group and suggests using one of the Ds when feeling the urge to smoke:

Delay acting on the urge,
Take **Deep** breaths,
Drink some water,
Or **Do** something else [54].

SUGGESTIONS FOR PRACTICE

- *Improve identification of smokers.*
- *Optimise cessation services: the evidence supports the use of behavioural therapy as the best method in achieving quit attempts. Likelihood of success increases when accompanied with NRT.*
- *Personalise care and address personal factors: smoking is seen as a way to reduce stress and provides escapism. If services can help reduce the stress in patients' lives it will reduce the emotional triggers to smoke and then tackling the biochemical addiction is more likely to be successful.*
- *Target specific populations.*

- *Make services more accessible: examples include evening sessions, drop-in sessions and services located more conveniently for public transport.*
- *Improve health literacy: services provided by GPs and local councils highlighting the harms of smoking and promoting the benefits of cessation must have their funding continued to sustain impact on smoking-related harm.*
- *Deliver brief interventions: the National Centre for Smoking Cessation and Training offers e-learning including videos of very brief interventions with pages for England, Northern Ireland, Wales, UK Armed Forces and the rest of the world. It also includes specific advice on interventions in pregnancy and for people with mental health problems. For detailed advice on how to quit, look online at* **https://elearning. ncsct.co.uk/** *[55].*

REFERENCES

1. Davey Smith G, Egger M. Socioeconomic differentials in wealth and health. *BMJ.* 1993;307(6912):1085–1086.
2. Rejineveld S. The impact of individual and area characteristics on urban socioeconomic differences in health and smoking. *International Journal of Epidemiology.* 1998;27(1):33–40.
3. Ritter J, Flower R, Henderson G, Loke Y, MacEwan D, Rang H. *Rang and Dale's Pharmacology.* 7th ed. Elsevier, London; 2012
4. West R. Tobacco smoking: Health impact, prevalence, correlates and interventions. *Psychology & Health.* 2017;32(8):1018–1036.
5. Wilkinson I. *Oxford Handbook of Clinical Medicine.* Oxford: Oxford University Press; 2017.
6. Zafeiridou M, Hopkinson N, Voulvoulis N. Cigarette smoking: An assessment of tobacco's global environmental footprint across its entire supply chain. *Environmental Science & Technology.* 2018;52(15):8087–8094.
7. Allender S, Balakrishnan R, Scarborough P, Webster P, Rayner M. The burden of smoking-related ill health in the UK. *Tobacco Control.* 2009;18(4):262–267.
8. Reid J, Hammond D, Boudreau C, Fong G, Siahpush M. Socioeconomic disparities in quit intentions, quit attempts, and

smoking abstinence among smokers in four western countries: Findings from the International Tobacco Control Four Country Survey. *Nicotine & Tobacco Research.* 2010;12(Supplement 1):S20–S33.

9. Adult smoking habits in the UK: 2017 [Internet]. GOV.UK. 2019 [cited 21 April 2019]. Available from: https://www.gov.uk/government/statistics/adult-smoking-habits-in-the-uk-2017

10. Szatkowski L, Lewis S, McNeill A, Coleman T. Is smoking status routinely recorded when patients register with a new GP? *Family Practice.* 2010;27(6):673–675.

11. Taggar J, Coleman T, Lewis S, Szatkowski L. The impact of the Quality and Outcomes Framework (QOF) on the recording of smoking targets in primary care medical records: Cross-sectional analyses from The Health Improvement Network (THIN) database. *BMC Public Health.* 2012;12(1).

12. Nwaru B, Simpson C, Sheikh A, Kotz D. External validation of a COPD prediction model using population-based primary care data: A nested case-control study. *Scientific Reports.* 2017;7(1).

13. Simpson C, Hippisley-Cox J, Sheikh A. Trends in the epidemiology of chronic obstructive pulmonary disease in England: A national study of 51 804 patients. *British Journal of General Practice.* 2010;60(576):e277–e284.

14. Gershon A, Dolmage T, Stephenson A, Jackson B. Chronic obstructive pulmonary disease and socioeconomic status: A systematic review. COPD: Journal of Chronic Obstructive Pulmonary Disease. 2012;9(3):216–226.

15. Ayers S. *Psychology for Medicine.* Los Angeles: Sage Publications; 2017.

16. Talhout R, Schulz T, Florek E, Van Benthem J, Wester P, Opperhuizen A. Hazardous compounds in tobacco smoke. *International Journal of Environmental Research and Public Health.* 2011;8(2):613–628.

17. West R. Tobacco smoking: Health impact, prevalence, correlates and interventions. *Psychology & Health.* 2017;32(8):1018–1036.

18. Penña V, Miravitlles M, Gabriel R, Jiménez-Ruiz C, Villasante C, Masa J et al. Geographic variations in prevalence and underdiagnosis of COPD. *Chest.* 2000;118(4):981–989.

19. Overview | Chronic obstructive pulmonary disease in over 16s: Diagnosis and management | Guidance | NICE [Internet]. Nice.org.uk. 2019. Available from: https://www.nice.org.uk/guidance/ng115 [Accessed 26th April 2019].

20. Miravitlles M, Naberan K, Cantoni J, Azpeitia A. Socioeconomic status and health-related quality of life of patients with chronic obstructive pulmonary disease. *Respiration.* 2011;82(5):402–408.

21. Prescott E, Godtfredsen N, Vestbo J, Osler M. Social position and mortality from respiratory diseases in males and females. *European Respiratory Journal.* 2003;21(5):821–826.

22. Baird B, Charles A. *Understanding Pressures in General Practice.* 2016.

23. Sin D, Wu J. Improved patient outcome with smoking cessation: When is it too late? *International Journal of Chronic Obstructive Pulmonary Disease.* 2011;259–267.

24. Anthonisen N, Connett J, Enright P, Manfreda J. Hospitalizations and mortality in the lung health study. *American Journal of Respiratory and Critical Care Medicine.* 2002;166(3):333–339.

25. Eberly L, Ockene J, Sherwin R, Yang L, Kuller L. Pulmonary function as a predictor of lung cancer mortality in continuing cigarette smokers and in quitters. *International Journal of Epidemiology.* 2003;32(4):592–599.

26. Lawder R, Whyte B, Wood R, Fischbacher C, Tappin D. Impact of maternal smoking on early childhood health: A retrospective cohort linked dataset analysis of 697 003 children born in Scotland 1997–2009. *BMJ Open.* 2019;9(3):e023213.

27. Mohsin M, Bauman A, Forero R. Socioeconomic correlates and trends in smoking in pregnancy in New South Wales, Australia. *Journal of Epidemiology & Community Health.* 2010;65(8):727–732.

28. Cui Y, Shooshtari S, Forget E, Clara I, Cheung K. Smoking during pregnancy: Findings from the 2009–2010. Canadian Community Health Survey. *PLoS ONE.* 2014;9(1):e84640.

29. Renfrew M, McAndrew F, Thompson J, Fellows L, Large A, Speed M. [Internet]. Sp.ukdataservice.ac.uk. 2010. Available

from: https://sp.ukdataservice.ac.uk/doc/7281/mrdoc/pdf/7281_ifs-uk-2010_report.pdf [Accessed 4th May 2019].

30. Manzano C, Castellano M, Roman L. Maternal smoking during pregnancy and its impact on postnatal neurodevelopment. *Clinics in Mother and Child Health*. 2016;13(3).

31. Cornelius MD, Leech SL, Lidu M. Prenatal tobacco exposure: Is it a risk factor for early tobacco experimentation? *Nicotine & Tobacco Research*. 2000;2(1):45–52.

32. Chen J, Millar WJ. Age of smoking initiation: Implication for quitting. *Health Reports*.1998;9:39–46.

33. Lancaster T, Stead L. Individual behavioural counselling for smoking cessation. *Cochrane Database of Systematic Reviews*. 2017.

34. Stead L, Koilpillai P, Fanshawe T, Lancaster T. Combined pharmacotherapy and behavioural interventions for smoking cessation. *Cochrane Database of Systematic Reviews*. 2016.

35. Free C, Knight R, Robertson S, Whittaker R, Edwards P, Zhou W et al. Smoking cessation support delivered via mobile phone text messaging (txt2stop): A single-blind, randomised trial. *The Lancet*. 2011;378(9785):49–55.

36. Taylor G, Dalili M, Semwal M, Civljak M, Sheikh A, Car J. Internet-based interventions for smoking cessation. *Cochrane Database of Systematic Reviews*. 2017.

37. Gómez-Coronado N, Walker A, Berk M, Dodd S. Current and emerging pharmacotherapies for cessation of tobacco smoking. *Pharmacotherapy: The Journal of Human Pharmacology and Drug Therapy*. 2018;38(2):235–258.

38. Cahill K, Lindson-Hawley N, Thomas K, Fanshawe T, Lancaster T. Nicotine receptor partial agonists for smoking cessation. *Cochrane Database of Systematic Reviews*. 2016.

39. Anthenelli R, Benowitz N, West R, St Aubin L, McRae T, Lawrence D et al. Neuropsychiatric safety and efficacy of varenicline, bupropion, and nicotine patch in smokers with and without psychiatric disorders (EAGLES): A double-blind, randomised, placebo-controlled clinical trial. *The Lancet*. 2016;387(10037):2507–2520.

40. Bryant J, Bonevski B, Paul C, O'Brien J, Oakes W. Developing cessation interventions for the social and community service setting: A qualitative study of barriers to quitting among disadvantaged Australian smokers. *BMC Public Health*. 2011;11(1).

41. Hoek J, Smith K. A qualitative analysis of low income smokers' responses to tobacco excise tax increases. *International Journal of Drug Policy*. 2016;37:82–89.

42. Vangeli E, Stapleton J, Smit E, Borland R, West R. Predictors of attempts to stop smoking and their success in adult general population samples: A systematic review. *Addiction*. 2011;106(12):2110–2121.

43. Zhou X, Nonnemaker J, Sherrill B, Gilsenan A, Coste F, West R. Attempts to quit smoking and relapse: Factors associated with success or failure from the ATTEMPT cohort study. *Addictive Behaviors*. 2009;34(4):365–373.

44. Smit E, Hoving C, Schelleman-Offermans K, West R, de Vries H. Predictors of successful and unsuccessful quit attempts among smokers motivated to quit. *Addictive Behaviors*. 2014;39(9):1318–1324.

45. Chaiton M, Diemert L, Cohen J, Bondy S, Selby P, Philipneri A et al. Estimating the number of quit attempts it takes to quit smoking successfully in a longitudinal cohort of smokers. *BMJ Open*. 2016;6(6):e011045.

46. Chesterman J, Judge K, Bauld L, Ferguson J. How effective are the English smoking treatment services in reaching disadvantaged smokers? *Addiction*. 2005;100:36–45.

47. West R, McNeill A, Raw M. Smoking cessation guidelines for health professionals: An update. *Thorax*. 2000;55(12):987–999.

48. Russell M, Wilson C, Taylor C, Baker C. Effect of general practitioners' advice against smoking. *BMJ*. 1979;2(6184):231–235.

49. Stead L, Buitrago D, Preciado N, Sanchez G, Hartmann-Boyce J, Lancaster T. Physician advice for smoking cessation. *Cochrane Database of Systematic Reviews*. 2013.

50. Catley D, Goggin K. A randomized trial of motivational interviewing: Cessation induction among smokers with low desire to quit. *American Journal of Preventive Medicine*. 2016;50(5):A4.

51. Lee E. The effect of positive group psycho-therapy and motivational interviewing on smoking cessation. *Journal of Addictions Nursing*. 2017;28(2):88–95.

52. Rollnick S, Butler C, Kinnersley P, Gregory J, Mash B. Motivational interviewing. *BMJ*. 2010;340(apr27 2):c1900–c1900.

53. Butler C, Rollnick S, Cohen D, Bachmann M, Russell I, Stott N. Motivational consulting versus brief advice for smokers in general practice: A randomized trial. *British Journal of General Practice*. 1999;49(445):611–616.

54. Belfast Health and Social Care Trust Public Health Agency. *Pregnancy and nicotine replacement therapy (NRT): What you need to know*. Available from: https://www.publichealth.hscni.net/sites/default/files/Smoking%20Pregnancy%20A5_Leaflet_02_16.pdf [Accessed 1st June 2019].

55. National Centre for Smoking Cessation and Training. *NCSCT Online Training*. Available at: https://elearning.ncsct.co.uk/ [Accessed 1st June 2019].

11

Safer Prescribing: The Threat and Challenge of Caring for People with Chronic Pain

CLARISSA HEMMINGSEN AND JAMES MATHESON

One of the most significant causes of human suffering.

Prior to 1986 stigma surrounding the prescription and taking of opioids meant people often suffered unnecessarily and died in pain. Then came the World Health Organisation (WHO) analgesic ladder, an easy-to-follow model advocating the introduction and incremental titration of analgesics, dosed ever upwards as required to relieve the burden of terminal cancer pain [1]. The resulting mercy of comfortable effective palliation legitimised opioid use and set the scene for the moral imperative of pain control to extend to the issue of chronic pain.

Research, however, has since shown these tools to be unsuited and lacking in consistent good quality evidence for use with these complex and sometimes lifelong problems [2]. Since then, UK guidance on prescription of opioids for chronic pain management has become increasingly standardised. Evidence is still lacking for clinical benefit over the 12-week period separating acute to chronic as defined by the British Pain Society [1–3],

and evidence is mounting on issues of tolerance, dependence and harm as doses escalate. Growing concern has led to calls for greater monitoring and a renewed understanding of the risks of long-term opioid use [1, 4–6].

Chronic pain itself responds well to opioids in the early treatment stages, but unlike acute or cancer pain, it has neither a predictable nor a linear trajectory. The experience of that pain and associated factors can be vastly different, altered by a person's cognitive and affective circumstances and their environment [7].

The *Opioids Aware* collaboration [6] launched as a resource to provide guidance on potential hazards. Evaluation of the evidence, however, is limited by factors such as short duration of clinical trials and the majority of studies reviewing prescription number rather than oral morphine equivalency, meaning that the extent of the UK's own opioid problem may be severely underestimated [2, 6]. Once oral morphine equivalency is corrected for, the increase in prescribed opioids between 1998 and 2016 rose from the previously estimated and frequently cited 34% by items prescribed, to a 127% increase by total volume of oral morphine [6].

MORBIDITY AND MORTALITY

Research indicates direct correlation of opioid-related harm with dose and continued use. The most at-risk user group are those already suffering the greatest distress and most in need of pain relief. They are most likely to experience significant adverse effects through drug-drug and drug-disease interaction [1, 2, 8]. The adverse consequences of high dose and prolonged opioid use (equivalent to 120mg morphine daily) include tolerance, dependence, addiction, abuse, cognitive impairment, immune suppression, hormonal disruption, gastrointestinal disturbance, nausea, headaches, somnolence, increased fracture risk, acute myocardial infarction, respiratory depression, increased pain and reduced quality of life through opioid-induced hyperalgesia and generally increased mortality [5, 7–10].

A CAUTIONARY TALE

Despite mortality figures in the UK being substantially lower than those seen in the US, trends have risen concerningly over the last 15 years in all regions. Tramadol, for example, was related to one death in England and Wales in 1996, rising to 208 in 2014 [2], prior to reclassification as a Schedule 3 controlled drug [5], and opioid-related deaths across the UK rose from almost 500 in 2001 to almost 900 in 2011 [9].

With the tripling of global opioid prescription use since 1986 [2, 11] nowhere have the resultant harms been more discussed than in the United States and Canada, with the Centre for Disease Control (CDC) reporting annual US sales of prescribed opioids quadrupling between 1999 and 2014 [2], and mortality trends showing a startling threefold increase in unintentional opioid-related deaths [3].

Significant differences exist between the US and UK healthcare systems in prescription regulation and pharmaceutical company influence, as well as wider drug policies [2,9]. With the pattern of increased opioid prescription being reproduced elsewhere, including in the UK, the US experience of subsequent opioid-related harm stands as a cautionary tale.

Risks of harm may be exacerbated by use of over-the-counter (OTC) opioids, which are perceived as comparatively safe by the public, but may increase a person's overall opioid dosage through unmonitored use [12]. OTC opioid usage is unregulated by trained professionals or guidelines, and dramatically increases the risk long-term harms and further adverse events [9, 13].

Studies of general samples from 2013 population statistics estimate reported chronic pain prevalence in the UK to be at around 43% (28 million adults), steadily rising with age to 62% of those over 75 years [1, 2]. There are also concerns about a 'hidden' population of high-functioning chronic pain sufferers who self-medicate through degenerative and inflammatory conditions with little interaction with health services [1]. Of those who receive opioids from their GP, research suggests an average 12% of patients with chronic pain receive strong long-acting classes of opioid [13] with prescription of these increasing substantially across the last 15 years (although beginning to decline from 2016), particularly morphine, oxycodone and fentanyl [6, 8].

Although these prescription increases have occurred nationally, one of the most significant driving characteristics for patient and area-level increase in strong opioid prescription has been socioeconomic deprivation [6, 9, 11]. Deprivation is associated with a much higher prevalence of pain, depression, drug misuse and mixed physical and mental multi-morbidities, with an increase in barriers to recovery both at individual and group levels [14–19]. The association between socioeconomic deprivation, indices of multiple deprivation (IMD) and pain is consistent across various countries [9, 16, 18, 23].

The Health Survey for England 2011 found that 44% of women and 40% of men in the lowest socioeconomic quartile met the criteria for chronic pain compared to 30% to 24% of those in the highest quartile [9]. The most common cited type of non-cancer pain is musculoskeletal, including chronic backpain – the largest cause of disability in working-age adults [18]. Several studies have cited deprivation as the greatest impacting factor on musculoskeletal chronic pain, severity and disability [18].

THE PAIN PROBLEM

Pain itself is complex, with deeply entrenched variables and underlying mechanisms across biological, psychological, emotional and social dimensions with risk factors including female sex, occupational factors, depression and anxiety, trauma, history of abuse or violence, lower socioeconomic and education level, obesity, smoking, older age, geographic and cultural background and deprivation as a whole [20, 21]. Chronic pain is understood not just to be a symptomatic element of other more identifiable morbidities, but a defined condition in its own right.

According to population estimates, around a quarter of adults globally suffer moderate to severe chronic pain with new, chronic, non-malignant pain developing in over 5 million people in the UK every year [22], the vast majority supported primarily by their general practitioner [1, 11, 13]. *The Global Burden of Disease Study* in 2015 ranked chronic pain as one of the most significant causes of human suffering and it remains particularly challenging to treat, occurring often with and can be further impacted by anxiety, depression and poor social outcomes [2].

THE PAIN EXPERIENCE

Pain reporting is always a subjective measure with psychosocial consequences and confounding variables playing a significant part in the experience, as well as response and participation in treatment types, overall quality of life and potential for disability, multimorbidity and mortality [24]. How the individual processes the sensory information of pain, interprets it, then experiences it and subsequently appraises it again may all be influenced by cognitive and biopsychosocial factors such as beliefs, unconscious processes, their pain history, social context, maladaptive coping strategies and psychological resources [2, 18, 20, 24, 25]. Particularly when pain becomes a chronic process, how the individual copes and adapts will determine a significant part of the overall outcome. In the UK approximately 49% of patients with chronic pain also experience depression, anxiety disorders and emotional distress [2] These people are twice

as likely to become chronic pain patients than the general population [24].

Individuals reporting depressive symptoms and pain exhibit greater negative thought processes, as well as a greater propensity for pain to advance from acute to chronic [18, 20, 24, 25] and poorer prognosis [21]. Pain can result in negative outcomes, including limitation of daily activities, loss of function, loss of relationships and job loss [2].

There is also increasing evidence from large-scale national research that pain may be reported 2 to 3 times more frequently in those with a documented history of trauma, post-traumatic stress disorder (PTSD), violence at any age and domestic abuse, unrelated to associated physical injuries [21, 25, 26, 27]. This adds to the well-established association between early adverse experiences, trauma, PTSD and chronic pain [2].

Regional differences are prominent across the UK, with 'severely limiting' chronic pain 37% more likely in the north than the south [10], and a positive association of higher opioid use in line with an established north-south health divide linked to socioeconomic deprivation [10]. An increase in high dose, long-term opioid prescription prevalence has been most positively established in patients with lower socioeconomic status and higher general deprivation scores [6, 9, 23, 29]. Similar trends in use and prescription variation have been found across multiple countries and populations [10, 28, 29].

IT'S NOT JUST THE OPIOIDS

Rates of opioid prescription map well to areas of drug-related deaths in England, with the north east consistently highest and the north west a close second [30]. Both map well to levels of deprivation [30]. The problem of risky medications is, however, not simply about single opioids. Ashaye et al.'s analysis of 132 patients on opioids for chronic musculoskeletal pain found multiple links between different opioids with patients on combinations of codeine, tramadol, morphine, oxycodone, buprenorphine and fentanyl [31]. The ONS's 2018 examination of drug-related deaths reported a cohort of vulnerable, at-risk people taking drugs but often using multiple drugs in combination with alcohol [32]. The reality for our most at-risk and chaotic patients is that they will use prescribed medications alongside unprescribed medication and street drugs. They may pay little heed to dosing recommendations and where one medication or tablet is ineffective, they may try increasing doses and medications way beyond any limits seen in the *British National Formulary*. There is a high likelihood of their being smokers and drinkers too. A recent review of deaths examined by the coroner at our practice revealed all had, at the time of death or recently before, been prescribed combinations of dependency-forming medications (DFMs) including opioids, gabapentinoids, benzodiazepines or other hypnotics, antidepressants and antipsychotics, each with their own risks individually and in combination.

NHS Digital figures show pregabalin prescriptions grew from less than half a million in 2006 to over 5.5 million by 2016 [33]. Over a similar period, gabapentin prescriptions have risen by over 400% from just over 1 million to 6.5 million, many outside of its licensed indication for neuropathic pain [33]. Again, the north east has the highest spending on pregabalin with the north west closely behind. The highest spending CCGs rank high in levels of deprivation [34]. As prescription rates rise, so do the drug-related deaths. In 2012 there were just 4 deaths related to pregabalin and 8 to gabapentin, but by 2016 these had risen to 111 and 59 respectively, most as a result of combining them with heroin or other opioids [35]. By 2017, 24% of those receiving a gabapentinoid had a co-prescription, most commonly with an opioid but increasingly also with a benzodiazepine [36].

Benzodiazepines are licensed for short-term use in anxiety. Their longer-term use is associated with worsening depression. Prescribing pattern differences are seen between affluent and deprived areas. In affluent areas a similar number of people are prescribed benzodiazepines, but in deprived areas courses are longer with many more people staying on them long term [37]. Benzodiazepines share some metabolic pathways with opioids and gabapentinoids, contributing to increased risks when used together. In addition, there is a growing presence in the illicit drug market of stronger benzodiazepines and substances marketed as benzodiazepines but containing other, often harmful, ingredients [38]. Due to issues of rapid tolerance, users of benzodiazepines commonly use high doses or 'megadoses' to achieve the desired effects – these doses may be up to 10 times the maximum recommended dose [38]. The exact extent

of increased risk of death with benzodiazepines is hard to define with mixed results in the literature due to research on different drugs and different populations with different risks and morbidities. The overall picture, however, suggests increased risks with their use, especially in combination with other centrally depressant medications and especially when there is a risk of pneumonia, in which benzodiazepines clearly increase both the risk of contracting the disease and of dying from it [38].

Over the last 5 years, spending on hypnotics like zopiclone and zolpidem has decreased but the rates of prescription have remained similar [39]. The number of deaths involving zopiclone and zolpidem continue to rise, from 96 in 2016 to 127 in 2017 and, as with benzodiazepines, in 8 out of 10 deaths, mixing with other drugs was implicated [30]. Higher levels of anxiolytic and hypnotic medications have long been understood to be associated with areas of deprivation [40]. In the UK there has been a widespread perception among doctors that z-drugs are safer than benzodiazepines though they share similar risks of respiratory effects including respiratory depression, especially when taken with alcohol [41]; addiction, with evidence of withdrawal symptoms after 3 weeks, less than its licensed duration of treatment [42], tolerance and misuse potential [43]. There is a high risk of rebound insomnia when stopped after longer-term use. Pharmacologically, zopiclone is known for its low index of fatal toxicity [44], as low or lower than benzodiazepines [45, 46]. One American review found the mortality risk associated with taking a hypnotic to be equivalent to smoking a pack of cigarettes a day [47]. In the US the Food and Drug Administration has placed a high-risk warning on the z-drugs after multiple reports of people being injured or killed by unconscious behaviours whilst on the medications including through activities such as cooking, driving and shooting themselves [48].

Antipsychotics are another class of risky medication that are more commonly prescribed in disadvantaged areas. They are prescribed around 3.5 times more frequently in the most deprived than the least deprived areas, and are often prescribed for non-psychotic reasons including depression, anxiety and insomnia [49]. In recent years there has been increased awareness of the risks of using antipsychotics in patients with dementia but more recent evidence suggests the doubled risk of all-cause mortality applies equally to people without dementia, rises with dose and shows little difference between typical and atypical forms [50]. Deaths from antipsychotics increased by 5% between 2016 and 2017 [30].

Antidepressant related deaths are also increasing, especially those involving tricyclic antidepressants [30]. Antidepressants are not always thought of as a risky medication but a systematic review of studies demonstrated a substantial increase in all-cause mortality (HR=1.33, 95% CI 1.14-1.55) consistent when controlling for the confounding effects of depression [51]. Davies and Read's systematic review challenged the general view that antidepressant withdrawal effects are infrequent and generally mild, reporting that more than half (56%) of people coming off these medications experienced withdrawal effects, and in almost half (46%) of these the symptoms were severe [52, 53].

Nor does the list of risky medications end there. Other medications which can contribute synergistically to central nervous system depression and risk of death include anti-epileptics and sedating antihistamines [38].

As clinicians working in areas of multiple and concentrated disadvantage we are increasingly aware of the risks of medications but our prescribing decisions are attempts to do something, anything, to alleviate the symptoms of our patients in the most desperate conditions. It is a tough challenge to tell a patient in chronic pain that you won't prescribe a medication when they have tried it and it helped, or when they know you have prescribed it for others in the past. Increasingly we find ourselves using these medications to treat the physical and mental manifestations of emotional, physical and social distress. What then should be done?

SUGGESTIONS FOR PRACTICE

- *Identify patients at high risk due to their prescribed (and unprescribed) medications, especially those taking an equivalent opioid dosage over 120mg of morphine daily or those taking multiple risky medications, and engage them in a process of reduction or rationalization [5].*

The Oxford Pain Management Centre has offered 5 tips for tackling opioid reduction in primary care including:

1. Education of the importance of opioid reduction.
2. Engagement of the patient and involving them as far as possible in decision-making.
3. Having a plan for weaning patients off.
4. Managing the impact in anxiety and depression.
5. Managing expectations and providing support

In reality, clinicians know that these consultations can be very difficult. It is important to take an individualised approach, taking into account each person's needs and barriers to care [4, 20, 53–57]. It is hard to practice person-centred care in a consultation where the person's agenda is the exact opposite of the clinician's and achieving patient buy-in and attendance at the necessary follow-up appointments is a huge challenge. The process may actually threaten the patient-doctor therapeutic relationship. Examples of successful good practice do exist in this area – see Grosvenor Road Surgery in Belfast's RCGP Bright Ideas write-up of their CBT pain management group as a very useful example [58].

Psychological medicine pain clinics have become more prevalent in the UK, employing cognitive behavioural therapy (CBT), behavioural therapy (BT) or mindfulness-based techniques alongside advice on pacing and avoiding boom-or-bust behaviours. These techniques have been shown to have small to moderate benefits for patients but more in terms of reducing the impacts of pain i.e. secondary suffering, depression and disability, than pain itself [59]. Research on accessibility and coverage of these services showed that the infrastructure lacks sufficient capacity, waiting times are long and the majority of patients remain under their GP. A common complaint from patients who do attend but leave disgruntled is that, 'they made out it was all in my head'. Some research has suggested that those who live in deprivation may not benefit to the same extent, if at all, due to various psychosocial differences [18].

SUGGESTIONS FOR PRACTICE

- *Provide holistic multidisciplinary care alongside non-pharmacological techniques.*

Exercise and physical therapies have also yielded promising results for pain reduction in some populations, but barriers to access and resources have been shown as well as limited uptake and continuation across studies involving patients within areas of deprivation.

SUGGESTIONS FOR PRACTICE

- *Not doubling up opioids e.g. codeine with tramadol.*
- *Not doubling up benzodiazepines and not pairing them with z-hypnotics.*
- *Not prescribing over BNF doses.*
- *Starting doses low.*
- *Rotating opioids to reduce tolerance and prevent escalation.*
- *Stopping an ineffective medication before starting another.*
- *Not placing risky medications on repeat.*
- *Regular formal medication reviews to monitor harm, escalation, management and side effects.*

With the difficulties in managing and reducing dependency-forming medications the best approach may be not to start them in the first place. In prison medicine a pro-active approach is taken to *de*-prescribing medications which are risky in terms of danger to the patient and potential for diversion and misuse. In addition, clear guidance is available for doctors working in secure environments in the RCGP's Secure Environments Group's publication, *Safer Prescribing in Prisons: Guidance for Clinicians. Second edition* [60] as to what those levels of risk are by way of a traffic light system and preferred options for treatment in common presentations such as pain, depression, anxiety and insomnia. Reviews and guidance are expected imminently from a number of national bodies on the prescribing issues discussed in this chapter. In anticipation of these or the creation of a guide to safer prescribing in the community given the similar problems experienced by the populations of deprived areas and by people who come into contact with the criminal justice system, primary care teams may consider utilising this very useful tool before initiating treatment in these scenarios.

Rising prescriptions of potentially harmful medications and their unequal distribution, biased towards deprived areas, risks the creation of a new, iatrogenic health inequality caused by patterns of prescribing our riskiest medications, frequently in combination, to our most at-risk patients. To prevent this tragedy, reduction of avoidable harms caused by overuse of opioids and other risky medications should be considered a priority and a matter of social equity for policymakers nationally and locally, as well as individual practitioners.

REFERENCES

1. Fayaz A, Croft P, Langford R, Donaldson L, Jones G. Prevalence of chronic pain in the UK: A systematic review and meta-analysis of population studies. *BMJ Open.* 2016; 6(6): e010364.
2. *Chronic pain: Supporting safer prescribing of analgesics* [Internet]. London: The BMA; 2017 [cited 2 April 2019]. Available from: https://www.bma.org.uk/-/media/files/pdfs/collective%20voice/policy%20research/public%20and%20population%20health/analgesics-chronic-pain.pdf?la=en
3. *Opioids for Persistent Pain.* London: British Pain Society; 2010. Available from: http://www.britishpainsociety.org/static/uploads/resources/files/book_opioid_patient.pdf [Accessed 2nd April 2019].
4. Sandhu H, Underwood M, Furlan A, Noyes J, Eldabe S. What interventions are effective to taper opioids in patients with chronic pain? *BMJ.* 2018; k2990.
5. Ponton R, Sawyer R. Opioid prescribing in general practice: Use of a two-stage review tool to identify and assess high-dose prescribing. *British Journal of Pain.* 2017; 12(3): 171–182.
6. Curtis H, Croker R, Walker A, Richards G, Quinlan J, Goldacre B. Opioid prescribing trends and geographical variation in England, 1998–2018: A retrospective database study. *The Lancet Psychiatry.* 2019; 6(2): 140–150.
7. Ballantyne J, Kalso E, Stannard C. WHO analgesic ladder: A good concept gone astray. *BMJ.* 2016; i20.
8. Ruscitto A, Smith B, Guthrie B. Changes in opioid and other analgesic use 1995–2010: Repeated cross-sectional analysis of dispensed prescribing for a large geographical population in Scotland. *European Journal of Pain.* 2014; 19(1): 59–66.
9. Mordecai L, Reynolds C, Donaldson L, de C Williams A. Patterns of regional variation of opioid prescribing in primary care

in England: A retrospective observational study. *British Journal of General Practice.* 2018; 68(668): e225–e233.

10. Todd A, Akhter N, Cairns J, Kasim A, Walton N, Ellison A et al. The Pain Divide: A cross-sectional analysis of chronic pain prevalence, pain intensity and opioid utilisation in England. *BMJ Open.* 2018; 8(7): e023391.

11. Kennedy M, Pallotti P, Dickinson R, Harley C. 'If you can't see a dilemma in this situation you should probably regard it as a warning': A metasynthesis and theoretical modelling of general practitioners' opioid prescription experiences in primary care. *British Journal of Pain.* 2018; 204946371880457.

12. Cooper R. 'I can't be an addict. I am.' Over-the-counter medicine abuse: A qualitative study. *BMJ Open.* 2013; 3(6): e002913.

13. Seamark D, Seamark C, Greaves C, Blake S. GPs prescribing of strong opioid drugs for patients with chronic non-cancer pain: A qualitative study. *British Journal of General Practice.* 2013; 63(617): e821–e828.

14. Jordan K, Thomas E, Peat G, Wilkie R, Croft P. Social risks for disabling pain in older people: A prospective study of individual and area characteristics. *Pain.* 2008; 137(3): 652–661.

15. The English Indices of Deprivation 2015 – Frequently Asked Questions (FAQs) [Internet]. London: Department for Communities and Local Government; 2016. Available from: https://assets.publishing. service.gov.uk/government/uploads/system/uploads/attachment_data/file/579151/ English_Indices_of_Deprivation_2015_-_ Frequently_Asked_Questions_Dec_2016. pdf [Accessed 3rd April 2019].

16. Poleshuck E, Green C. Socioeconomic disadvantage and pain. *Pain.* 2008; 136(3): 235–238.

17. Health state life expectancies by national deprivation deciles, England and Wales: 2015 to 2017. Office for National Statistics; 2019. Available from: https://www.ons. gov.uk/peoplepopulationandcommunity/ healthandsocialcare/healthinequalities/bulletins/healthstatelifeexpectanciesbyindex ofmultipledeprivationimd/2015to2017/pdf [Accessed 6th April 2019].

18. Carr J, Klaber Moffett J. The impact of social deprivation on chronic back pain outcomes. *Chronic Illness.* 2005; 1(2): 121–129.

19. McLean G, Gunn J, Wyke S, Guthrie B, Watt G, Blane D et al. The influence of socioeconomic deprivation on multimorbidity at different ages: A cross-sectional study. *British Journal of General Practice.* 2014; 64(624): e440–e447.

20. Reid M, Eccleston C, Pillemer K. Management of chronic pain in older adults. *BMJ.* 2015; 350(feb13 2): h532.

21. van Hecke O, Torrance N, Smith B. Chronic pain epidemiology and its clinical relevance. *British Journal of Anaesthesia.* 2013; 111(1): 13–18.

22. Toye F, Seers K, Tierney S, Barker K. A qualitative evidence synthesis to explore healthcare professionals' experience of prescribing opioids to adults with chronic non-malignant pain. *BMC Family Practice.* 2017; 18(1).

23. Leue C, Buijs S, Strik J, Lousberg R, Smit J, van Kleef M et al. Observational evidence that urbanisation and neighbourhood deprivation are associated with escalation in chronic pharmacological pain treatment: A longitudinal population-based study in the Netherlands. *BMJ Open.* 2012; 2(4): e000731.

24. Turk D, Fillingim R, Ohrbach R, Patel K. Assessment of psychosocial and functional impact of chronic pain. *The Journal of Pain.* 2016; 17(9): T21–T49.

25. Meints S, Edwards R. Evaluating psychosocial contributions to chronic pain outcomes. *Progress in Neuro-Psychopharmacology and Biological Psychiatry.* 2018; 87: 168–182.

26. McWilliams L, Cox B, Enns M. Mood and anxiety disorders associated with chronic pain: An examination in a nationally representative sample. *Pain.* 2003; 106(1): 127–133.

27. Ellsberg M, Jansen H, Heise L, Watts C, Garcia-Moreno C. Intimate partner violence and women's physical and mental health in the WHO multi-country study on women's health and domestic violence: An observational study. *The Lancet.* 2008; 371(9619): 1165–1172.

28. Williams D, Teljeur C, Bennett K, Kelly A, Feely J. Influence of material deprivation on prescribing patterns within a deprived population. *European Journal of Clinical Pharmacology.* 2003; 59(7): 559–563.

29. Chen T, Chen L, Kerry M, Knaggs R. Prescription opioids: Regional variation and socioeconomic status – evidence from primary care in England. *International Journal of Drug Policy.* 2019; 64: 87–94.

30. Office for National Statistics. Deaths related to drug poisoning in England and Wales: 2017 Registrations. 2018. Available from: https://www.ons.gov.uk/peoplepopulation-andcommunity/birthsdeathsandmarriages/deaths/bulletins/deathsrelatedtodrugpois oninginenglandandwales/2017registrations [Accessed 28 April 2019].

31. Ashaye T, Hounsome N, Carnes D et al. Opioid prescribing for chronic musculo-skeletal pain in UK primary care: Results from a cohort analysis of the COPERS trial. *BMJ Open.* 2018; 8:e019491. doi: 10.1136/bmjopen-2017-019491.

32. Office for National Statistics. Drug-related deaths "deep dive" into coroner's records. 2018. Available from: https://www.ons.gov.uk/peoplepopulationandcommunity/birthsdeathsandmarriages/deaths/articles/drugrelateddeathsdeepdiveintocoronersre-cords/2018-08-06 [Accessed: 25 April 2019].

33. NHS Digital Prescriptions Dispensed in the Community: Statistics for England, 2007–2017. Available from: NHS Digital figures show pregabalin prescriptions grew from less than half a million in 2006 to over 5.5 million by 2016 [Accessed 1st June 2019].

34. Open Prescribing. Prescribing of Pregabalin by all CCGs. Available from: https://open-prescribing.net/measure/pregabalin/ [Accessed 1st June 2019].

35. Iacobucci G. UK Government to reclassify pregabalin and gabapentin as deaths rise. *BMJ.* 2017; 358: j4441.

36. Montastruc F, Loo SY, Renoux C. Trends in first gabapentin and pregabalin prescrip-tions in primary care in the United Kingdom, 1993–2017. *JAMA.* 2018; 320(20): 2149–2151.

37. Open Prescribing. Anxiolytics and hypnotics: Average daily quantity per item by all CCGs. Available from: https://openprescribing.net/measure/bdzadq/ [Accessed 22nd June 2019].

38. Johnson CJ, Barnsdale LR, McCauley A. *Investigating the Role of Benzodiazepines in Drug-Related Deaths: A Systematic Review Undertaken on Behalf of The Scottish National Forum on Drug-Related Deaths.* Edinburgh: NHS Scotland; 2016.

39. Open Prescribing. Available from: https://openprescribing.net/ [Accessed 2nd June 2019].

40. The Pharmaceutical Journal. Mental health prescribing higher in more deprived parts of the UK. *The Pharmaceutical Journal.* 3rd June 2009. Available from: https://www.pharmaceutical-journal.com/news-and-analysis/news/mental-health-prescribing-higher-in-more-deprived-areas-of-the-uk/10965975.article [Accessed 2nd June 2019].

41. Chung W-S, Lai C-Y, Lin C-L, Kao CH. Adverse respiratory events associated with hypnotics use in patients of chronic obstruc-tive pulmonary disease. *Medicine.* 2015; 94(27): e1110.

42. Cimolai N. Zopiclone: Is it a pharmaco-logical agent for abuse? *Canadian Family Physician.* 2007; 53(12): 2124–2129.

43. Agravat A. 'Z'-hypnotics versus benzodi-azepines for the treatment of insomnia. *Progress in Neurology and Psychiatry.* 2018; 22.

44. Lunesta E. Assessment of Zopiclone. World Health Organisation. https://www.who.int/medicines/areas/qual-ity_safety/4.6ZopicloneCritReview.pdf Accessed [2nd June 2019].

45. Reith DM, Fountain J, McDowell R, Tilyard M. Comparison of the fatal toxicity index of zopiclone with benzodiazepines. *Journal of Toxicology: Clinical Toxicology.* 2003; 41(7): 975–980.

46. Gunja N. The clinical and forensic toxicity of Z-drugs. *Journal of Medical Toxicology.* 2013; 9(2): 155–162.

47. Kripke DF. Hypnotic drug risks of mortality, infection, depression, and cancer: But lack of benefit. *F1000 Research.* 2016; 5: 918.

48. Dyer O. FDA issues black box warnings on common insomnia drugs. *British Medical Journal.* 2019; 365: l2165.

49. Marston L, Nazareth I, Petersen I, Walters K, Osborn DPJ. Prescribing of antipsychot-ics in UK primary care: A cohort study. *BMJ*

Open. 2014; 4(12). Available from: https://bmjopen.bmj.com/content/4/12/e006135 [Accessed 2nd June 2019].

50. Ralph SJ, Espinet AJ. Increased all-cause mortality by antipsychotic drugs: Updated review and meta-analysis in dementia and general mental health care. *Journal of Alzheimers Disease Reports.* 2018; 2(1): 1–26.

51. Maslej MM. The mortality and myocardial effects of antidepressants are moderated by pre-existing cardiovascular disease: A meta-analysis. *Psychotherapy and Psychosomatics.* 2017; 86: 268–282.

52. Davies J, Read J. A systematic review into the incidence, severity and duration of antidepressant withdrawal effects: Are guidelines evidence-based? *Addictive Behaviors.* 2018. S0306–4603(18)30834-7.

53. Oxford Pain Management Centre. *Guidance for Opioid Reduction in Primary Care.* Oxford: Oxford University Hospitals NHS Foundation Trust; 2017.

54. Foy R, Leaman B, McCrorie C, Petty D, House A, Bennett M et al. Prescribed opioids in primary care: Cross-sectional and longitudinal analyses of influence of patient and practice characteristics. *BMJ Open.* 2016; 6(5):e010276.

55. Cherkin D. How can the intractable problem of chronic musculoskeletal pain (CMP) be effectively managed? The need for a well-integrated systems approach. *Journal of General Internal Medicine.* 2018; 33(S1): 4–6.

56. McCrorie C, Closs S, House A, Petty D, Ziegler L, Glidewell L et al. Understanding long-term opioid prescribing for non-cancer pain in primary care: A qualitative study. *BMC Family Practice.* 2015; 16(1).

57. Lozier C, Nugent S, Smith N, Yarborough B, Dobscha S, Deyo R et al. Correlates of use and perceived effectiveness of non-pharmacologic strategies for chronic pain among patients prescribed long-term opioid therapy. *Journal of General Internal Medicine.* 2018; 33(S1): 46–53.

58. McCullagh R. CBT pain management course. Royal College of General Practitioners. Bright Ideas. Available from: https://www.rcgp.org.uk/clinical-and-research/resources/bright-ideas/cbt-pain-management-course.aspx [Accessed 2nd June 2019].

59. Williams ACDC, Eccleston C, Morley S. Psychological therapies for the management of chronic pain (excluding headache) in adults. *Cochrane Database of Systematic Reviews.* 2012; 11. Art. No.: CD007407. doi: 10.1002/14651858.CD007407.pub3.

60. Bicknell M. Farmer D. Watson C. *Safer Prescribing in Prisons: Guidance for Clinicians.* Second Edition. Available from: https://www.convenzis.co.uk/wp-content/uploads/2018/09/SPIP_Liverpool_010219.pdf [Accessed 2nd June 2019].

12

Persistent Physical Symptoms

JULIA HOSE AND SUSAN HARRIS

The organs weep the tears the eyes refuse to shed.

Persistent physical symptoms (PPS) is an enormous topic, taking up over a fifth of GP appointments. Persistent physical symptoms are exactly that: physical symptoms, which may or may not have an organic cause, and which are also chronic and distressing. Medically unexplained symptoms (MUS) are physical symptoms which are not accounted for by organic disease. In practice we try to use the term PPS, as it is more acceptable to patients [1] and avoids placing medical explanation or intervention at the heart of the experience, although we will also use MUS when this term is used in research or guidelines to which we refer.

Nomenclature around PPS is uncertain and changeable, which is frustrating to both clinicians and patients [2]. Many of the labels used are not acceptable to patients, as they attribute most, or all, of the suffering to an underlying mental disorder [1]. Secondly, lack of clear labelling can lead to diagnostic confusion and lack of clarity not only between doctor and patient, but between clinicians themselves. This presents challenges for research, as some studies include patients with formal diagnostic labels and some do not.

Some syndromes such as fibromyalgia, chronic fatigue syndrome and irritable bowel syndrome (IBS), for which the aetiology is poorly understood, can be helped by the approaches we will discuss [3].

International Classification of Diseases (ICD) 11 and Diagnostic and Statistical Manual of Mental Disorders (DSM) 5 have tried to move to more positivistic diagnoses as this is associated with better outcomes [4]. Absence of pathology is therefore not the key issue, rather the presence of overwhelming distress. This encourages early consideration of PPS as a possible diagnosis, rather than diagnosis by exclusion. The new diagnosis, body distress disorder (BDD), encompasses most of the previous terms, such as somatoform disorder, apart from dissociative neurological disorder which is coded elsewhere [5, 6].

CASE STUDY

Alex

Alex is 48 years old and lives with his partner, Phil (unemployed due to depression), and their 16-year-old daughter, Alison. He works as a carer in a nursing home. Alex has chronic obstructive pulmonary disease (COPD), and although he has quit smoking and complies with his medication, he regularly reports to A&E with increased breathlessness. Little is found objectively, but he is often prescribed antibiotics and steroids. He quit smoking immediately after his diagnosis two years ago, after smoking 30 per day since age 17. Alex regularly presents with breathlessness to his GP, complaining his COPD medication is unhelpful. Over the last 6 months, he has developed non-specific abdominal pain with no associated features other than some altered sensation in his abdomen and legs. Alex attributes this to adhesions from an appendicectomy 20 years ago, which he thinks has been worsened by breathing difficulties affecting his abdominal muscles. Alex was admitted at the onset of this symptom as an emergency, as it was very severe although nothing significant was found on CT or exploratory laparotomy. Alex complained about the surgery afterwards, feeling the surgeon was incompetent in not finding anything. Alex has been off work for three weeks now due to abdominal pain and is very worried about the financial implications. Alex was briefly prescribed tramadol and is now asking to have this reinstated as the only thing which helps. Prior to his COPD diagnosis, Alex attended the surgery fairly frequently with various non-specific symptoms but could always be reassured. The COPD was initially attributed to anxiety, and Alex moved GP practices following this as he was very angry about the missed diagnosis.

Identification

PPS are very common, with at least 20% of GP appointments concerning physical symptoms without clear underlying cause, but over 75% of those who visit with such conditions will be limited to a single consultation [7]. This rises to 25–50% in secondary-care settings [8]. Of those presenting with PPS some patients may have underlying pathology, accounting for some of the symptoms, but other symptoms may not fit or the degree of symptom experienced by the patient may appear out of proportion to the degree of pathology found. Where PPS are suspected, they are best assessed in a spirit of collaboration and curiosity and within a biopsychosocial framework. This facilitates the exploration of all factors affecting people's lives, in order to better understand the whole clinical presentation and what goals the individual with these symptoms has. We need to move towards understanding 'what matters' to people rather than 'what is the matter' with someone.

While clinicians may worry about missing a physical diagnosis, it is just as important not to miss a mental health diagnosis or social factors which are contributing to symptoms. Teasing out aetiological factors can be difficult. The diagnosis of PPS should always be reviewed and reviewable. People with PPS are just as likely as everyone else to develop physical disease, and studies have suggested that up to 4–10% of people initially diagnosed with MUS are later diagnosed with a disease that could have accounted for their symptoms [7, 9].

For most patients the prognosis is good, with approximately 75% improving back to their baseline within 12 months. Around 25–33% of people may develop chronic symptoms, with around a 1% prevalence of severe disorder [7, 10]. A recent study found that parental psychopathology, number of co-morbid medical conditions and physical functioning were associated with prognosis, emphasising the role of both medical illness and early environment [10].

CASE STUDY CONTINUED

Alex has no history of mental health difficulties. He has been in a relationship with Philip for around 20 years, and they adopted Alison when she was two. Alison is doing well at school but has had occasional trouble with bullying. She is due to go to sixth form soon and plans to go to university to be a nurse. Alex worked various retail jobs until he was in his late 20s, when he started work as a carer, a job he loves. Alex was born in London and left with his mum, age 14, following repeated periods of physical abuse from his dad. Mum worked multiple jobs and was rarely at home. Alex acted in a parental role to his younger two siblings. He has little contact with his mum and brother as they are unhappy about his relationships, but is close to his sister, Anna, who is three years younger. Alex has a wide circle of friends and used to go out regularly but has reduced his activity since his diagnosis of COPD. He used to binge drink, but this has reduced. Alex used stimulants heavily in his early 20s, but stopped at the start of his relationship with Phil. On reflection he feels that this helped him to cope.

Aetiology

There are many theories about the causes of PPS. A common understanding is summarised by the 18th century physician, William Osler, in his quote,

'The organs weep the tears the eyes refuse to shed'. This frames physical symptoms without physical cause as a direct result of unexpressed emotional distress. Freud and his peers elaborated on this concept introducing ideas about repressed trauma manifesting directly into the body (hysteria), forming the classical basis of terms such as psycho-somatic symptoms, or somatisation [11, 12].

Although helpful, these ideas miss the complexity and nuance in PPS. What about people without childhood trauma? Or when symptoms are partially explained? Why do different cultures experience symptoms differently? What role do deconditioning, polypharmacy and iatrogenic effects play for these symptoms? We have divided known aetiological factors into biological, psychological and social as a well-recognised framework, although we recognise that this is somewhat artificial given the interplay between the three.

Biological Factors

Biological factors must be considered, and there is increasing evidence of the contribution of various physiological processes which contribute to the development and maintenance of unexplained symptoms, perhaps most robustly in chronic pain. Central sensitisation was initially theorised from animal models as a method by which pain may be perpetuated without ongoing stimulus. However, recent neuroimaging has demonstrated grey matter changes in pain processing regions and altered resting brain connectivity between pro-nociceptive and anti-nociceptive regions alongside immune changes which are implicated in widespread pain and allodynia, and other symptoms such as sleep disturbance and cognitive changes [13]. This should be seen as a spectrum, rather than simply absent or present, and can be a result of a bottom-up process with ongoing nociceptive input (e.g. rheumatoid arthritis) or top down (e.g. fibromyalgia). Autonomic dysfunction may help to explain many physical symptoms [14] when taken in combination with individual psychological and social issues. This can also help people to understand how deconditioning and prior trauma may have affected their processing of information and sensation by affecting filter systems of perception [15] and now contribute to their experience in a way which avoids blame or a purely psychological explanation which people often find unacceptable.

Another possible contributory factor is dys-regulation of the hypothalamic pituitary (HPA) axis, with increased arousal and inappropriate triggering of the fight-or-flight response, resulting in chronic hyper-vigilance and exaggerated stress response [16]. These are particularly relevant for people who have been subject to early life deprivation or abuse, where the body's ability to manage stress has been demonstrably affected, but it must be noted that the data is very variable between studies. There does appear to be a genetic component to many functional syndromes, though this is hard to separate from health beliefs common to families and learned health behaviours [17, 18]. Individual symptoms, or functional syndromes, may also be associated with peripheral changes, e.g. intestinal flora in IBS [19].

Lastly, in relation to biological considerations, we must remember drugs, prescribed or otherwise, as either causative or maintaining factors in PPS. Through direct harm, side effects or withdrawal syndromes many medications can worsen symptoms. Looking at timings of medication prescription, or dose changes, may help to understand symptom progression. Equally, non-prescribed drugs may worsen or relieve symptoms and must be enquired about. Cannabis in particular is often used by people for pain relief.

Psychological Factors

No single psychological model appears to fully explain the experience of people with PPS, and detailed discussion of cognitive or dynamic theories is outside the scope of this chapter. Risk factors, such as childhood abuse or early death of a loved one, predispose us to multiple mental and physical health conditions, including PPS [8]. The importance of the meaning of the physical symptom for the individual cannot be overemphasised, as there are often associations with difficult life experiences or fears for the future [20]. The symptom or illness can also be a form of interpersonal communication, particularly when people struggle to express their own needs or feelings [21]. Symptoms can also occur without any of these factors or be secondary to health anxiety. It is helpful to know about difficult life experiences, as this may be a way of understanding an individual's coping methods, or attachment styles (templates for relating to others, specifically caregivers in this context) [22, 23]. Such a detailed investigation may not be essential for a primary care clinician, so only ask about areas you feel comfortable helping with. If you see a lot of interpersonal factors or meaning for the individual, perhaps in terms of their history or help-seeking style, then referral for a relational therapy may be warranted.

People may also struggle with 'cognitive errors', such as catastrophising, where symptoms are interpreted in a negative manner producing significant distress. You may note these already, observing someone who 'is a worrier' or 'is really black and white about the world'. These 'errors' can exacerbate symptoms and even help to explain symptoms in the absence of any clear predisposing factors [24, 25]. We all have different ways of thinking and may revert to less helpful or more reactive ones when stressed, but if this is significant for your patient then a referral for a cognitive therapy may be helpful.

Consider perpetuating factors such as selective attention, where the person becomes focused on a symptom or bodily area – perhaps repeatedly touching it – magnifying the symptom experience [26]. We can readily demonstrate how this works by concentrating on a body part, and repeatedly tapping it to sensitise the skin. This is a useful way to introduce distraction techniques as a tool addressing both the immediate experience and long-term symptom prognosis.

Social Factors

Socioeconomic deprivation is strongly associated with PPS development and severity [27]. With people who have complex needs, it's very important to see them as part of their wider social and cultural system. Consider their role within the family – how does the symptom affect that? How do family members react to their condition? Awareness of this social milieu helps you understand why things have developed, and perhaps how to manage situations such as including family in education and care planning. Similarly, people who are very isolated may struggle to regulate their distress or have few people outside of healthcare to turn to for support.

We know that there can be many social obstacles to recovery, such as financial issues arising

from the benefits system, especially where people perceive their condition as not being legitimised by medical and social organisations [28]. These can be hard to ask or talk openly about, but it's important to understand any potential positive gain from symptom experience, or the anxiety associated with change.

LEARNING EXERCISE

- *What risk factors does Alex have for complex health needs?*
- *How would you speak to him about these issues?*
- *Could any of Alex's experiences be attributed to a mental health condition? Why/why not?*

Treatment in Primary Care

Having identified patients with PPS, and with an understanding of how these patients and their symptoms can develop, we now move on to how we can help these patients. A recent update of a systematic review suggested that patient-involving and central-acting interventions are more likely to be successful [4]. Kroenke [29] developed a stepped care model for MUS, which can helpfully be adapted here into three stages:

1. Determine severity (assessment).
2. Assess and treat functional syndromes and psychiatric syndromes.
3. Develop plan for managing in primary care.

Determine Severity

Most people's symptoms naturally resolve with brief explanation and reassurance. Try to avoid cycles of repetitive reassurance, as these can become problematic in their own right [30]. In 20–25% of people, symptoms do not resolve, and the clinician should move to step two. Need for progression can be detected by having a follow-up visit at around six weeks which can be cancelled by the patient if they feel better. This approach helps people to feel that concerns have been heard and taken into account. Use of PHQ-15 may identify multiple troubling symptoms early [30]. Bear in mind all the symptom domains (somatic, cognitive, emotional, behavioural and social) when exploring symptoms to help develop an illness narrative for each patient. Clinicians have a key role in helping people make sense of their experiences [31].

In a few studies professionals talk of patients not wanting to think about psychosocial factors, yet analysis of audio-recordings of appointments and patient interviews suggests that patients almost always cue to emotional distress, but that this is either not recognised or dismissed [32–34]. Patients may then 'ramp up' their symptom description, for example using emphatic language to describe symptoms and learn that attention is paid to somatic complaints. Helping patients to develop co-constructed illness narratives can be hugely powerful and avoids the one-size-fits-all approach which patients often find unhelpful.

SUGGESTIONS FOR PRACTICE

- *Although the full schedule is not pragmatic in primary care, concepts from the McGill Illness Narrative Interview (MINI) [35] may be of help to structure the assessment:*
- *Basic exploration of symptoms including timeline and other events (consider doing over several appointments, could use a diary) which may not be causal but are linked in any way.*
- *Relevant experiences of the individual or those they know, and impact of the symptom/illness has had on them.*
- *Any explanatory models, including cultural. Try linking to the biopsychosocial aetiological factors above, remembering to keep them relevant to the individual.*
- *This helps clinicians to develop an explanatory framework with their patients, which can then be used to build new understandings to provide relief from uncertainty and identify possible strategies for improvement which are based on the individual formulation. Try to develop a few ways of explaining the body-mind link and how symptoms can be produced without identifiable lesions, so you feel confident when faced with a person in distress.*
- *Consider using patient information leaflets or other professionally written sources e.g. from the Royal College of Psychiatrists or neurosymptoms.org or service user resources, such as FND hope. This can be immensely helpful for helping*

people to not feel alone with their experience and in developing a shared narrative between clinician and patient.

Assess and Treat Functional or Psychiatric Syndromes

Anxiety and depression are common complicating factors in all chronic health conditions and a significant proportion of people with PPS will also have depression or anxiety, although their presence does not predict overall outcome [8]. Consider also PTSD and complex trauma presentations, for example, following a difficult health experience such as ITU [36]. Pertinent symptoms can be elicited using standard history taking or through the use of questionnaires (e.g. PHQ-9), however, these can have limitations in this setting, as those patients with PPS often have nuanced presentations where the somatic symptoms of depression (e.g. appetite change) could be a direct expression of the PPS.

It is easy to miss, or dismiss, the possibility of underlying mood disorder in these patients, as they can often be complicated and seem difficult to communicate with. There is a risk of over-normalisation by clinicians ('well of course they'd be depressed if they have all this pain all the time'). Remember, a good proportion of these patients don't develop any significant mood disruption. Evidence also shows that patients with MUS can be reluctant to reveal an underlying mental disorder to clinicians, for fear of their symptoms being solely attributed to that and being dismissed as 'it's all in their head'. Careful discussion with the patient can help, covering how commonly the two problems present together (appropriate normalisation by the clinician) and how treating one may help the other using previous ideas around central sensitisation and sensation processing.

Patients with PPS can be particularly sensitive to medication side effects and commencement/withdrawal effects. They will often have tried various medications in the past, and a careful history is needed to unpick what has been tried, how the patient got on and why it was stopped. In our experience, this often reveals that the patient may not have tried a medication for long enough to see maximum effects (up to ten weeks) due to initial agitation or nausea, or because they had not been appropriately counselled prior to commencement.

Develop Plan for Managing in Primary Care

Care plans can be hugely powerful documents, allowing clinicians and patients to collaborate in developing personalised treatment plans, helping everyone feel more in control and improving the interpersonal dynamic. Additionally, they demonstrate to the patient that they are valued rather than dismissed as not being ill. Plans should be as specific as possible to the individual and any advice or guidance should be unambiguous and symptom-focused. There may need to be agreements about targeted physical examinations, which should not become overly ritualised but can be hugely powerful when used in conjunction with clear explanatory frameworks and symptom-based care.

Involving family members or other carers is vital, as if they do not agree with or understand the care plan, it is likely to be unsuccessful. Additionally, their own beliefs may need to be challenged, for example in allowing the person to be alone more often rather than relying on their family for support.

Consideration of onward referrals, or triggers for referrals, e.g. change in symptoms, should be factored into the patient care plan. A balance needs to be struck between the significant risk of over investigation, such as direct complications, incidental findings, false positives or reinforcing unhelpful health beliefs, and that of missing a major pathology [37]. No one will ever get this totally right and recognising and acknowledging this is hugely powerful, as is sharing your own concerns and uncertainty openly with the individual – the optimal outcome is collaboration even in the face of major unknowns [38].

SUGGESTIONS FOR PRACTICE

Tips for onward referrals and investigations

- *Explain why you are recommending **this** test/ referral to the patient and be open about what a negative result would mean e.g. no further tests. It is important to manage people's expectations in a positive way.*
- *Avoid delivering negative tests as good news – remember that this may be hugely distressing. Use phrases like 'we've ruled out anything*

sinister, however, you remain profoundly affected ... could we agree to think about how to help you in a different way?'
- *Be open with secondary-care colleagues in referrals – ask that patients are sent back to you rather than passed around the secondary-care system to avoid ongoing iatrogenic harm.*

The Clinician as Intervention

Agreeing to see people in a regular and predictable way can help to avoid some of the conflict and frustration which can come from patients calling ad hoc for appointments and is a cornerstone of treatment in primary care. A therapeutic alliance is composed not only of rapport – the warm, caring part of a relationship – but a working togetherness, which is an effective working of one patient with ideally one clinician (with support). These patients can present a challenge within the healthcare environment, with clinicians often reporting feelings of frustration, irritation and helplessness in such consultations [39]. Clinicians find patients with PPS challenging, often because they challenge the classic model of medical training and because of the need to tolerate a high degree of challenge and uncertainty [40]. In addition, patients with PPS may have other complex issues, such as personality and attachment difficulties, which can influence the quality of the doctor-patient relationship and influence patient attitudes towards treatment, as well as their ability or desire to attend follow-up sessions. All of this risks feeding into a clinician's sense of frustration and helplessness.

Clinicians are challenged in all the above ways, and their perception of being in control during the consultation is lost. In order to regain some power, and (as the clinician sees it) 'help' the patient, they often feel the need to do something for these patients. Studies suggest that while clinicians think patients want a diagnosis, treatment and a cure, most patients with PPS want to be listened to, treated with compassion and understanding [32]. Additionally, patients themselves tend to demonstrate an innate understanding that nothing will be found on assessment, that tests and investigations may not be necessary, and that they may not be cured. Instead patients seek explanation and support through difficult episodes.

Clinicians' anxiety can lead to inappropriate or over-prescribing, over investigation and inappropriate referral, all of which can themselves cause considerable harm. Additionally, a confrontational or combative consultation can risk important symptoms being missed. Clinicians are left feeling worried and practising even more defensively, the patient experiences the clinician as persecutory, and the relationship breaks down, increasing the risk of error and poor outcomes.

Specific Treatment Options

MEDICATION

In patients with functional syndromes encompassed under the MUS umbrella (e.g. IBS), there may be some role for a number of medications. Existing guidelines are primarily symptom-based [41].

Antidepressants have been used as neuromodulating agents for people with PPS, rather than for their mood-lifting effects. This is a somewhat contentious issue, as some meta-analyses have been supportive [4, 42] while Cochrane advised there was no evidence for their use above placebo in 2014. In practice, they are not licensed, but are used pragmatically and at times to good effect for people without mental disorder with significant symptom burden.

Many patients with MUS may have been to various doctors (GPs and specialists) and tried multiple medications over the years. They are often on long lists of tablets with minimal or no benefit. Additionally, these patients demonstrate management challenges in part due to difficulties with attachment and personality which can influence their ability to concord with medications, follow-up arrangements and treatment regimes. Clinicians will often find themselves responding urgently to changes in function or symptoms without a clear rationale apart from a desire to help someone in distress. In desperation, the clinician may give the patient a medication to try – in order to simply do something as discussed above. If enough clinicians adopt this strategy, patients end up on lots of medications. Side effects from medications can also cause new or worsen existing physical symptoms, and repeated prescribing can reinforce ideas about the nature of the individual's condition and become a source of conflict in the future. Despite this, changes can be a great source of anxiety for both patient and practitioner.

Specific medications which can be problematic are painkillers and benzodiazepines. These medications may form part of a considered treatment regime but can also produce significant side effects. Dosing should be clearly titrated against symptom relief, with a plan for cessation if doses are escalating without clear benefit. Opiates in particular are associated with numerous negative long-term consequences, and evidence of their use in chronic pain is mixed at best [43]. Where pain is not consistently controlled, consider a dose reduction or stopping altogether. This can be a hard conversation, but clearly advising people of the long-term effects and issues around the potential for opiates to even increase pain perception can be immensely helpful.

Given the complex issues around medication it may become apparent that a patient's concordance with prescribed medication regimes has been variable. Simple engagement strategies can improve concordance and strengthen the therapeutic alliance [44]. Realistic counselling about what to expect in terms of timeframe for change following commencement of a medication, side effects and expected degree of improvement can help. In addition, organised pre-booked follow-up sessions, ideally with the same clinician, can go a long way to making headway with these patients.

LEARNING EXERCISE

- *How would you use the stepped care model and your own understanding of Alex's situation to develop a co-constructed illness narrative and care plan? Who else may need to be involved here?*

Lifestyle and Social Prescribing

As with (almost) everything in medicine, getting more exercise, eating better, drinking less alcohol, smoking less, not taking illicit substances, getting more sleep and undertaking meditation or other stress-reduction activity is likely to make someone feel better in general, and can be advocated for everyone. However, there are a multitude of steps and barriers to each of these changes, especially in this cohort of patients who, for a variety of reasons already discussed, may not have the tools to easily improve these areas of lifestyle without guidance. Familiarity with local charities and health programmes in your area that provide lifestyle change programmes can be beneficial. Maybe also consider debt advice and back-to-work programmes? Thinking about the history you have taken and what you know about the individual, try to target specific areas of need for that individual.

Psychological Treatments

Psychotherapeutic approaches have a reasonable evidence base, although they are not currently specified by Cochrane or other guidance bodies. Meta-analysis [45] demonstrated a moderate effectiveness for cognitive-behavioural therapy (CBT), but emphasised the need for longer appointment duration and attention to interpersonal aspects, in addition to the core CBT techniques. Many other approaches have been demonstrated to be helpful, such as psychodynamic interpersonal therapy [46], and some are available in local Improving Access to Psychological Therapy (IAPT) services, who now have a specific mandate to work with people with PPS and long-term health conditions. There is an emerging evidence base for GPs holding symptom clinics in primary care [47], however, GP interventions which focus on symptom reattribution alone have not demonstrated benefits and should not be used without combination with other approaches [48].

Some areas are developing community-based liaison mental health services, often called psychological medicine services, which work either from a local hospital, or with primary care, to support management of people with highly complex and distressing needs. Early referral to such services can be beneficial in preventing further deterioration or worsening of distress.

Involving the Wider Healthcare Organisation

WHOLE PRACTICE APPROACH

Although GPs generally consult alone, primary care clinicians work as part of a team from medical peers to reception staff; all of whom can be affected by complex patients.

Common issues encountered within practices are:

- Continuity of Care
  At a time when resources are stretched it can be difficult to maintain continuity of care

due to issues with appointment availability and nuances of booking systems. Sometimes patients will actively avoid continuity – so-called 'doctor shopping' – preferentially seeing a different doctor each time, perhaps where contentious medication or inappropriate (in the eyes of the GP) referral is sought, but underlying patient needs haven't been met. Whatever the cause, lack of continuity of care has a big impact on patients, as all of the historical learning about that individual is lost. New clinicians may go back through the investigation cycle with a similarly disappointing outcome.

- Waiting Room Difficulties
  Complex patients often have difficulties with attachment, interpersonal skills and struggle to tolerate distress for all the reasons discussed in section one. Given that waiting rooms and receptions are hectic places, it is unsurprising that situations can escalate, and heated conversations can occur in the waiting room. Patients may also find themselves in distress or having significant physical symptoms in waiting areas which can interrupt their planned care as different clinicians get involved.

SUGGESTIONS FOR PRACTICE

- *Care Plans*
  We suggest that just as people with brittle asthma should have easy-to-access care plans, so should people with debilitating physical symptoms, especially where there may be multiple people or agencies involved. We suggest including reception staff in this plan. This may include writing a small script for how to respond to particularly distressing situations or people who contact the clinic very frequently.
- *Case Discussion/Peer Support*
  Some primary care practices advocate using case discussion to alert all clinicians to complex people, whether as part of their regular meetings or case by case. This also allows people to get some support from peers and demonstrates teamwork which can be helpful if there is a complaint or other difficult outcome.
- *Named Clinician/Coding*
  Evidence supports allocating a named clinician to see people for regular follow-up. This should be indicated on your computer system so

everyone knows to book in with only this clinician. If possible, try not see people between regular appointments unless they are acutely unwell, encouraging them to use their own coping skills.

- Training
Understanding the basics of what makes complex patients complex is useful for all healthcare staff and helps reduce barriers to treatment and improve therapeutic alliance. Design training sessions aimed at all staff to avoid either overly compliant or high conflict relationships with patients.

REFERENCES

1. Marks EM, Hunter MS. Medically unexplained symptoms: An acceptable term? *British Journal of Pain*. 2015 May;9(2):109–14.
2. Toft T, Fink PE, Oernboel EV, Christensen KA, Frostholm L, Olesen F. Mental disorders in primary care: Prevalence and co-morbidity among disorders. Results from the functional illness in primary care (FIP) study. *Psychological Medicine*. 2005 Aug;35(8):1175–84.
3. Henningsen P, Zipfel S, Herzog W. Management of functional somatic syndromes. *The Lancet*. 2007 Mar 17;369(9565):946–55.
4. Henningsen P, Zipfel S, Sattel H, Creed F. Management of functional somatic syndromes and bodily distress. *Psychotherapy and Psychosomatics*. 2018;87(1):12–31.
5. Price JR, Okai D. Functional disorders and 'medically unexplained physical symptoms'. *Medicine*. 2016 Dec 1;44(12):706–10.
6. Fink P, Schröder A. One single diagnosis, bodily distress syndrome, succeeded to capture 10 diagnostic categories of functional somatic syndromes and somatoform disorders. *Journal of Psychosomatic Research*. 2010 May 1;68(5):415–26.
7. Peveler R, Kilkenny L, Kinmonth AL. Medically unexplained physical symptoms in primary care: A comparison of selfreport screening questionnaires and clinical opinion. *Journal of Psychosomatic Research*. 1997 Mar 1;42(3):245–52.
8. Olde Hartman TC, Borghuis MS, Lucassen PL, van de Laar FA, Speckens AE, van Weel C. Medically unexplained symptoms, somatisation disorder and hypochondriasis: Course and prognosis. A systematic review. *Journal of Psychosomatic Research*. 2009 May 1;66(5):363–77.
9. Katon WJ, Walker EA. Medically unexplained symptoms in primary care. *The Journal of Clinical Psychiatry*. 1998; 59:15–21.
10. Stone J, Smyth R, Carson A, Lewis S, Prescott R, Warlow C, Sharpe M. Systematic review of misdiagnosis of conversion symptoms and "hysteria". *BMJ*. 2005 Oct 27;331(7523):989.
11. van Eck van der Sluijs J, ten Have M, De Graaf R, Rijnders CA, Van Marwijk HW, van der Feltz-Cornelis CM. Predictors of persistent Medically Unexplained physical Symptoms: Findings from a general population study. *Frontiers in Psychiatry*. 2018;9:613.Freud and somatisation.
12. Ursin H. Sensitization, somatization, and subjective health complaints. *International Journal of Behavioral Medicine*. 1997 Jun 1;4(2):105.
13. Harte SE, Harris RE, Clauw DJ. The neurobiology of central sensitization. *Journal of Applied Biobehavioral Research*. 2018 Jun;23(2):e12137.
14. Martínez-Martínez LA, Mora T, Vargas A, Fuentes-Iniestra M, Martínez-Lavín M. Sympathetic nervous system dysfunction in fibromyalgia, chronic fatigue syndrome, irritable bowel syndrome, and interstitial cystitis: A review of case-control studies. *JCR: Journal of Clinical Rheumatology*. 2014 Apr 1;20(3):146–50.
15. Rief W, Broadbent E. Explaining medically unexplained symptoms-models and mechanisms. *Clinical Psychology Review*. 2007 Oct 1;27(7):821–41.
16. van Ravenzwaaij J, Olde Hartman TC, Van Ravesteijn H, Eveleigh R, Van Rijswijk E, Lucassen PL. Explanatory models of medically unexplained symptoms: A qualitative analysis of the literature. *Mental Health in Family Medicine*. 2010 Dec;7(4):223.
17. Holliday KL, Macfarlane GJ, Nicholl BI, Creed F, Thomson W, McBeth J. Genetic variation in neuroendocrine genes associates with somatic symptoms in the general

population: Results from the EPIFUND study. *Journal of Psychosomatic Research.* 2010 May 1;68(5):469–74.

18. Landmark-Høyvik H, Reinertsen KV, Loge JH, Kristensen VN, Dumeaux V, Fosså SD, Børresen-Dale AL, Edvardsen H. The genetics and epigenetics of fatigue. *PM&R.* 2010 May 1;2(5):456–65.

19. Salem AE, Singh R, Ayoub YK, Khairy AM, Mullin GE. The gut microbiome and irritable bowel syndrome: State of art review. *Arab Journal of Gastroenterology.* 2018 Jun 20. genetics of functional syndromes

20. Maunder R, Hunter J. An integrated approach to the formulation and psychotherapy of medically unexplained symptoms: Meaning-and attachment-based intervention. *American Journal of Psychotherapy.* 2004 Jan;58(1):17–33.

21. Kirmayer LJ. *Rhetorics of the Body: Medically Unexplained Symptoms in Sociocultural Perspective.* Somatoform Disorders 1999 (pp. 271–286). Springer, Tokyo.

22. McWilliams LA. Adult attachment insecurity is positively associated with medically unexplained chronic pain. *European Journal of Pain.* 2017 Sep;21(8):1378–83.

23. Adshead G, Guthrie E. The role of attachment in medically unexplained symptoms and long-term illness. *BJPsych Advances.* 2015 May;21(3):167–74.

24. Deary V, Chalder T, Sharpe M. The cognitive behavioural model of medically unexplained symptoms: A theoretical and empirical review. *Clinical Psychology Review.* 2007 Oct 1;27(7):781–97.

25. Brown RJ. Medically unexplained symptoms: A new model. *Psychiatry.* 2006 Feb 1;5(2):43–7.

26. Salkovskis PM, Gregory JD, Sedgwick-Taylor A, White J, Opher S, Ólafsdóttir S. Extending cognitive-behavioural theory and therapy to medically unexplained symptoms and long-term physical conditions: A hybrid transdiagnostic/problem specific approach. *Behaviour Change.* 2016 Dec;33(4):172–92.

27. Creed F, Tomenson B, Chew-Graham C, Macfarlane G, McBeth J. The associated features of multiple somatic symptom complexes. *Journal of Psychosomatic Research.* 2018 Sep 1;112:1–8.

28. Rossen CB, Buus N, Stenager E, Stenager E. Identity work and illness careers of patients with medically unexplained symptoms. *Health.* 2017 Nov 1:13.

29. Kroenke K. Patients presenting with somatic complaints: Epidemiology, psychiatric co-morbidity and management. *International Journal of Methods in Psychiatric Research.* 2003 Feb;12(1):34–43.

30. van Ravesteijn H, Wittkampf K, Lucassen P, van de Lisdonk E, van den Hoogen H, van Weert H, Huijser J, Schene A, Van Weel C, Speckens A. Detecting somatoform disorders in primary care with the PHQ-15. *The Annals of Family Medicine.* 2009 May 1;7(3):232–8.

31. Edwards TM, Stern A, Clarke DD, Ivbijaro G, Kasney LM. The treatment of patients with medically unexplained symptoms in primary care: A review of the literature. *Mental Health in Family Medicine.* 2010 Dec;7(4):209.

32. Salmon P, Ring A, Dowrick CF, Humphris GM. What do general practice patients want when they present medically unexplained symptoms, and why do their doctors feel pressurized? *Journal of Psychosomatic Research.* 2005;59(4):255–60.

33. Wileman L, May C, Chew-Graham CA. Medically unexplained symptoms and the problem of power in the primary care consultation: A qualitative study. *Family Practice.* 2002;19(2):178–82.

34. Johansen ML, Risor MB. What is the problem with medically unexplained symptoms for GPs? A meta-synthesis of qualitative studies. *Patient Education and Counselling.* 2017;100(4):647–54.

35. Groleau D, Young A, Kirmayer LJ. The McGill Illness Narrative Interview (MINI): An interview schedule to elicit meanings and modes of reasoning related to illness experience. *Transcultural Psychiatry.* 2006;43(4):671–91.

36. Jackson JC, Hart RP, Gordon SM, Hopkins RO, Girard TD, Ely E. Post-traumatic stress disorder and post-traumatic stress symptoms following critical illness in medical intensive care unit patients: Assessing the magnitude of the problem. *Critical Care.* 2007 Feb;11(1):R27.

37. Nimnuan C, Hotopf M, Wessely S. Medically unexplained symptoms: How often and why are they missed?.*QJM*. 2000 Jan 1;93(1):21–8.

38. NHS PlymouthMedically Unexplained Symptoms: a whole systems approach in Plymouth 2009. Available from: https://serene.me.uk/helpers/mus-plymouth.pdf [Accessed 30th May 2019]

39. Stone L. Blame, shame and hopelessness: Medically unexplained symptoms and the'heartsink'experience. *Australian Family Physician*. 2014 Apr;43(4):191.

40. Shattock L, Williamson H, Caldwell K, Anderson K, Peters S. 'They've just got symptoms without science': Medical trainees' acquisition of negative attitudes towards patients with medically unexplained symptoms. *Patient Education and Counselling*. 2013 May 1;91(2):249–54.

41. Hookway C, Buckner S, Crosland P, Longson D. Irritable bowel syndrome in adults in primary care: Summary of updated NICE guidance. *BMJ*. 2015 Feb 25;350:h701.

42. Ford AC, Talley NJ, Schoenfeld PS, Quigley EM, Moayyedi P. Efficacy of antidepressants and psychological therapies in irritable bowel syndrome: Systematic review and meta-analysis. *Gut*. 2009 Mar 1;58(3):367–78.

43. Chou R, Turner JA, Devine EB, Hansen RN, Sullivan SD, Blazina I, Dana T, Bougatsos C, Deyo RA. The effectiveness and risks of long-term opioid therapy for chronic pain: A systematic review for a National Institutes of Health Pathways to Prevention Workshop. *Annals of Internal Medicine*. 2015 Feb 17;162(4):276–86.

44. Conn VS, Ruppar TM, Enriquez M, Cooper PS, Chan KC. Healthcare provider targeted interventions to improve medication adherence: Systematic review and meta-analysis. *International Journal of Clinical Practice*. 2015 Aug;69(8):889–99.

45. Liu J, Gill NS, Teodorczuk A, Li ZJ, Sun J. The efficacy of cognitive behavioural therapy in somatoform disorders and medically unexplained physical symptoms: A meta-analysis of randomized controlled trials. *Journal of Affective Disorders*. 2018 Oct 22.

46. Kleinstäuber M, Witthöft M, Hiller W. Efficacy of short-term psychotherapy for multiple medically unexplained physical symptoms: A meta-analysis. *Clinical Psychology Review*. 2011 Feb 1;31(1):146–60.

47. Burton C, Weller D, Marsden W, Worth A, Sharpe M. A primary care Symptoms Clinic for patients with medically unexplained symptoms: Pilot randomised trial. *BMJ Open*. 2012 Jan 1;2(1).

48. Gask L, Dowrick C, Salmon P, Peters S, Morriss R. Reattribution reconsidered: Narrative review and reflections on an educational intervention for medically unexplained symptoms in primary care settings. *Journal of Psychosomatic Research*. 2011 Nov 1;71(5):325–34.

13

Social Prescribing: Connecting People for Health and Well-Being

TIM ANFILOGOFF

Looking at what matters <u>to</u> people, not just what is the matter <u>with</u> them.

Social prescribing is a practical response to a simple reality. Many people, especially those with limited education or social networks, do not know how to seek help with the problems they face other than visiting their GP. A CAB and CommRes survey of GPs in 2015 found that 19% of GP face-to-face time was spent on issues other than health and 72% of GPs said this had risen in the previous year [1]. The Low Commission estimated that 15% of GP time is spent on issues around welfare benefits alone [2]. That the GP does not necessarily know how to respond (or have time to research non-medical issues) is frustrating for both doctor and patient and can lead to further frustrating visits. Only 31% of GPs in the CAB survey felt able to advise patients on non-medical matters – and, of course, that tells us nothing about the quality of the advice they did feel able to give. Helping people access the right support is a skill in itself.

The risk of pathologising social problems is also very real, where a hard-pressed, but freely accessible clinician, is met with a frequently attending patient with, for example, low mood and non-specific aches and pains. Many services to which patients can be referred onto are predicated on people meeting a threshold of ill health or need which actively undermines the concept of prevention.

Much has been said about the social and environmental determinants of health [3, 4]. It is intuitively obvious, but supported also by research, that poverty and debt can be both a consequence and a catalyst of mental health problems [5]. While there is always the risk of a busy GP erring towards prescribing medication to help people with anxiety and low mood, in the words of one GP in the vanguard of social prescribing, 'Why prescribe Prozac to someone who has lost his job when you may be able to prescribe work?'

It is obvious that the higher the level of disadvantage, the higher the likely level of input is needed to help someone turn their lives around. This can rarely be done in a ten-minute consultation however well conducted and is why social prescribing is so necessary and potentially so powerful.

WHAT IS SOCIAL PRESCRIBING?

NHSE has provided a best practice summary guide [6] for those seeking to develop social prescribing to accompany the new resources announced in the NHS plan (January 2019) [7].

The key elements of the link worker model are set out there and in the National Social Prescribing

Network's publication *Making Sense of Social Prescribing* [8] and are broadly:

- **Agencies who know how to refer** (often GPs and other primary care staff, but it does not have to be health professionals – though this is where social prescribing started in a desire to make good the gap between primary care and the community).
- **Link workers who take those referrals** and have time and skills to hear where people are and where they want to be and then help them come up with a plan that will work for them.
- **Link workers matching people** with a range of support in their communities to break social isolation, ensure access to benefits and services, prevent eviction and help people take control of their health, as appropriate to the person. They work with the person until the outcomes they have agreed are achieved or this no longer becomes possible.
- **Link workers supporting asset-based community development**, that is helping create new links across sectors and communities and supporting new groups to develop in partnership with communities.

The link worker role had sprung up all over the country organically, which must say something about its value. While the Bromley by Bow Centre is internationally famous for the work it has been undertaking since 1984 [9], the national social prescribing network only held its first national conference in January 2016, pulling together practitioners, clinicians and commissioners' views of what social prescribing is and what it achieves. Accordingly, the link worker role has been and is still called many different things, including well-being adviser, community connector, community navigator, community health worker, community (health) agent and health adviser, to name but a few. NHSE and the national network use link worker as the generic term.

WHO IS SOCIAL PRESCRIBING FOR?

While it is perfectly possible and reasonable to have target groups for social prescribing services (homeless people, people with mental health problems, family carers, type 2 diabetics), some of the preventive quality of social prescribing can be lost if a service isn't generic. In Hertfordshire , when the Community Navigator Service was set up it chose not to have eligibility criteria other than the following:

- The professional has someone in front of them about whom they are concerned, but
- There is no obvious solution or service to which to refer them or which they will be able to use.

There are a range of situations where this open, generic approach can be very helpful. Family carers may often reject the label 'carer' (*I am just his wife, mother, etc.*) and therefore may not easily accept referral to a carers' organisation. People who are already stigmatised, for example, type 2 diabetics often feel blamed for their illness [10], may respond better to a service where other people without that label are doing exercise and losing weight together (although some will particularly value the de-stigmatising support of peer groups). Many people will have a range of issues both medical and social. In particular, social isolation/loneliness is now understood to be a major public health issue [11]. Moreover, loneliness actively militates against patient activation and undermines people's motivation to improve their health. There is evidence that lonely people are more likely to visit a GP or A & E and more likely to enter local authority funded residential care, while 76% of GPs report that one to five patients a day come to their surgery because they are lonely (the classic 'ill for which there is not a pill') [12].

Good social prescribing referrals to some extent rely on referrers understanding the potential of the open conversation with the link worker. This can tease out issues which the GP may never become aware of in a ten-minute consultation, but which matter most to the particular person. A home visit is usually the starting point and this can reveal the iceberg that lies invisible below the water. It is enough for the GP to see its tip in the consulting room and so make the referral.

WHY IS SOCIAL PRESCRIBING TRANSFORMATIVE?

There is clear evidence that social prescribing can have a very positive impact [13, 14]. As to why it works, the feedback from practitioners, clinicians and people who use the service seems fairly straightforward. Generally, link workers hear that the people they work with now feel (back) in control of their lives, have a reason to get up in the morning, feel listened to and (re)connected to their community [15]. GPs talk about people being deflected to services or support that prevents the need for clinical interventions and makes it easier to work on their clinical issues. The consensus appears to be that these solutions stick, in a way that previous attempts to help people may have failed, because of some simple key elements:

1. Link workers can take the *time* to find out what is most important to the person (this may not always be the issue that led to the referral) – not what is the matter *with* them but what matters *to* them. This is key in terms of building trust and supporting motivation around change.
2. Link workers can work with the person at a speed and in a way that makes sense to the person. Not assuming that a particular type of prescription is appropriate, for example, but understanding that the person may want to do *some* exercise but hates the idea of a gym or a health walk or any kind of sport. So the

link worker works on the person's interest in environmental volunteering which can then address both the agreed need for exercise and create an easy way of developing a social life with other volunteers, digging out ponds in the local park.
3. Link workers do not create a dependency relationship but stick with the person until the plan agreed with them has led to the required outcomes. This may include taking them to a support group for the first couple of times; reassuring and encouraging them when they think they can't stick to the plan they agreed; helping them understand and remember the money advice from the CAB until they no longer need such hand-holding; knowing when the person is integrated to a social group and doesn't need the Link Worker's help to *stay* engaged.
4. Link workers can help co-ordinate and navigate when the complexity of the system gets too much.

The first-ever national social prescribing conference, January 2016, produced the following summary of how good social prescribing works [16] (Figure 13.1).

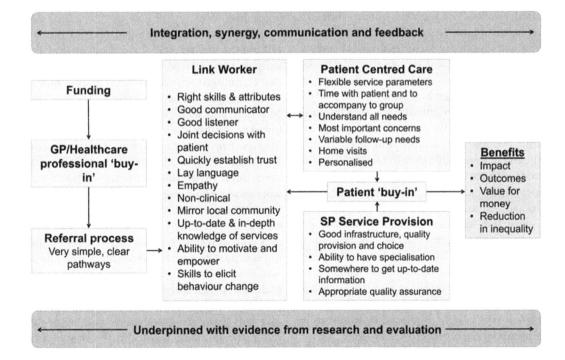

Figure 13.1 Summary of how good social presribing works.

CASE STUDY

Case Study One: Jim

The GP senses there is an unmet need, but can't easily find out what it is or treat it.

An elderly male in one of the area's most deprived wards was socially isolated. His frequent attendances at the GP surgery were not improving his health and well-being (and were presenting problems for the reception staff because of his behaviour). Feeling there was more going on than she could tease out of him in their consultations, the GP got Jim to agree to contact from a local community navigator who arranged to visit him at home.

Jim was a hoarder and his house was full of heaps of paper, boxes and rubbish. The drains had been blocked for some time, and his solution to having lost the landlord's phone number was to stop paying his rent, assuming that would get the landlord to visit. Meanwhile, sanitation had become a problem not just for him but increasingly for his neighbours with whom he was becoming more and more unpopular. Jim's increasingly bizarre behaviour had meant his sisters had disassociated themselves from him, feeling powerless to help.

The community navigator, Alicia, finally helped Jim find the landlord's phone number under a pile of hoarded junk. She made contact and issues around rent and drains were resolved. Alicia now helped Jim to get a local service to declutter his house and took him to the local community café a couple of times, to get him back into interacting with people in his community. He then began to attend the café regularly on his own.

Jim's outlook and attitude improved significantly, and he gradually began to make better connections with the people around him. One crucial moment was when his neighbour let him hold her young baby. He told his sisters about the help Alicia had given him and that Christmas, for the first time in years, his sisters took the risk of inviting him to spend the day with them. They had a pleasant day and he proudly showed them a blanket he had been given by a local charity, which Alicia had linked him to, as a Christmas present. One of the sisters was particularly impressed by it and so he then presented the blanket to her as a gift.

The GP found this improvement in his social connectedness meant he was now prepared to work with her on reducing his historical polypharmacy. When Jim told her about giving his sister the blanket, his pride made him seem six inches taller.

Sadly, Jim recently died. But he would have told you – and his family and friends agreed – that the last two years were the best of his adult life, not least because people in his community now said hello to him when he was out and about. He felt better physically and emotionally and found friendship and a sense of community that made all the difference to his later years. He visited the GP less often and was now polite and friendly with the reception staff.

People come up against problems with the system as it requires form-filling, waiting lists, repeat visits and a range of other things that make bureaucratic sense but are very difficult for some citizens to comply with. This creates additional health inequalities – the people who most need help can lose it simply because of difficulties complying. Social prescribing has the power to change this.

CASE STUDY

Case Study Two: Jean

Holistic response means understanding people's whole lives.

The psychiatrist discharged Jean to the local talking therapy service. She did not answer their calls or their letters. Fortunately, they knew of the community navigator service and had got Jean's consent to make a referral. The navigator, Miriam, rang Jean. Jean did not reply. Miriam knocked on her door. Jean did not answer the first few times she visited. But Miriam persisted. Eventually Jean let Miriam in. The first long conversation revealed that at the top of Jean's many worries was a huge pile of correspondence she was too terrified to open. With Jean's consent Miriam read and sorted the correspondence. Jean's benefits had been stopped because she was not opening her post and had missed interviews and she was about to be evicted. Working with the CAB and others, Miriam helped Jean sort out these practical matters which relationship-breakdown and her sense of hopelessness had made simply insurmountable for her. If the situation had persisted, Jean would have become more ill and homeless, her suffering would have increased and cost the health service and local authority more in time and money. Without social prescribing, the local NHS would not have been geared up to prevent this happening.

Jean said, 'Once the threat of eviction was removed…I felt a weight had lifted and I could now concentrate on me and on tackling the depression… I still feel that I have something to give and ultimately, I want to get back into work and I would like to look at volunteering as a way of doing this'. She said she still had bad days, but now there was hope; she rated her mental health at 6/10 when it had previously been 1/10.

Linking to the Local Assets in your Community and Voluntary Sector

THE IMPORTANCE OF INFORMATION AND ADVICE INFRASTRUCTURE

Part of the sample link worker's job description [17], is to 'forge strong links with local VCSE organisations, community and neighbourhood level groups, utilising their networks and building on what's already available to create a map or menu of community groups and assets. While research skills will often be really important in this role, especially around micro-groups and informal, very local assets, a lot will depend on the local information and advice infrastructure.'

CASE STUDY

Case Study Three: HertsHelp

In Hertfordshire social prescribing arrangements are underpinned by HertsHelp, a single point of access to the 12,000 or so entries on the HertsDirect community database. Most people call on the phone, but they are accessible in a range of ways including online. HertsHelp provide skilled triage to people who self-refer, or who are referred by GPs (or 'active signposting' receptionists) or other professionals. A simple online form helps GPs refer at the touch of a button, allowing them to say 'Would it be okay if I get HertsHelp to give you a ring, Mrs Bloggs?' As well as being simple for the very busy GP, this recommendation helps when HertsHelp calls, if Mrs Bloggs has forgotten the referral or is unsure she wants to talk. 'Your doctor/practice suggested I give you a call', is a very

useful tool in helping get a conversation going. If it becomes clear that Mrs Bloggs cannot manage to discuss her issues over the phone, because of their complexity, her hearing, emotional distress or confusion, a community navigator can be sent to visit her at home.

It is hoped that where communities have not yet networked the different sources of support into a cohesive, integrated offer, the role of the new link workers funded by NHSE will be key catalysts in joining this all up. The 'no wrong door' principle is generally regarded as the ideal end state for a community wishing to support its most marginalised, even if it is not always easy to achieve perfectly on the ground. Social prescribing is part of making people's journey around the different types of support less random. The language of navigation is often used by professionals (who find the system confusing enough themselves) and citizens often talk about the sense of being lost in a maze when having to deal with housing, benefits, social care and the health service.

What is particularly interesting about onward referrals is their variety. The majority were to well-known organisations (though even this shows that many people have never heard of Age UK, or the CABx) but some small, very local, or very specialised groups received only one or two referrals in the month. The fear expressed by some small groups is often that such systemic access may lead to them being overwhelmed. But they are also keen to ensure they get the right sort of referrals from those people who they can best help.

It is imperative for considerable stakeholder engagement prior to commissioning the navigator service. In particular, it was made clear that the community navigators were not there to do anyone else's job (some agencies were very concerned that it would take commissioned work away from them and they would fail to meet targets) but rather to ensure agencies got the right referrals at the right time. Some agencies were concerned they would get too many referrals.

There is at least some anecdotal evidence that this systemic approach supports people to access help *before* they are in crisis, and with skilled input that makes the referral easier to manage for the receiving services and makes prescriptions more likely to stick. But this is not to underplay the serious resource restraints much of the community and voluntary sector currently faces.

The navigators have also proved great problem-solvers, often finding ways around gaps in services, matching agencies together to create solutions for individuals, creating new assets in the community, rather than, as some commissioners feared, endlessly demanding new services be commissioned.

All of this serves to underline how important it is that new social prescribing roles are built sensitively onto the foundations of what each locality already has to offer in terms of community groups and voluntary organisations. This requires a lot of open discussions. Otherwise there is a huge risk of alienating some of the key assets that the link workers will need to work with, or of duplicating and causing confusion to referrers, providers and citizens alike. For two helpful checklists on what to consider when developing a new scheme see Chapter 9 and the Summary Guide at Annex C.

Social Prescribing Link Workers Do not Exist in a Vacuum

There are a range of services and ways of working that overlap with the social prescribing link worker model discussed above. Sometimes other workers can take on the link worker role with an occasional client – perhaps where they know that without that extra bit of input the 'prescription' simply won't work or where they have developed a relationship with someone who cannot usually sustain a positive relationship with services. Sometimes health champions or social prescribing volunteers can engage them, especially where their needs are less complex and they don't need so many agencies co-ordinated and navigated. Altogether Better is one model of 'health champions' that has been shown to reduce the reliance on primary care contact without a paid link worker model [18].

How to Get Involved Locally

Projections from the first-ever NHSE survey of CCGs about social prescribing suggest that there were already hundreds of link workers in England in the spring of 2018 and 50% of CCGs appear to have been commissioning some level of social prescribing. We also know that local authorities are sometimes sole or co-commissioners of similar schemes.

NHSE and the National Social Prescribing Network are committed to building up the skills

and resilience of this developing network nationally, helping projects share best practice, mentor each other and develop the best possible services, building on what we are all learning about what works.

Significant New Resources

We know that the new resources coming to social prescribing are substantial: about 1,000 workers, one per primary care network (PCN) funded at 100% of cost, for five years, with money coming on stream from July 2019, direct to PCNs.

Lastly, and very positively for the future of social prescribing in creating the much needed bridge between clinicians and communities, medical student activists in England have recently developed their own National Social Prescribing Student Champion Scheme so local medical students will be able to access peers with an interest in creating medical practices that works in full synergy with the health-promoting possibilities of connected communities [19].

SUGGESTIONS FOR PRACTICE

- *The summary guide is the key tool that will help you (and partners) think through what is needed locally.*
- *Your CCG should have a lead officer, identified by NHSE, who will be looking to work with primary care networks (PCNs), local authorities and the voluntary sector in your area. They will be seeking to help PCNs deliver your local allocation of the 1,000 new additional social prescribing link workers being funded through the long term plan. You can find that list via the NHSE SP platform [20].*
- *The best way to ensure your patients have access to existing or developing social prescribing (if they don't already) is to find the key contacts in the CCG, PCNs, local authorities and voluntary sector organisations to ensure that your patients are part of an integrated referral process which ensures access for those who need it most.*
- *You can find out about the regional networks which are facilitated by NHSE SP facilitators via the NHSE platform or the national social prescribing network website [21]. The regional facilitators will provide support in accessing best practice and help you network with practitioners*

and commissioners in the region (or nationally) who may have most in common with what you are locally trying to achieve.

REFERENCES

1. A very general practice: Citizens Advice policy briefing based on a CommRes Survey of 1,002 GPs in the UK, May2015
2. Low Commission Report, 2014
3. The Social Determinants of Health, The Facts, WHO, 2003
4. Health foundation Infographics www.health.org.uk/infographic/what-makes-us-healthy
5. *Still in the red: update on debt and mental health*, MIND, 2011: www.mind.org.uk/media/273468/still-in-the-red.pdf
6. www.england.nhs.uk/wp-content/uploads/2019/01/social-prescribing-community-based-support-summary-guide.pdf
7. www.england.nhs.uk/long-term-plan/
8. westminsterresearch.westminster.ac.uk/item/q1v77/making-sense-of-social-prescribing
9. www.bbbc.org.uk/wp-content/uploads/2018/06/Unleashing-Healthy-Communities_Summary-Report_Researching-the-Bromley-by-Bow-model.pdf
10. www.hyms.ac.uk/about/news/2017/hull-york-medical-school-research-helps-drive-innovation-in-diabetes-treatment
11. www.campaigntoendloneliness.org/
12. www.gov.uk/government/news/pm-launches-governments-first-loneliness-strategy
13. A review of the evidence assessing impact of social prescribing to healthcare demand and cost implications (2017) Polley, M. et al. www.socialprescribingnetwork.com/resources
14. www4.shu.ac.uk/research/cresr/ourexpertise/evaluation-rotherham-social-prescribing-pilot
15. Workshop notes, EoE regional conference workshop November 2017
16. Westminster University, January 2016 – national social prescribing website
17. See NHSE Sample Job Description https://www.england.nhs.uk/publication/social-prescribing-and-community-based-support-summary-guide/
18. www.altogetherbetter.org.uk/
19. https://collegeofmedicine.org.uk/national-prescribing-student-champion-scheme/
20. To join the platform, please contact england.socialprescribing@nhs.net
21. www.socialprescribingnetwork.com/

14

Why Do People Not Engage With Healthcare?

AUSTIN O'CARROLL

It is impossible to provide quality care if people cannot access that care.

We know people in areas of deprivation have extremely poor health indices and reduced lifespans when compared to their wealthier counterparts, and despite the obvious need these communities have poorer access to primary and secondary health services, so affirming Tudor Hart's highly predictive law that the provision of services is inversely proportional to the need for such services [1–16]. We know those on the margins of deprivation (people who are homeless, migrants, using drugs, from the travelling community and more) experience even worse health and have even less access to healthcare [17–22]. Access has been recognized as a key indicator of quality service – it is impossible to provide quality care if people cannot access that care [23, 24]. We know that inaccessible primary care results in increased hospitalization for people in areas of deprivation [25].

A number of models exist to identify the factors that influence access [26–28]. Here we are using a model developed from research by the author into barriers faced by homeless people when accessing health services. This model is preferred as it focuses on barriers which allows individual service providers examine their own service for potential

barriers. It adopts Levesque's journey from when health need emerges to when the patient accesses the healthcare they require. Hannay's symptom iceberg, which has been floating round since 1979, identified that the vast majority of symptoms experienced by patients do not actually end up being proffered to a health professional but are dealt with by either ignoring the symptom, self-treating or obtaining management advice from family, friends or (in the modern era) the Internet. The potential patient will decide that some of these symptoms require the attention of a healthcare professional. They then need to access a primary care provider. Depending on the seriousness of the medical condition underlying the symptom, they will require either multiple attendances or referral to other primary or secondary care professionals.

Not all journeys are initiated by the patient. As health systems seek to improve population health through preventative medical interventions, there are a growing number of interactions where the health professional initiates the consultation through invitation either by leaflet, poster, in person, by letter, telephone or e-mail. Along this continuum lurk a series of potential barriers. It is through understanding the range and nature of these barriers that we can identify why people from deprived areas or marginalized communities have such poor access to healthcare. Different barriers take effect at particular stages of the medical journey (Figure 14.1).

doctor either through the effects of the illness on their reasoning or due to fear of health professionals deriving from their experiences of prior treatment.

PSYCHOLOGICAL INFLUENCES

Psychological influences are usually personal ways of dealing with medical symptoms that deter an individual from accessing healthcare. Some of these are individual idiosyncratic thoughts/feelings, while others derive from their familial/friendship/cultural background. An individual may value stoicism and tolerate symptoms that indicate a treatable medical condition rather than go to the doctor. This stoicism may relate to their age [29, 30]; their familial background beliefs [31]; their sense of gender identity (men being less likely to consult) [32]; their work colleagues (e.g. doctors tend to avoid attending health professionals); or their cultural background. Mental illness is a particular individual affliction which can act as a barrier to individuals attending a

INTERNALIZED BARRIERS

Internalized barriers are thoughts or feelings that have been internalized from one's interaction with society at large. Thus, a patient who uses drugs may face stigmatizing attitudes when they attend a health service and this may make it difficult for them to access that surgery. If, as a result of that experience, they internalize any of the following cognitions or emotions, those same thoughts and feelings may effectively prevent them from attending that same or similar services:

- I will face similar prejudice if I attend.
- I will not receive appropriate and quality treatment if I attend.
- Attending that health service makes me uncontrollably angry or depressed.

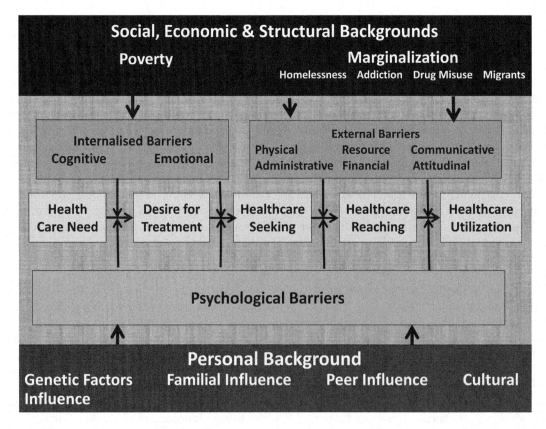

Figure 14.1 Barriers to accessing healthcare.

- They do not like me as I use drugs so it is my own fault and I should not bother them further.

Internalized barriers are probably the most effective barrier as the person does not even turn up to obtain a service. There are a range of internalized barriers that have been identified in the literature (Figure 14.2). Many of these apply particularly to certain marginalized groups (e.g. homeless, drug users, ethnic minorities and more).

- The fatalistic cognition deters usage of health services as, if one is going to die young why try to prevent it: 'I don't care about me life…I can see death, in me… And it is going to happen someday. I think it's going to be very soon…I didn't expect to live very long either'.
- Denial similarly interferes with patients making healthy decisions: 'It's way pushed at the back of me head. I will not let that fuckin' disease beat me. I do think about it too and I do say "stop thinking about it. Don't let this take over"'.

EXTERNAL BARRIERS

External barriers are elements that either prevent or significantly deter patients from attending health services; these are often disproportionately experienced by certain social groups (e.g. those from marginalized or deprived backgrounds). Such barriers can be best understood through analysis under the subheadings of physical, communication, resource, administrative and attitudinal barriers.

PHYSICAL BARRIERS

Universal design ensures that a building and its services are accessible to everyone. Any structure that impedes access to a person with a disability has created a physical barrier e.g. steps, lack of accessible toilet facilities, dangerous premises for people who are blind etc. Geographic barriers are also created by distance from a surgery. Such barriers will disproportionally affect those with low mobility and poor access to private or public transport (e.g. older infirm people on social welfare; homeless people).

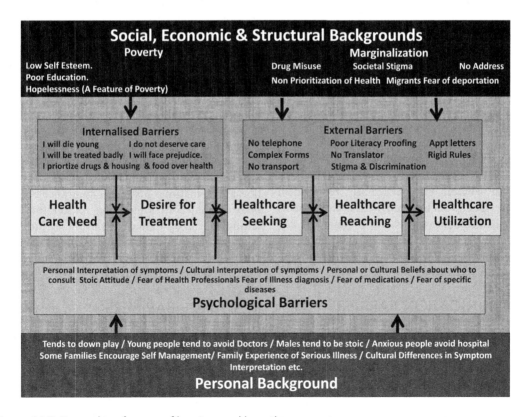

Figure 14.2 Examples of range of barriers and how they operate.

ADMINISTRATIVE BARRIERS

Administrative barriers are those administrative processes that interfere with patients obtaining access to their doctor. Many of these are faced by all people (e.g. filling in an application form for the right to free primary care). However, they act as particular barriers for those who are uncomfortable with such processes due to poor literacy, language or intellectual difficulties or who have competing priorities (e.g. homeless people or drug misusers). 'And as well, I should have [registered], which is my responsibility to have, but…. it was just…how to go about [doing it] and I didn't know what to do because…I didn't know [how to fill in the forms]'.

Health service providers often know that these administrative processes result in certain groups (e.g. homeless people) not being able to exercise their right to free healthcare, but do not take action (e.g. homeless people continue to be sent hospital appointments by letter when they are unlikely to receive them).

Rules of service usage are a particularly thorny administrative barrier especially when dealing with patients who have challenging behaviours. Rigid rule systems (e.g. removing people from a service's lists as they have missed appointments etc.) and barring policies will often result in excluding some of the unhealthiest people from our practices. As one homeless patient who was barred for using drugs on the premises noted, 'I'm a drug addict for f**k's sake'.

FINANCIAL BARRIERS

Financial barriers are particularly relevant in countries that do not have universal health systems e.g. the United States or Ireland. They are also relevant in the UK where access to a private health system can improve access to diagnostic and secondary care treatment.

COMMUNICATION BARRIERS

Communication barriers arise when the patient has a difficulty communicating with the health service. This occurs with ethnic minorities and migrants who have a need for interpreters and translated health documents/signage. It is also an issue for people with disabilities with communicative issues such as deaf/blind people, people with voice impairments, dyslexia and patients with learning difficulties. Illiteracy (which affects predominantly those from areas of deprivation and marginalized groups) not only interferes with understanding signage or information leaflets but can also make the language of health professionals impossible to understand. Lastly, discomfort with technology (including the phone) can interfere with access. Many older people are not comfortable making appointments over the phone or downloading and filling in application forms from the Internet. Sending appointments by post is useless for homeless people or those who change address often due to insecure housing. Patients also report not opening medical post in fear of what news they might be receiving [1].

ATTITUDINAL BARRIERS

Attitudinal barriers exist where health professionals and/or their staff hold prejudicial attitudes towards potential patients that results in those patients either feeling uncomfortable or experiencing actual discrimination. It is well established that drug users, homeless people and ethnic minorities/migrants can experience discrimination when seeking to access care. 'They told me in the A&E that they couldn't take me in because I was a drug addict and I made my own choices'. As one drug user eloquently summarized, 'I think that we generalize too much towards each other as addicts and as doctors. There's too much - you've done this to yourself… And as regards the drug thing, a lot of addicts get into it ridiculously young, there's a lack of education and sometimes just plain ignorance because there's usually an underlying reason for them taking that drug. Usually to avoid or hide bad memories from their lives or childhood or whatnot, because usually there are broken homes or socio-economic things involved'.

RESOURCE BARRIERS

A critical issue is that even if patients have full access to local healthcare facilities, those facilities may not have the necessary resources to meet demand. We know that areas of deprivation and marginalized groups in particular have significantly higher health needs yet they are not automatically allocated extra resources to meet these needs. The reality on the ground is that many of the positions for health professionals are not filled, and thus augments the existing inequity.

The full range of barriers faced by patients in areas of deprivation is exhaustive. These barriers are further augmented for members of marginalized groups. All these groups face significantly worse attitudinal barriers. Many of them (in particular homeless people and drug users) exist in chaotic and uncertain circumstances that amplify administrative barriers. Language difficulties and illiteracy also add to the disenfranchisement of these groups.

HOW DOES ONE REDUCE THE BARRIERS FOR ALL PATIENTS?

The best method to address barriers is to adopt an ethos consistent with a low-threshold and high-fidelity service. It should be noted, however, that many of the causes of poor access (in particular structural barriers) are outside the control of individual practices [33–39].

Low-threshold services recognize that barriers are always present and it is not a case of removing barriers but rather of minimizing them to as low a barrier as possible and maintaining alertness that the barriers do not propagate due to inattention. This requires vigilance from all staff members.

SUGGESTIONS FOR PRACTICE

There are several ways to break down the barriers.

Physical Barriers

- *Physical barriers require the implementation of universal design. Geographic barriers may need to be addressed though a house call or advocating for public transport in the area. Reducing walking distances also improves geographic accessibility [40, 41].*

Administrative Barriers

- *All administrative processes should be constantly reviewed to ensure they have minimum questions; are easily understood and are translated into languages common in the surgery.*

- *Where complex administrative forms are required, staff should make themselves available to help patients fill them in (while respecting patient confidentiality). Appointment systems may need to be made more flexible with available drop in or 'emergency' slots protected [42].*
- *Affording extra time to patients in areas of deprivation where the complex interaction of psychological, clinical and social issues need focus to untangle has also improved patients' willingness to attend.*

Communicative Barriers

- *Availability of information in common languages and the presence of interpreting services can help break down these barriers.*
- *Provide literacy proofed materials.*
- *Invest in communication skills training for professionals and staff.*
- *Provide loop systems for deaf people and Braille for blind people.*

Attitudinal Barriers

- *Develop an open and accepting culture in the practice. The simple display of non-judgemental and respectful behaviours has been shown to improve access [42].*
- *Adopting a clear written value document that is constantly referred to (and not merely sitting on a computer) is particularly important.*
- *Addressing attitudes may require disability or cultural awareness training.*

Resource Allocation Barriers

- *Although a health systems issue, individual practices can advocate to ensure maximum resources are both assigned and delivered to their practice.*

Internalized Barriers

- *First the factors in a practice that created such issues (e.g. prejudicial attitudes of staff, excessive administrative barriers etc.) need to be rectified [43].*
- *The provision of a truly quality service will help develop a reputation for accessibility.*

- *Practices need to reach out from the practice. Reaching out may include the advertising of the service as being friendly and accessible; the development of a local reputation for openness; and/or a whole practice involvement in engagement of patients into care [44, 45].*
  - *Hope Citadel Healthcare achieved phenomenal rates of cervical screening for a practice in an area of high deprivation (in the top 4% of UK practices) through whole practice enthusiastic recruitment of patients. Developing a name for advocating on behalf of marginalized patients also helps improve access.*
- *Some marginalized groups, such as the homeless, have very poor access to GP care due to the range and potency of the barriers they encounter. Overcoming barriers for these groups may require the development of an outreach service to homeless services. This may be particularly so in urban areas with large numbers of homeless people.*

High-fidelity services seek to maintain relationships with patients to maximize the possibility of continuity of care. The maintenance of relationships with all patients will be achieved by the quality of care and communication as well as ease of use of administrative processes of the practice. However, how the practice addresses challenging behaviours will also play a part. Many patients from dysfunctional backgrounds find rigid rules difficult and tend to assert themselves in manners that cause fear for staff and can create dangerous situations. Learning the skills to manage challenging behaviours can prevent such behaviours escalating to the point where barring becomes inevitable. Furthermore, practices can arrange to temporarily bar a patient from one practice and put them on probation for a period of time at a partner practice. This ensures such patients, who often face significant poor health, do not lose access to health advice and care.

Access is a key component of quality. The creation of a beautiful shiny new practice that is inaccessible for many potential patients means one has developed a low-quality service. If we truly wish to address accessibility we need to understand the complex dynamics of the barriers that prevent our patients obtaining the care they need and deserve.

REFERENCES

1. Jani B, Bikker AP, Higgins M, Fitzpatrick B, Watt G, Mercer S. Patient centredness and the outcome of primary care consultations with patients with depression in areas of high and low socioeconomic deprivation. *Br J Gen Pract.* 2012; 62(601):e576–e581.
2. Macintyre S. *Inequalities in Health in Scotland: What Are They and What Can We Do About Them?* Occasional Paper No. 17. Glasgow, UK: MRC Social & Public Health Sciences Unit; 2007.
3. Barnett K, Mercer SW, Norbury M, Watt G, Wyke S, Guthrie B. Epidemiology of multimorbidity and implications for health care, research, and medical education: A cross-sectional study. *Lancet.* 2012;380(9836):37–43.
4. Marmot M. *Fair Society, Healthy Lives. Strategic Review of Health Inequalities.* London: HMSO Publications; 2010.
5. Goodwin N, Dixon A, Poole T, Raleigh V. *Improving the Quality of Care in General Practice.* London: The King's Fund; 2011.
6. Mackenbach J, Van De Mheen H, Stronks K. A prospective cohort study investigating the explanation of socio-economic inequalities in health in the Netherlands. *Soc Sci Med.* 1994; 38: 299–308.
7. Power C, Matthews S. Origins of health inequalities in a national population sample. *Lancet.* 1997; 350: 1584–1589.
8. Mercer SW, Watt GC. The inverse care law: Clinical primary care encounters in deprived and affluent areas of Scotland. *Ann Fam Med.* 2007; 5(6): 503–510.
9. NHS England. Urgent and Emergency Care Review - Evidence Based Engagement Document. 2013.
10. Simeons S, Hurst J. The Supply of Physician Services in OECD Countries OECD Health Working Papers No 21. 2006 France.
11. Benzeval M, Judge K, Whitehead M. *Tackling Inequalities in Health.* London: King's Fund; 1995.
12. Van de Mheen H, Stronks K, Looman CWN, Mackenbach JP. Does childhood socioeconomic status influence adult health through behavioural factors? *Int J Epidemiol.* 1998; 27: 431–437.

13. Lundberg O. The impact of childhood living conditions on illness and mortality in adulthood. *Soc Sci Med.* 1993; 36: 1047–1052.

14. Sturm R, Gresenz CR. Relations of income inequalities and family income to chronic medical conditions and mental health disorders: National survey. *Br Med J.* 2002; 324: 1–5.

15. Field K, Cart FB, Briggs J. Socio-economic and locational determinants of accessibility and utilization of primary healthcare. *Health Soc Care Community.* 2001; 9: 294–308.

16. Alter DA, Naylor CD, Austin P, Tu JV. Effects of socioeconomic status on access to invasive cardiac procedures and on mortality after acute myocardial infarction. *N Engl J Med.* 1999; 341: 1359–1367.

17. O'Carroll A, O'Reilly F. Health of the homeless in Dublin: Has anything changed in the context of Ireland's economic boom? *European Journal of Public Health.* 2008; 18(5): 448–453. doi: 10.1093/eurpub/ckn038. Epub 2008 Jun 25.

18. O'Reilly F, Barror S, Hannigan A, Scriver S, Ruane L, McFarlane A, O'Carroll A. *Homelessness: An Unhealthy State. Health Status, Risk Behaviours and Service Utilisation among Homeless People in Two Irish Cities.* Dublin: The Partnership for Health Equality; 2015.

19. All Ireland Traveller Health Study Team; School of Public Health, Physiotherapy and Population Science, University College Dublin. *All-Ireland Traveller Health Study Summary of Findings.* Dublin: Department of Health and Children; 2010.

20. Baggett TP, O'Connell JJ, Singer DE, Rigotti NA. The unmet health care needs of homeless adults: A national study. *Am J Public Health.* 2010; 100(7): 1326–1333. doi: 10.2105/AJPH.2009.180109. Epub 2010 May 13.

21. Lebrun-Harris LA, Baggett TP, Jenkins DM, Sripipatana A, Sharma R, Hayashi AS, Daly CA, Ngo-Metzger Q Health status and health care experiences among homeless patients in federally supported health centers: Findings from the 2009 patient survey. *Health Services Research.* 2013; 48(3): 992–1017. doi: 10.1111/1475-6773.12009. Epub 2012 Nov 7.

22. Ware J, Mawby R. *Patient Access to General Practice: Ideas and Challenges from the Front Line.* London: Royal College of General Practitioners; 2015.

23. Shengelia B, Murray CJL, Adams OB. Beyond access and utilization: Defining and measuring health system coverage. In *Health Systems Performance Assessment. Debates, Methods and Empiricism.* Edited by Murray CJL, Evans DB. Geneva: World Health Organization; 2003:221–234.

24. Levesque JF, Harris MF, Russell G. Patient-centred access to health care: Conceptualising access at the interface of health systems and populations. *Int J Equity Health.* 2013; 12: 18. http://www.equity-healthj.com/content/12/1/18

25. Erny-Albrecht K, Bywood P. Expert Plus. *Barriers to primary health care access—an update.* PHCRIS Adelaide: Primary Health Care Research & Information Service; 2016.

26. Penchansky R, Thomas WJ. The concept of access: Definition and relationship to consumer satisfaction. *Med Care.* 1981; 19: 127–140.

27. Gelberg L, Andersen RM, Leake BD. The behavioral model for vulnerable populations: Application to Medical Care use and outcomes for homeless people. *Health Serv Res.* 2000; 34(6): 1273–1302.

28. Levesque JF, Harris MF, Russell G. Patient-centred access to health care: Conceptualising access at the interface of health systems and populations. *Int J Equity Health.* 2013; 12: 18. http://www.equity-healthj.com/content/12/1/18

29. D'Avolio D, NE Strumpf, Feldman J, Mitchell P, Rebholz C. Barriers to primary care: Perceptions of older adults utilizing the ED for nonurgent visits. *Clin Nurs Res.* 2013; 22. 10.1177/1054773813485597

30. Campbell SM, Roland MO. Why do people consult the doctor? *Fam Pract.* 1996;13(1):75–83.

31. Dowrick C. Why do the O'Sheas consult so often? An exploration of complex family illness behaviour. *Soc Sci Med.* 1992;34(5):491–497.

32. O'Brien R, Hunt K, Hart G. 'It's caveman stuff, but that is to a certain extent how guys still operate': Men's accounts of masculinity and help seeking. *Soc Sci Med.* 2005;61(3):503–516.

33. O'Donnell P, Tierney E, A O'Carroll, Nurse D, MacFarlane A. Exploring levers and barriers to accessing primary care for marginalised groups and identifying their priorities for primary care provision: A participatory learning and action research study. *Int J Equity Health.* 2016; 15: 197.

34. Van Cleemput P, Parry G, Thomas K, Peters J, Cooper C. Health-related beliefs and experiences of Gypsies and Travellers: A qualitative study. *J Epidemiol Commun Health.* 2007;61(3):205–210.

35. Greenfields M, Brindley M. Impact of insecure accommodation and the living environment on Gypsies' and Travellers' health. Traveller Movement & Bucks New University. 2016. https://www.gov.uk/government/uploads/system/uploads/attachment_data/file/490846/

36. Schanzer B, Dominguez B, Shrout PE, Caton CLM. Homelessness, health status, and health care use. *Am J Publ Health.* 2007; 97(3): 464–469.

37. Noël L, Fischer B, Tyndall MW, Bradet DR, Rehm J, Brissette S et al. Health and social services accessed by a cohort of Canadian illicit opioid users outside of treatment. *Canadian Journal of Public Health.* 2006; 97(3): 166–170.

38. *Barriers and Facilitating Factors in Access to Health Services in the Republic of Moldova.* Copenhagen: WHO Regional Office for Europe; 2012.

39. Dahlgren G, Whitehead M. European strategies for tackling social inequities in health – Levelling up Part 2. WHO Regional Office for Europe. 2006. http://www.euro.who.int/__data/assets/pdf_file/0018/103824/E89384.pdf. Accessed 10 Nov 2015.

40. Adams J, White M. Socio-economic deprivation is associated with increased proximity to general practices in England: An ecological analysis. *J Public Health.* 2005;27:80–81.

41. Pearce J, Witten K, Hiscock R et al. Are socially disadvantaged neighbourhoods deprived of health-related community resources? *Int J Epidemiol.* 2007; 36: 348–355.

42. SE LHIN. Understanding Health Inequities and Access to Primary Health Care in Southeastern Ontario. 2015.

43. Stewart M, Reutter L, Makwarimba E, Rootman I, Williamson D, Raine K,Wilson D, Fast J, Love R, McFall S, Shorten D, Letourneau N, Hayward K, Masuda J, Rutakumwa W. Determinants of health-service use by low-income people. *CJNR.* 2005; 37(3): 104–131.

44. Atterbury J. Fair Access for All? Gypsies and Travellers in Sussex, GP Surgeries and Barriers to Primary Healthcare. 2010 FFT http://www.gypsy-traveller.org/pdfs/fair_access_health.pdf Accessed 3rd March 2018.

45. Ross LE, Vigod S, Wishart J, Waese M, Spence JD, Oliver J, Chambers J, Anderson S, Shields R. Barriers and facilitators to primary care for people with mental health and/or substance use issues: A qualitative study. *BMC Fam Pract.* 2015; 16: 135.

15

Managing Difficult Conversations

HELEN BARCLAY

This healthcare culture is alienating and non-intuitive.

Primary care involves managing people as well as managing disease; clinicians are experts in communication and most clinicians derive enormous satisfaction from enabling their patients to live healthier lives.

But there are some conversations that even clinicians struggle with. Perhaps the patient does not listen to your advice, they don't understand the way the health system works, they miss appointments, they present frequently in crisis but refuse help, they don't seem to respond to questioning as expected. They may be labelled a 'vague historian' (giving a poor account of their medical past), be aggressive or agitated, not attend hospital appointments, have unrealistic expectations, have safeguarding issues, have addiction, mental health problems, personality disorder, traumatic histories– the list of difficult conversations is potentially unlimited.

There are entire books dedicated to managing each type of difficult conversation, from consultation models to psychological techniques, and it is beyond the scope of this chapter to address all of them or provide a definitive guide. Additionally, each clinician will find their own unique style that works for them – simply showing some of your personality, letting the patient see that you are

human and are responding as a person as well as a doctor, can have a positive impact on the dynamic of a difficult consultation.

Figure 15.1 gives an idea of the types of consultation that can be difficult – but it is not exhaustive. Note that most of these consultations require addressing multiple factors. Additionally, patients who attend with difficult problems and non-compliant attitudes often have a history of trauma, which might affect their ability to engage with services that try to help them [1]. These situations can disrupt our surgeries, health outcomes tend to be worse despite high use of resources, and they can be a source of considerable stress and burnout in healthcare staff.

Despite the difficulties, it really must be emphasised these can be some of the most rewarding patients to work with when things go well – but it might require a shift in gear, a more considered approach, or a long-term strategy rather than relying on a single conversation.

THE CULTURE OF HEALTHCARE

Humans are social beings and we naturally respond to others within a cultural framework, helping us to navigate social interactions and

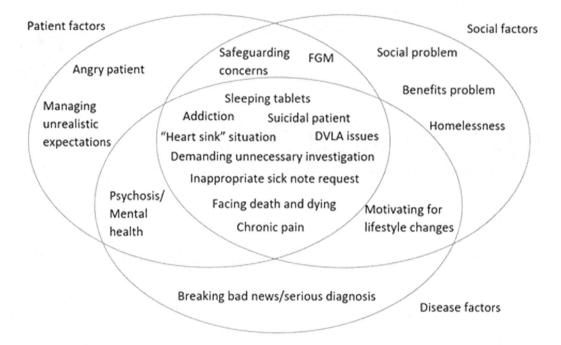

Figure 15.1 Examples of difficult conversations with underlying factors.

the surrounding environment [2, 3]. A familiar or shared culture makes communication easy when all participants understand it. But it makes things harder when you are acting in a culture that is not your own [4]. A process of acculturation can take place over time [2], but patients would need to engage with the service during this time to enable this to happen.

Consider the steps required for a straightforward clinician appointment. They include (but are not limited to):

- Recognising that there is a problem.
- Recognising that a clinician could help with it.
- Being registered with a clinician and knowing how to book an appointment.
- Calling/arriving at the designated time to book an appointment.
- Attending at the designated time and booking in.
- Navigating the waiting room (sometimes there is a lengthy wait which may be intimidating).
- Spending 10 minutes with a clinician and explaining the problem, feeling listened to, finding out what is wrong and how to fix it.

- Remembering the content of the consultation and the plan.
- Picking up the script from the pharmacy and potentially arranging repeat scripts.
- Making and keeping any necessary lifestyle changes.
- Repeating the above steps as necessary, until the problem is resolved.

Most people navigate all these steps seamlessly, because they understand the culture of our healthcare system and how to interact with it. They know that they must prepare what they need to say in advance, and roughly what sort of treatment they might expect. They have a general awareness of how the NHS works and understand that they are one patient of many, and that the clinician will try their best to help them within the timeframe offered, but that they must also take some responsibility for looking after their own health – a form of social contract between the patient and clinician [5].

For some people, however, this healthcare culture is alienating and non-intuitive [6] and patients are not empowered to manage their health or seek help [4, 7]. A frequently noted response to multiple deprivations is low expectations for one's future health [8] and it is a clinician's role to challenge and help patients to change this. Some of the most important medicine that clinicians provide may not involve medications or specific treatments, but rather involves listening to patients and helping to change habits or health attitudes – conversations rather than lectures.

Patients who are from disadvantaged groups have more health problems and use health services less effectively than patients who are from more affluent groups [7]. It can be harder to communicate effectively due to different speaking styles, culture, or health literacy [9]. Health beliefs vary widely between groups and equally between individuals, and it's important to use the tools we have learned to explore these and to build health literacy [9]. This may take multiple consultations and need tailoring to individual ability [10].

People who have undergone multiple traumas are often living in a perpetual state of high alert; in unwelcoming environs (and when worried about their health enough to come see a doctor) their pre-existing stress levels can escalate to a point where they cannot function normally. Rather than focus on the outcome of the medical consultation, we first must consider how we can help the patient relax. The importance of building trust cannot be understated [11]. To encourage engagement in people like this with our services, we must be prepared to meet them partway across the cultural divide.

BARRIERS TO AN EFFECTIVE CONVERSATION

Barriers to communication come in many forms. They might include:

- Cultural divides (In both UK patients and new arrivals).
- Language (both in English-speaking and non-English-speaking patients).
- Intimidation.
- Shame.
- Addiction.
- Multiple forms of social exclusion.

- Fear of rejection.
- Fear of illness.
- Difficulty with accessing appointment.
- Fear of deportation.
- Mental illness.

One way of overcoming these barriers is to consider what we can do *before* we get patients into the consultation room to improve their ability to engage comfortably with our services. This might include efforts to improve access arrangements, build trust, reduce fear of coming to the clinician, provide support with appointments and follow-up arrangements, outreach medicine and help to manage expectations to enable a constructive relationship with their healthcare team [12].

Sometimes, difficult conversations can be anticipated and planned for. It may be useful to plan in extra time or flexibility e.g. a double appointment or using the last slot in a session. Some surgeries even plan for a few longer appointments each week, to enable deeper conversations without interruption [7].

Another very useful strategy is making clinician surgeries into 'psychologically informed environments' (PIEs) [13].

PSYCHOLOGICALLY INFORMED ENVIRONMENTS

This concept from a primary care perspective means all practice staff are encouraged to consider, from a psychological angle, how patients perceive the environment in the surgery, and how they can best enable patients to accept help and think about their own health [6, 14]. All patients who see the clinician have come through the waiting room first – it is an important part of their experience.

There is no box-ticking exercise for this.

The definitive marker of a PIE is simply that, if asked why the unit is run in such and such a way, the staff would give an answer in terms of the emotional and psychological needs of service users, rather than giving some more logistical or practical rationale [13].

LEARNING EXERCISE

Have you spent time in the public areas of your surgery recently? What features might make it a psychologically informed environment? What could be improved? What impact do you think this would have on the patients when they are upset, worried or angry?

Calming an Agitated Patient

When someone is standing, pacing, shouting or otherwise demonstrating their agitation physically, they are not in a state where they can respond to verbal information [11]. Sometimes, the only safe response is to call for police assistance, but if you feel safe enough and there is an opportunity, there are some techniques which might help get a patient to the point where you can help them.

John Conolly, a London-based counsellor who leads a counselling service for the homeless, suggested a 6-step assertion process to help in this situation in his speech at the Pathways from Homelessness conference 2019 [11]:

SUGGESTIONS FOR PRACTICE

- *Using non-verbal communication whilst delivering an assertive message (e.g. 'please sit down so that we can talk'). Maintaining a gentle voice, repeating reassuring phrases, open body language and a calm facial expression will do far better than anything else you can say. This might take some time.*
- *Allowing silence for the message to sink in.*
- *Restating the assertion whilst acknowledging the patient's agitation.*
- *Reflecting their feelings and the content of their speech e.g. 'I know you feel annoyed but when you pace, I find it hard to concentrate – please sit down so that we can talk'. Avoid being sidetracked into an argument but use empathy, attention and respect to help the patient trust you and feel that you are listening.*
- *Repeat the cycle until the patient calms down – it is likely to take 3–4 cycles. Some doctors might stop at 2 cycles which is usually ineffective.*
- *Focus on a solution, paraphrase it several times. Finally, it is important to thank the person for calming down and, if indicated, apologise on behalf of the service.*

The patient is likely to try and bait you into an argument, but it is essential you aren't distracted by this. They may blame you for their problems and the verbal attacks can seem quite personal. It is important to remember this is an unconscious behaviour, blame is a part of the high conflict cycle of thinking – it is their long-term problem and it is not personal [11].

Once they are calmer, you can try to look at the available options and work out how to proceed.

The Dysfunctional Consultation – 'We are Getting Nowhere'

Early in a consultation, it is often obvious if the patient and doctor are going to disagree. Once this becomes clear, the doctor's demeanour can unconsciously change, the patient will notice, and they feel they are not being listened to. The consultation becomes dysfunctional; the patient will continue to express their needs repeatedly and will not listen to the doctor until they themselves feel they have been heard. This scenario will resonate with many clinicians. These consultations can be very dissatisfying.

During a busy surgery, the doctor's mind will inevitably search for a way to get a speedy conclusion, and to explain to the patient how they need to move forward. But to the patient, their overriding priority is usually simply to be heard. For this reason, it is essential to show the patient you are listening, show compassion and empathise with their difficult situation. Without this key step, the conversation will remain dysfunctional.

It is undoubtedly challenging to deal with disagreement in a 10-minute consultation. It is a normal human response to be affected by the patient's state of mind – they may be unconsciously (or consciously) drawing you into a conflict, pushing your buttons to get a response [5]. Sometimes, that patient may have learned this behaviour as a way of not being ignored, and of having their needs met. It might have started in childhood in people who have had unreliable or inappropriate caregivers [11, 12] or may have been learned later in life through unfortunate circumstance.

When faced with disagreement or a patient's burning issue that you know will result in disagreement, remember that they need to feel that you are listening to them – using empathy, attention and respect can dismantle their barriers [15], being interested in what they are thinking and why.

If there is one issue that they keep coming back to confront this directly and early on (a classic example would be a request for sleeping tablets). Explain that you have heard their concern and will address this issue, but first need to find out more details about the problem. Handled well, the doctor can take a step back and avoid getting embroiled in the demands of the patient, remain calm and through this, can calm the patient down too.

Once the patient accepts that you are listening to them, and want to help them, a huge hurdle is overcome and agreeing on a way forward becomes possible.

The next step is analysing the problem with the patient and starting to consider possible ways forward. At this stage, you are still likely to be in disagreement with the patient, but with a foundation of trust you can start to unpick their health beliefs or their expectations for the consultation – it is important not to just dismiss them as this may well result in a significant backwards step. Trust and mutual respect are essential to coming to a shared management plan.

The patient may have some quite unrealistic expectations and it will be necessary to set limits on what you can achieve, and probably to apply some boundaries. This might involve negotiating trial periods with medications, writing symptom diaries or signposting to other services so you can focus on the medical issues, and the patient can receive help in other areas from a more appropriate provider.

Trauma-informed Care

Many patients with intractable symptoms, or frequent attenders, have a history of trauma relating to the physical symptoms they are experiencing. This can be true for almost any condition, from heart disease, obesity, diabetes and hypertension, right through to more obviously trauma-linked conditions like depression, sexual dysfunction or chronic pain. Although they may be requesting physical treatments and investigations, treating the underlying post-traumatic symptoms could have a much greater likelihood of success [16]. However, it takes a considered and careful conversation to elicit the possibility of underlying trauma, and clinician training in the UK does not routinely include modules on trauma-informed care. Clinicians are best placed in the health service to provide this continuity, and there is evidence that providing clinicians with education in trauma-based care improves outcomes for patients [17]. For those working in areas of higher socioeconomic deprivation, considering further training in this area could be worthwhile.

Minimising Detrimental Effects on Yourself as a Clinician

Difficult conversations can have a profound effect on the professional, not only the patient. When your communication skills are tested, and if you do not get to the outcome you had hoped for, it is disheartening.

When a person makes you feel frustrated, or angry, or upset, it can be helpful to realise that often the feelings you are having reflect the patient's own state of mind – a case of transference and counter-transference. This should be recognised.

SUGGESTIONS FOR PRACTICE

- *Reflecting and responding appropriately, speaking to colleagues and ensuring you can take a step back can make managing patients that are difficult to consult with much less likely to result in burnout [6, 18].*
- *Participation in a Balint group has been found to be particularly effective for this [19].*

It is normal to find some conversations challenging, but clinicians should not underestimate their expertise in getting through to patients experiencing complex difficulties.

CASE STUDY

A Message of Hope

A clinician colleague saw a very vulnerable patient in an outreach clinic with many serious unmet health needs. The patient was not registered with a clinician practice. After a long and difficult conversation, the patient started shouting and left. The clinician was left upset, feeling that she had not done a good job that day. Over a year later, the patient saw the clinician again in passing whilst in the surgery, waiting to see a different doctor. She called the clinician over and thanked her for that outreach consultation – she felt the clinician had listened to her, and even thought she couldn't remember the content of the consultation it had left a positive impression and was the catalyst for her registering with a clinician and starting to address some of her problems.

This example should serve as a message of hope for clinicians on those days when difficult conversations remain difficult, despite our best efforts. We may not be able to easily fix the issues, but by putting some thought into our communication, and treating patients as individuals and listening to their concerns, clinicians have huge potential to improve health outcomes.

REFERENCES

1. Raja S, Hasnain, M, Hoersch M, Gove-Yin S, Rajagopalan C (2015) Trauma informed care in medicine. *Family and Community Health* 38(3):216–226 (11).
2. Samovar L (2017) The challenges of intercultural communication: Managing differences. Chapter 11 from *Communication Between Cultures*.
3. Burley A (2017) Choking up-Relationships, Multiple Exclusion Homelessness and Psychologically-Informed Environments. *Homeless in Europe, Trauma and Homelessness*, pp. 8–10.
4. Joyce M (2007) Non-verbal communication, culture and consumption, Chapter 5 from *Key Themes in Interpersonal Communication*.
5. Hughes P, Kerr I (2000) Transference and countertransference in communication between doctor and patient. *Advances in Psychiatric Treatment*. 6(1):57–64. doi:10.1192/apt.6.1.57.
6. Johnson R (2017) Principles and practice in psychology and homelessness: Core skills in pretreatment, trauma informed care and psychologically informed environments. Chapter 3 from *Cross-cultural Dialogues on Homelessness: From Pretreatment Strategies to Psychologically Informed Environments*. Ann Arbor, MI: Loving Healing Press.
7. Mercer SW et al. (2016) The CARE Plus study – a whole-system intervention to improve quality of life of primary care patients with multimorbidity in areas of high socioeconomic deprivation: exploratory cluster randomised controlled trial and cost-utility analysis. *BMC Medicine*. 14:88.
8. Mcleod U, Gill P (2014) General practice, health inequalities and social exclusion, Chapter 1 from *Working with Vulnerable Groups*. Royal College of General Practitioners.
9. Coulter A (2011) Building health literacy, Chapter 3 from *Engaging Patients in Healthcare*. McGraw-Hill Open University Press.
10. Keller D, Sarkar U, Schillinger D (2014) Health literacy and information exchange in medical settings, Chapter 3 from the *Oxford Handbook of Health Communication, Behaviour Change and Treatment Adherence*.
11. Conolly J (2019) Trauma-Informed Communication Skills and Setting Limits – lecture at Pathways from Homelessness conference, March 2019 Video available at https://vimeo.com/325173923
12. Levy JS (2013) *Pretreatment Guide for Homeless Outreach and Housing First*. Loving Healing Press: Ann Arbor, Michigan.
13. Johnson R, Haigh R (2010) 'Social psychiatry and social policy for the 21st century – new concepts for new needs: The 'psychologically-informed environment. *Mental Health Soc Inclusion*. 14(4):30–35.
14. Breedvelt JF (2016) *Psychologically Informed Environments: A Literature Review*. Mental Health Foundation: London.
15. Eddy B, Calming Upset People Fast with EAR (2018) Jan 02 [cited 01/05/2019] In: Psychology Today. 5 types of people who can ruin your life [internet blog]. Sussex Publishers LLC. Available at: https://www.psychologytoday.com/us/blog/5-types-people-who-can-ruin-your-life/201801/calming-upset-people-fast-ear; Machtinger EL et al. (2015) From treatment to healing: The promise of trauma-informed primary care. *J Women's Health*. 25(3):193–197.
16. Machtinger EL et al. (2015) From treatment to healing: The promise of trauma-informed primary care. *J Women's Health*. 25(3):193–197. Green BL, Saunders PA, Power E et al.

(2015) Trauma-informed medical care: CME communication training for primary care providers. Fam Med. 47(1):7–14.

17. Green BL, Saunders PA, Power E et al. (2015) Trauma-informed medical care: CME communication training for primary care providers. Fam Med. 47(1):7–14; Moscrop A (2011) 'Heartsink' patients in general practice: a defining paper, its impact, and psychodynamic potential. Br J Gen Pract. 61 (586):346–348.

18. Moscrop A (2011) 'Heartsink' patients in general practice: A defining paper, its impact, and psychodynamic potential.

Br J Gen Pract. 2011;61(586):346–348; Kjeldmand D, Holmström I (2008) Balint groups as a means to increase job satisfaction and prevent burnout among general practitioners. *The Annals of Family Medicine.* 6(2):138–145.

19. Kjeldmand D, Holmström I (2008) Balint groups as a means to increase job satisfaction and prevent burnout among general practitioners. *The Annals of Family Medicine.* 6(2):138–145.

16

Motivational Interviewing

DOT MUNDT-LEACH

'It is possible to guide patients to their own decisions without imposing or suggesting anything yourself'.

Encouraging patients to make changes that may improve their health and quality of life can be a complex journey for everyone involved. One approach designed to make this process more effective is motivational interviewing (MI), an interpersonal style of facilitating change within individuals. It is based around the principle that behaviour change is elicited not through confrontation or the imposition of ideas, but through guided self-motivation [1]. Originally developed in the early 1980s in the United States as a treatment approach for alcohol dependency, the practice of MI has since spread across the globe and into a range of different fields, particularly those of health and social care [2].

THE ORIGINS OF MOTIVATIONAL INTERVIEWING

Motivational interviewing was first developed by William R. Miller in 1983 [1] as a one-to-one counselling style for alcohol dependency. MI challenged the conventional 'disease model' for alcohol addiction that suggested it results from a specific 'denial type' personality. Instead, Miller proposed, 'denial is not inherent in the alcoholic individual, but rather is the product of the way

in which counsellors have chosen to interact with problem drinkers'.

MI built on the social psychological principle that opposing someone's viewpoint by directly arguing with him or her is counteractive. This is because through direct argumentation with someone, you are likely to elicit from him or her the opposing argument. As a person verbally defends a position that you have argued against, he or she becomes more committed to that position.

MI is not based on any one theory but has its origins in a number of different social psychological models of behaviour. Miller and clinical psychologist Stephen Rollnick [3], who co-developed MI, stress that studying its theoretical basis is not essential to practising MI with someone. Instead, it should be understood as a method of communication which is learned over time.

Given the robust evidence base that links socioeconomic disadvantage, negative health behaviours and excess morbidity and mortality [4–7], an MI approach is well worth considering in practice. Research has shown that MI can produce significant clinical improvements amongst patients, regardless of who (doctor, nurse, psychologist, midwife, dietician) is providing the counselling, delivered in sessions as short as fifteen minutes [8]. Increased positive outcomes from adopting the MI approach, above traditional counselling styles, have been demonstrated in multiple fields, not limited to smoking cessation [9, 10], problem gambling [11], physical inactivity [12] and dental health [13]. There is also evidence that MI may be particularly effective for promoting healthy behaviour changes in low-income groups [12] and ethnic minorities [14].

THE ELEMENTS OF MOTIVATIONAL INTERVIEWING

The full MI approach can be broken down into two parts of four components. First is the consideration of the underlying 'spirit' of MI, and its four guiding principles. Second are the practical methods through which these concepts can be enacted: OARS, and change talk. Figure 16.1.

THE SPIRIT OF MOTIVATIONAL INTERVIEWING

- **Collaboration** (rather than confrontation). Instead of an unequal power dynamic in which the clinician directs the patient to make changes, patient and clinician should actively work together in a partnership that addresses the specific situation.

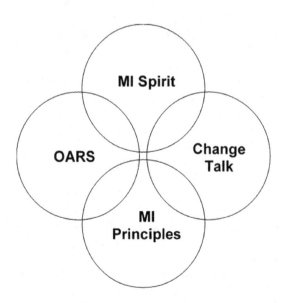

Figure 16.1 The elements of MI.

- **Evocation** (rather than imposing ideas). By eliciting patients' goals, concerns and pre-existing ideas, they will bring forward their own arguments for change. This is far more effective than didactically imparting clinical knowledge as a method of persuasion.
- **Autonomy** (rather than authority). A clinician must recognise that no matter their input, it is the patient who ultimately makes decisions about his or her own life. Mutual acknowledgement of this can be the key step in facilitating healthy behaviour change [15].

THE FOUR PRINCIPLES OF MI (RULE)

The guiding principles of MI can be remembered by the acronym 'RULE': Resist, Understand, Listen and Empower.

R: Resist the righting reflex. Rather than the clinician giving their own suggestions or corrections to problems, patients should be guided through their own ambivalence so that they produce their own reasons for change.

U: Understand your patient's motivations. In a time-limited consultation, asking a patient about their own reasons for making a change can be more useful than imposing your own.

L: Listen to your patient. In the MI approach, listening well is a key part of showing empathy, improving clinicians' understanding of their patients' concerns and improving rapport and trust.

E: Empower your patient. Engaging in the above steps with a patient, whilst actively engaging them in the decision-making process, helps to reinforce that it is they who are in control of their actions and must enact the changes they wish to make. [15, 16].

OARS

The acronym OARS is a way of remembering the collection of core micro-counselling skills through which MI can be adopted.

Open-ended questions: These encourage patients to elaborate on what they have said and explore their own motivations for change more deeply.

Affirmations: These statements recognise patients' successes and encourage them to overcome any setbacks or concerns they encounter throughout the process.

Reflections: Reflective listening is a way of presenting back to patients the points they have put across, in order to guide them to resolve ambivalence.

Summaries: Providing summaries gives patients a chance to review what thoughts they have expressed and explore the different sides of the argument they may have elicited [17].

CHANGE TALK

Throughout a consultation, a clinician can strategically listen for, elicit and respond to 'change talk', a type of speech which has shown to be correlated with behavioural change outcomes [3]. MI proposes that when considering a change, it is normal for a patient to foster ambivalence towards enacting it, understanding why it may be beneficial to them, whilst negating it with a 'but' statement. Change talk consists of statements patients make in a consultation which reveal consideration of, motivation for, or commitment to the move away from the 'cons' and towards the 'pros' of a change [15].

DARN-CAT is a mnemonic for describing the different types of change talk:

PREPARATORY CHANGE TALK

Desire: 'I *wish* I could lose some weight'.
Ability: 'I *could* go for a walk every evening'.
Reason: 'I *should* have enough energy to play with my kids'.
Need: 'I really *have* to do something soon about this'.

IMPLEMENTING CHANGE TALK

Commitment: 'I *will try* and make some small changes to my diet'.
Activation: '*I am ready* to give this a go now'.
Taking steps: '*I've cooked a healthy dinner every day this week*'.

Classifying change talk is not as important as learning to recognise and affirm its multiple presentations. Through exploring patients' deeplyheld

values and reasons for making change, their motivation for doing so will be strengthened [15].

MOTIVATIONAL INTERVIEWING IN PRACTICE

Now that the elements of MI, and its relevance to clinical practice have been outlined, a fictional example of a consultation which engages with the approach is outlined below. The specific elements being used or evoked in each sentence are noted in brackets.

CASE STUDY

John is a 60-year-old man with a history of smoking 40 packs a year, poorly-controlled COPD, and a diagnosis of depression. He attends the clinic regularly complaining of shortness of breath and coughing, which severely limit his daily activities. After reviewing his medication, you would like to explore smoking cessation with John using an MI approach.

Practitioner: Could you tell me a little about your smoking at the moment John? [Open question].

John: Well it's a big part of my life, I've always done it, you know.

Practitioner: It's a big part of your life. [Reflection].

John: Yes, I'll smoke a few packs throughout the day really. It calms me down.

Practitioner: And how do you feel about it? [Open question].

John: It's alright. Otherwise I would drink or some other vice I suppose, and I don't really drink, so smoking is my thing.

Practitioner: [Resisting the righting reflex] Smoking is your thing, you say. [Reflection].

John: Yes, I mean I've tried to quit before, as you know. And I would like to, in an ideal world [Change talk --desire]. It's not as simple as that though, is it?

Practitioner: I know what you mean. [Empathy]. What do you like about smoking? [Eliciting the pros].

John: Well, it's addictive, isn't it? They calm me down and I don't think I could get through the day without one. There're people all round you doing it, too. You can't get away.

Practitioner: [Resisting the righting reflex, allowing for pauses].

John: But I do know it's bad for my chest. If I weren't smoking maybe I wouldn't be coming in here to see you all the time about all these inhalers. [The cons, change talk – reason].

Practitioner: You notice that smoking affects your chest? [Reflection, evocation, eliciting discrepancy].

John: Oh yes, without a doubt. I'm going the way my parents went, with the coughing. Both smoked for years. It's too late now.

Practitioner: You managed to give quitting a go a few years ago, didn't you? [Affirmation].

John: Yes, I stopped for a month. Went back to it though, didn't I.

Practitioner: One month of no smoking is pretty impressive. [Affirmation].

John: I don't know really. It was too hard in the end. I would like to try again but I just don't think I could at the moment. [Change talk – desire].

Practitioner: What would have to change to make you start thinking about giving quitting another go? [Open, hypothetical, question, promoting autonomy].

John: It's everything, isn't it? Those pills didn't agree with me last time though. They made me feel awful.

Practitioner: The pills weren't working for you.

John: No, that's why I stopped.

Practitioner: I see, ok. So, you've noticed that smoking is really troubling your chest at the moment. And you would like to try and quit again, but you're not sure how, because of the medication you were on last time? [Summary, understanding patient's motivations].

John: Yes, that's a lot of it, I think.

Practitioner: Ok, I think I've got that. You can tell me what you think of this idea, [Promotion of autonomy, resisting imposition] But there are a few other ways we can help you to give this another go that don't involve those pills. It might be of interest to you if I just talked you through some of your options. How would you feel about that? Open question].

John: Ok, go on then.

The above scenario shows how, as a clinician, it is possible to guide patients to their own decisions, conclusions and motivations for changing, without imposing or suggesting anything yourself. In utilising a combination of different elements of MI, patients who may at first seem highly unmotivated or resistant may start to autonomously engage with the early stages of healthy behaviour change and go on to enact it.

In clinical practice within a deprivation context, MI would ideally form part of a number of synergistic interventions to support behaviour change. A recent example of this, the 'Mam-Kind' intervention, addresses low breastfeeding-initiation rates at community maternity services in three areas of deprivation in England and Wales, where alongside breastfeeding advice from midwives, peer-supporters were trained to deliver one-to-one ante- and post-natal MI sessions to mothers [18]. The results of this pilot study, and many others from across the UK, suggest promising potential for the feasibility of incorporating MI into multi-disciplinary clinical interventions, particularly in areas of social deprivation [12, 18–20].

Systematic reviews of motivational interviewing have shown its success in facilitating patient-led, sustainable behaviour change in a range of clinical contexts [8, 12, 14]. Although certain elements of MI may already be naturally used within many clinical consultations, understanding its 'spirit' and learning to recognise change talk can help to optimise the time you have with patients, and more effectively achieve positive outcomes [15]. Considering an MI approach may be particularly pertinent when engaging with socioeconomically disadvantaged groups, where fostering healthy behaviour changes can reinforce autonomy, empower patients and go on to positively interact with other determinants of health.

REFERENCES

1. Miller WR. Motivational Interviewing with Problem Drinkers. *Behav Psychother* [Internet]. 1983 Apr 16 [cited 2019 May 8];11(02):147. Available from: http://www.journals.cambridge.org/abstract_S0141347300006583

2. Rollnick S, Miller WR, Butler CC, Aloia MS. Motivational Interviewing in Health Care: Helping Patients Change Behavior. COPD *J Chronic Obstr Pulm Dis* [Internet]. 2008 Jan 2 [cited 2019 May 8];5(3):203. Available from: http://www.tandfonline.com/doi/full/10.1080/15412550802093108

3. Miller WR, Rollnick S. Ten Things that Motivational Interviewing Is Not. *Behav Cogn Psychother* [Internet]. 2009 [cited 2019 May 9];37:129–40. Available from: https://www.cambridge.org/core/services/aop-cambridge-core/content/view/5E0C55EB86946986E573B9F4C0CAB795/S1352465809005128a.pdf/ten_things_that_motivational_interviewing_is_not.pdf

4. Nandi A, Glymour MM, Subramanian S V. Association Among Socioeconomic Status, Health Behaviors, and All-Cause Mortality in the United States. *Epidemiology* [Internet]. 2014 Mar [cited 2019 May 10];25(2):170–7. Available from: http://www.ncbi.nlm.nih.gov/pubmed/24487200

5. Stringhini S, Dugravot A, Shipley M, Goldberg M, Zins M, Kivimäki M et al. Health Behaviours, Socioeconomic Status, and Mortality: Further Analyses of the British Whitehall II and the French GAZEL Prospective Cohorts. Lopez AD, editor. *PLoS Med* [Internet]. 2011 Feb 22 [cited 2019 May 10];8(2):e1000419. Available from: https://dx.plos.org/10.1371/journal.pmed.1000419

6. Pampel FC, Krueger PM, Denney JT. Socioeconomic Disparities in Health Behaviors. *Annu Rev Sociol* [Internet]. 2010 Aug [cited 2019 May 10];36:349–70. Available from: http://www.ncbi.nlm.nih.gov/pubmed/21909182

7. Williams ED, Tapp RJ, Magliano DJ, Shaw JE, Zimmet PZ, Oldenburg BF. Health Behaviours, Socioeconomic Status and Diabetes Incidence: The Australian Diabetes Obesity and Lifestyle Study (AusDiab). *Diabetologia* [Internet]. 2010 Dec 26 [cited 2019 May 10];53(12):2538–45. Available from: http://link.springer.com/10.1007/s00125-010-1888-4

8. Rubak S, Sandbaek A, Lauritzen T, Christensen B. Motivational Interviewing: A Systematic Review and Meta-Analysis. *Br J Gen Pract* [Internet]. 2005 Apr 1 [cited 2019 May 10];55(513):305–12. Available from: http://www.ncbi.nlm.nih.gov/pubmed/15826439

9. Lindson-Hawley N, Thompson TP, Begh R. Motivational Interviewing for Smoking Cessation. *Cochrane Database Syst Rev* [Internet]. 2015 Mar 2 [cited 2019 May 10];(3). Available from: http://doi.wiley.com/10.1002/14651858.CD006936.pub3

10. Inaz Karatay G, lü mser Kublay G, Nuran Emirog O, Professor lu R. Effect of Motivational Interviewing on Smoking Cessation in Pregnant Women. *J Adv Nurs* [Internet]. 2010 [cited 2019 May 10];66(6):1328–37. Available from: https://onlinelibrary.wiley.com/doi/pdf/10.1111/j.1365-2648.2010.05267.x

11. Cowlishaw S, Merkouris S, Dowling N, Anderson C, Jackson A, Thomas S. Psychological Therapies for Pathological and Problem Gambling. *Cochrane Database Syst Rev* [Internet]. 2012 Nov 14 [cited 2019 May 10];(11). Available from: http://doi.wiley.com/10.1002/14651858.CD008937.pub2

12. Hardcastle S, Blake N, Hagger MS. The Effectiveness of a Motivational Interviewing Primary-Care Based Intervention on Physical Activity and Predictors of Change in a Disadvantaged Community. *J Behav Med* [Internet]. 2012 Jun 5 [cited 2019 May 10];35(3):318–33. Available from: http://link.springer.com/10.1007/s10865-012-9417-1

13. Harrison R, Benton T, Everson-Stewart S, Weinstein P. Effect of Motivational Interviewing on Rates of Early Childhood Caries: A Randomized Trial. *Pediatr Dent* [Internet]. 2007 [cited 2019 May 10];29(1):16–22. Available from: https://www.ingentaconnect.com/content/aapd/pd/2007/00000029/00000001/art00005

14. Hettema J, Steele J, Miller WR. Motivational Interviewing. *Annu Rev Clin Psychol* [Internet]. 2005 Apr [cited 2019 May 10];1(1):91–111. Available from: http://www.ncbi.nlm.nih.gov/pubmed/17716083

15. Rollnick S, Miller WR, Butler C. *Motivational Interviewing in Health Care: Helping Patients Change Behavior* [Internet]. New York: The Guilford Press; 2008 [cited 2019 May 9]. 210 p. Available from: https://ebookcentral.proquest.com/lib/manchester/reader.action?docID=406031

16. Haque SF, D'Souza A. Motivational Interviewing: The RULES, PACE and OARS. *Curr Psychiatr* [Internet]. 2019 [cited 2019 May 9];18(1):27–8. Available from: https://www.mdedge.com/psychiatry/article/191765/addiction-medicine/motivational-interviewing-rules-pace-and-oars

17. Miller WR, Rollnick S. *Motivational Interviewing: Preparing People for Change.* New York: Guilford Press; 2002. 428 p.

18. Paranjothy S, Copeland L, Merrett L, Grant A, Phillips R, Gobat N et al. A Novel Peer-Support Intervention using Motivational Interviewing for Breastfeeding Maintenance: A UK Feasibility Study. *Health Technol Assess (Rockv)* [Internet]. 2017 Dec [cited 2019 May 14];21(77):1–138. Available from: https://www.journalslibrary.nihr.ac.uk/hta/hta21770

19. Mitcheson L, Bhavsar K, McCambridge J. Randomized Trial of Training and Supervision in Motivational Interviewing with Adolescent Drug Treatment Practitioners. *J Subst Abuse Treat* [Internet]. 2009 Jul 1 [cited 2019 May 14];37(1):73–8. Available from: https://www.sciencedirect.com/science/article/pii/S0740547208002146

20. Craigie AM, Macleod M, Barton KL, Treweek S, Anderson AS, WeighWell team. Supporting Postpartum Weight Loss in Women Living in Deprived Communities: Design Implications for a Randomised Control Trial. *Eur J Clin Nutr* [Internet]. 2011 Aug [cited 2019 May 14];65(8):952–8. Available from: http://www.ncbi.nlm.nih.gov/pubmed/21559034

17

Person-centred Care

DEENA EL-SHIRBINY

Empowering individuals to self-manage chronic and complex conditions.

The landscape of the NHS has undergone considerable changes over the past few decades. The *Five Year Forward View* emphasises that NHS systems are increasingly under pressure as the population lives longer with more complex health issues [1]. Demands on primary care are also increasing at a time when funding and workforce resources are diminishing [2].

According to the Department of Health, people with long-term conditions are the most frequent users of healthcare services, accounting for 50% of all GP appointments and 70% of all inpatient bed stays [3]. Citizens Advice estimates that 20% of all GP appointments are for patients who need non-medical help or support [4]. With increased access to information via the internet and social media, there is also a drive from patients for greater involvement in decisions about their care.

All of these factors have increased the focus on a broader and holistic approach which takes into account the personal, environmental and social factors which impact on health and well-being while also empowering individuals to self-manage chronic and complex conditions.

PERSON-CENTRED CARE IN HEALTH POLICY

Over the past two decades, person-centred care has featured in health policy with increasing prominence. The 2000 NHS plan included a commitment to personalisation and stated:

'Step by step over the next 10 years the NHS must be redesigned to be patient-centred – to offer a personalised service...by 2010 it will be commonplace' [5].

In 2002, The Wanless report focused on enablement, empowerment and seeing patients as 'partners in care' [6]. It argued that only by people becoming 'fully engaged' in their own healthcare could the escalating costs of health and social care provision associated with the growing burden of disease remain in tandem with funding available.

Further to this, the 2008 Darzi report highlighted the importance of people collaborating in decisions [7], after which the Health and Social Care Act 2012 imposed a legal duty for NHS England and clinical commissioning groups to involve patients in their care [8]. More recently, NHSE launched their universal personalised care plan strategy in 2019 which outlined the changes required for a shift in approach to a system in which person-centred care would be 'business as usual' [9].

WHAT IS PERSON-CENTRED CARE?

Throughout this chapter we have used the term person-centred care. However, there are several other terms which are used to encapsulate this model of care including 'personalised care' and 'patient-centred care'. In recent years, there has been a move away from the use of 'patient' to 'person' to reflect a more holistic model which places the individual at the centre of their care. Person-centred care offers an alternative, more encompassing view on health, taking into account the wider aspects of an individual's well-being. It switches the focus to the individual in the context of their world rather than as a patient in the consulting room.

There is no single agreed definition despite many national and international organisations aspiring to deliver it. This reflects the evolving and multi-dimensional nature of care as well as the concepts that underpin it. Person-centred care may mean something different for each individual, health professional or organisation.

There are, however, several fundamental principles which underpin person-centred care [10]:

- Respect for the person's values, preferences and expressed needs.
- Personalised, coordinated and integrated health, social care and support.
- Equal partnership in the relationship between healthcare professionals and patients.
- Involvement of family, friends and carers.
- Supporting people to recognise and develop their own strengths and abilities to enable them to live an independent and fulfilling life.

Person-centred care is often referred to as asset-based. This refers to the philosophy around individual and community strengths and capabilities as the foundation for improving health and well-being. The concept of co-production or collaboration has also emerged in recent years as a fundamental aspect of personalised care. Rather than a health system which does things to or for people, co-production works with individuals and enables them to exercise choice and exert greater control over the types of support they need for better health and well-being outcomes.

In essence, person-centred care represents a move away from patients being passive recipients of healthcare to active partners. Given this partnership with individuals, families/carers and communities, it follows that there is no one-size-fits-all

model. Each individual or community will have its own resources, needs, preferences and values which must be taken into account. When considering the benefits of a person-centred approach in areas of socioeconomic deprivation, this tailored model becomes even more important given the stark differences in medical needs, community resources and challenges from one community or surgery to another.

PERSON-CENTRED CARE AND HEALTH INEQUALITIES

On average, people in disadvantaged areas have multiple long-term conditions 10–15 years earlier than those in better off neighbourhoods [11]. The abundance of chronic and complex conditions in areas of high need is challenging and often disheartening for health professionals, especially when the factors which contribute extend far beyond the consulting room. While a health professional may be addressing a patient's rising HbA1c (glycated hemaglobin), or compliance with a statin in a time-pressured appointment, the person's priorities may in fact be: housing, employment, financial difficulties or the fact that they are caring for someone else.

Furthermore, there is concern that clinicians in areas of deprivation face the disadvantage of less experience in person-centred consulting skills as patients can be less likely to engage in shared decision-making [12]. This has potential implications for professional clinical examinations (currently the Clinical Skills Assessment) and recruitment of GPs.

It is universally accepted that the causes of poor health and health inequality are systemic. A person-centred model counters this, offering an opposing systemic approach which mobilises services in a way that can be tailored to individuals and communities.

WHAT DOES PERSON-CENTRED CARE INVOLVE?

As discussed there is no standard way of providing person-centred care. However, there are several components and tools which are used which we will examine more closely:

SOCIAL PRESCRIBING

Social prescribing, sometimes referred to as community referral, is a means of enabling GPs, nurses and primary care professionals to refer people to a range of local, non-clinical services. Social prescribing can include a wide variety of services and activities including volunteering, parenting classes, art therapy, walking groups, advice about employment, debt management and housing.

There are several models for social prescribing, but most involve a link worker who liaises with individuals to access local and community support. Rather than looking at social prescribing as something health professionals do, many proponents consider it to be a holistic process which includes clinical, non-clinical and community organisations but is also embedded in the community as a whole in an organic manner. This systemic model extends beyond signposting: handing out leaflets and the passive direction of individuals to other organisations or groups. It enables the development of community infrastructure which promotes the growth of health-creating communities.

A review of the evidence assessing the impact of social prescribing on healthcare demand and cost implications found average reductions following referrals to social prescribing schemes of of 28% in GP services, 24% in attendance at A & E and statistically significant drops in referrals to hospital [13].

CASE STUDY

Rotherham Social Prescribing Service

The Rotherham Social Prescribing Service was set up in 2012 and is one of the largest schemes of its kind. The service is delivered by Voluntary Action Rotherham in partnership with more than 20 local and community organisations. A team of voluntary and community sector advisers provide a single gateway to voluntary and community support for GPs and service users. They receive referrals from GPs of eligible patients and carers and assess their support needs before referring them on to appropriate voluntary and community services. An evaluation of the service found that non-elective inpatient episodes reduced by 7% (19% when service users aged over 80 are excluded); accident & emergency attendances reduced by 17% (23% of those under 80). After three to four months, 82% of these people who use services with long-term conditions had experienced positive change in at least one well-being outcome area.

Shared Decision-making

Shared decision-making is another key component of person-centred care. 'It is a process in which health professionals and individuals work together to make decisions and select tests, treatments and care plans based on clinical evidence that balances risks and expected outcomes with patient preferences and values' [14].

Shared decision-making involves sharing information, including uncertainties, about options, and outcomes, and using this with the knowledge, views and experiences of the patient to make decisions. In certain forms it may consist of structured decision-making aids or programmes, which are designed to show information about different options, but can also occur through dialogue in a consultation, when the patient is involved in making choices about their healthcare such as starting a new medication.

In shared decision-making, the conversations between the health professional and patient are viewed as a meeting between experts which contrasts with other consultation models, for example, where the doctor makes a decision about treatment for the patient, or the patient makes their own decision, often based on their own independent research. This model is particularly relevant in chronic health conditions, where the patient may have many years of experience of their symptoms and responses to treatments.

Numerous studies have shown that shared decision-making improves patients' satisfaction with, and involvement in their own healthcare [15]. It has also been found to reduce the number of invasive procedures when individuals are educated on all the treatment options available to them [16].

CASE STUDY

MAGIC Project

Practices in Newcastle and Cardiff involved in the Health Foundation's MAGIC (Making Good Decisions in Collaboration) project distributed leaflets encouraging patients to ask three questions about their treatment:

- What are my options?
- What are the pros and cons of each option for me?
- How do I get support to make a decision that's right for me?

These were accompanied by a video in which patients talked about how they used these questions to understand their care and get more involved. The video could be accessed on Newcastle-upon-Tyne NHS Foundation Trust website and was played in practice waiting areas.

Health Coaching and Patient Activation

Health coaching is defined as 'helping people gain the knowledge, skills, tools and confidence to become active participants in their care so that they can reach their self-identified health goals' [17]. Rather than simply telling people they need to lose weight or stop smoking, health coaching encourages self-discovery and aims to inspire people to become more motivated and confident in managing their own health, making healthy lifestyle choices and more informed decisions in order to achieve the things that are important to them.

'Patient activation' is a behavioural concept which describes the knowledge, skills and confidence a person has in managing their own health and healthcare [18]. People who have low levels of activation are less likely to play an active role in staying healthy. They are less good at seeking help when they need it, at following a doctor's advice and at managing their health when they are no longer being treated. The patient activation measure (PAM) is a validated tool for measuring the level of patient engagement in their healthcare. It can be used to tailor support according to an individual's patient activation level through an individualised approach which takes into account their needs and capabilities.

CASE STUDY

The Cornwall Community Pharmacy Patient Activation Service

In December 2016 Cornwall and Isles of Scilly Local Pharmaceutical Committee and the South West Cardiovascular Clinical Network launched a developmental service in 20 community pharmacies across Cornwall. The project used the PAM and motivational interviewing in pharmacies to improve patient activation and self-management of type II diabetes over three months. Of the patients who completed the service, 98% achieved (72%) or partially achieved (26%) their goals after the three-month intervention.

Collaborative Care and Support Planning (CCSP)

Collaborative care and support planning are sometimes referred to as personalised care and support planning. It is a collaborative process that aims to determine what is important to individuals to allow treatment and care plans to be developed which align with their primary considerations. As with many constituents of person-centred care, CCSP is a systemic process which is based around good conversations between individuals and professionals. It is a continuous and proactive process which aims to move away from single-disease pathways and a 'tick box' approach to the management of complex and long-term conditions.

Shared decision-making and health coaching underpin the CCSP process. Areas explored include health and well-being outcomes, an action plan, goal setting, contingency/emergency plans, risk assessment, informal support from friends/family and resources in the local community.

Fundamental principles of CCSP include [19]:

- Individuals are an equal and active partner in developing their own care plans.
- The information in the plan must be meaningful, relevant and accessible to the person.
- It is designed to be portable and shared electronically when possible with whomever the person wishes and consents to share their plan with.
- One key worker should be identified to coordinate the process across services.

CASE STUDY

The Holmside Story

Holmside, a 9,000-person, inner-city practice in Newcastle implemented a personalised approach to their routine care based on a care and support planning process. This included all patients with any number or combination of long-term conditions into a single recall system. Rather than multiple reviews, patients were invited in for a single consultation. The surgery found that patient and staff satisfaction and engagement increased, there were less unplanned attendances at the practice, and no deterioration in QOF measures or increase in practice costs.

Health Literacy

The World Health Organisation has defined health literacy as 'the personal characteristics and social resources needed for individuals and communities to access, understand, appraise and use information and services to make decisions about health' [20]. Research has found that 43% of adults of working age in England cannot fully understand and use health information containing only text. This rises to 64% when numerical information is included [21].

There is significant evidence indicating a link between low health literacy and poorer health outcomes. It predicts poor diet, smoking and lack of physical activity and is associated with an increased risk of morbidity and premature death in older adults. Health literacy tends to be poorer in areas of socioeconomic deprivation and makes it harder for people to access appropriate services, communicate with health professionals, understand medication labelling and instructions and take part in decisions. It is associated with increased use of emergency and acute services rather than preventive services resulting in higher healthcare costs [22].

Traditionally, services have been set up with the expectation that patients will be able to navigate interactions with health professionals and the often complex structure of health services. Addressing the impact of poor health literacy requires a culture change in which the health service and health professionals are aware of and responsive to the individuals that use the service.

CASE STUDY

Healthy Gems

Healthy Gems was a course written in response to poor health literacy levels in Oldham which had been linked to higher levels of attendance to A & E for under fives and inappropriate use of GP appointments for minor ailments that could be treated at home. Parents and professionals recognised carers of young children often did not feel confident that they could make the right decision for their child's care especially around coughs, rashes, and high temperatures. The interactive course takes a couple of hours and is delivered in children's centres, schools, libraries, GP practices and other community settings. It teaches parents and carers the difference between a healthy child and a sick child and most importantly gives them the confidence to make decisions about where and when to ask for help with their child's health. Their confidence is measured with a pre- and post-course questionnaire, which showed an increase of confidence in all areas asked, including an increase from 65% to 97% for the statement 'I understand the signs/symptoms to look for when children are ill' and an increase from 62% to 93% for 'I feel confident in knowing how to access different services'.

REFERENCES

1. *The Five Year Forward View.* NHS England, October 2014.
2. Baird B et al. *Understanding Pressures in General Practice.* The Kings Fund, May 2016.
3. Department of Health. Report. Long-term conditions compendium of Information: 3rd edition, 2012.
4. Citizen's Advice Bureau. A very general practice. How much time do GPs spend on issues other than health? May 2015.
5. Department of Health. *The NHS Plan: A Plan for Investment, a Plan for Reform.* Cm 4818-I. Norwich: HMSO, July 2000.
6. Wanless D. *Securing Our Future Health: Taking a Long-Term View.* London: HM Treasury, April 2002.
7. Darzi A. *High Quality Care for All: NHS Next Stage Review Final Report.* Norwich: TSO, June 2008.

8. Department of Health. Health and Social Care Act, March 2012.

9. NHS England. Universal Personalised Care: Implementing the Comprehensive Model, January 2019.

10. Health Innovation Network. What is person-centred care and why is it important? Cited March 2019. Available from https://healthinnovationnetwork.com/wp-content/uploads/2016/07/What_is_person-centred_care_HIN_Final_Version_21.5.14.pdf

11. Kings Fund. Long term conditions and multi-morbidity. Cited March 2019. Available from https://www.kingsfund.org.uk/projects/time-think-differently/trends-disease-and-disability-long-term-conditions-multi-morbidity

12. Cunningham D, Yeoman L. Recently-qualified general practitioners' perceptions and experiences of General Practice Specialty Training (GPST) in deprived areas of NHS Scotland – a qualitative study. *Educ Primary Care*. 2019; 30(3): 158–164.

13. Polley M et al. Review of evidence assessing impact of social prescribing on healthcare demand and cost, June 2017. Available from https://www.westminster.ac.uk/file/107671/download

14. National Learning Consortium. Shared Decision Making, December 2013.

15. Swanson KA, Bastani R, Rubenstein LV et al. Effect of mental health care and shared decision making on patient satisfaction in a community sample of patients with depression. *Med Care Res Rev* 2007 Aug; 64(4):416–30. PMID: 17684110.

16. O'Connor AM, Llewellyn-Thomas HA, Flood AB. Modifying unwarranted variations in health care: Shared decision making using patient decision aids. *Health Aff(Millwood)* 2004; Suppl Variation:VAR63-72. PMID: 15471770.

17. Bennett HD et al. Health coaching for patients with chronic illness. *Fam Pract Manag* 2010 Sep-Oct;17(5):24–29.

18. Hibbard JH, Stockard J, Mahoney ER, Tusler M. Development of the Patient Activation Measure (PAM): Conceptualising and measuring activation in patients and consumers. *Health Serv Res* 2004;39(4 Pt 1):1005–1026.

19. Department of Health. Care and Support Statutory Guidance, 2014.

20. World Health Organisation. The Mandate for Health Literacy. Cited March 2019. Available from https://www.who.int/healthpromotion/conferences/9gchp/health-literacy/en/

21. NHS, Health Education England. Toolkit launched to tackle low health literacy. Cited March 2019. Available from https://www.hee.nhs.uk/news-blogs-events/news/toolkit-launched-tackle-low-health-literacy

22. Public Health England. Improving health literacy to reduce health inequalities, September 2015.

18

Trauma-informed Care

RUTH THOMPSON

'The change from a normal calm safety state to arousal and emotional dysregulation can be swift'.

With grateful thanks to Bessel Van Der Kolk and his book *The Body Keeps the Score* [1].

Traumatic events are, by definition, memorable: stressful events or situations (either short or long lasting) of exceptionally threatening or catastrophic nature, which are likely to cause pervasive distress in almost everyone (ICD-10 1994). In cases of public, mass number and large-scale traumatic events, the memory may be held collectively with annual events, symbols and occasionally parades. In 2017 a terrorist attack happened in my home city of Manchester. People are likely to know they have been part of traumatic event and ask for help if struggling with emotions.

Memory though, can be an inconstant and poor storage facility. The impact of many traumatic events may go unrecognised by patient and clinician though its legacy is played out in every interaction. The overwhelming neurophysiological impact of trauma and the adaptations people unconsciously take to cope can be seen by clinicians who are prepared to open the can of worms.

Our response then should be to enable patients to learn skills that enable them to cope with physical sensations so that they can feel secure in their bodies. We should also know enough about stages on the road to recovery in order to help people use appropriate medications and access therapy as required.

Since the early 1990s and the introduction of brain imaging of positron emission tomography (PET) and functional MRI, we have been able to watch brains respond to different stimuli as they 'light up' in different research settings. Our understanding of trauma has moved from observed behaviour and hypothesis to observable changes in brain activity.

HOW DO THE BRAIN AND BODY RESPOND TO THREATENING EVENTS?

The sensory perceptions entering the brain pass though the thalamus in the limbic system which communicates either at speed with the amygdala or more slowly with the neocortex. The amygdala, described by Van der Kolk as 'the smoke detector' of brain, decides if incoming data is relevant for survival and communicates with the body via the autonomic nervous system (ANS) to orchestrate whole-body response. The arousal of the body, which involves release of adrenaline, works at speed and not under the control of the neocortex, the higher-order, slower-thinking part of brain. Thus, in situations of danger the body may be moving before the neocortex is aware of the threat.

Porges [2] coined the word 'neuroception' to describe the capacity to evaluate relative danger and safety in one's environment. Together the limbic area of the brain and ANS regulate our physiological states at any particular moment. The emotional brain responds to our perceived level of safety and determines to what degree the fight-or-flight adrenaline is activated. A clinician about to take an exam may perceive a mild threat and have a low-level adrenaline release, which reduces after talking to colleagues, whereas a child witnessing domestic abuse, where the main caregiver is under threat, may respond with 'watchful frozenness'. If the perception of threat or actual danger increases, the emotional brain will escalate the response (Table 18.1).

LEARNING EXERCISE

- *Can you explain fight-or-flight adrenaline response to a threatening event?*
- *Consider a variety of threatening events and practise explaining the threat and the body's response, initially with a colleague then with patients e.g.*
  - *Visit to the dentist.*
  - *Motor traffic accident.*
  - *Terrorist event.*
  - *Mugging.*

For many people who have been in a traumatic event, neuroception will be set at high alert. Small stimuli, such as sounds or smells, will trigger the limbic and ANS system and cause hyperarousal. The person may then be flooded with difficult sensations and this state may take some time to pass. Cognitive and behavioural responses may include thought intrusions, emotional numbing and avoidance of people and situations. After a single-episode traumatic incident, these symptoms will be initially high and generally decrease over time,

as shown by McFarlane's study [3] of 50 Australian firefighters

How is Pathological Response to Traumatic Events Defined?

Of all the people affected by the Manchester bombing, the majority have recovered successfully. There has been a variation in responses from people, even from those standing next to each other. There has also been a pathological response from some people not directly involved but in the surrounding area. What differentiates people who develop post-traumatic stress disorder (PTSD) from people who are temporarily stressed is that they start organising their lives around the trauma. The National Vietnam Veterans Readjustment Study [4] shows that only 15.2% of Vietnam veterans developed prolonged PTSD, though this may be under-reporting as people may not link long-term emotions back to a traumatic event.

Over the years, 10,000s of people involved in retrospective and even prospective studies have given insight into conditions that predict whether a person will develop PTSD or other mental illnesses. Factors include:

- Pre-trauma vulnerability.
- Preparedness for the event.
- Magnitude of stressor.
- Quality of the immediate and short-term responses.
- Post-event recovery factors.

Narrative memory is when we recall the story of an event and how it fits into the narrative of our lives. Traumatic memories are when patients are plunged into the event and relive the arousal and sensations as if it was happening – a 'flashback'. How memory changes over time is shown in a 50-year prospective study [5] of 200 males who were recruited just prior to the onset of WW2. Between interviews in

Table 18.1 Perception of Threat and Response

Safety	Normal activities, able to concentrate, self-regulate body, interact with others with reciprocity.
Level 1 danger	Social response - call for help and support from people around us.
Level 2 danger	Fight or flight release of adrenaline which 'arouses' the body for activity.
Level 3 danger	Freeze - body preserves itself by shutting down and expending as little energy as possible.

1945 and 1990 those without PTSD had processed their traumatic experiences into narrative recall, whereas those with PTSD, reported wartime memories that were preserved essentially intact, with sound, smell and visceral sensations, over 45 years after the war had ended.

SUGGESTIONS FOR PRACTICE

- *Explain to patients what to expect over days, weeks and months following a traumatic event.*
- *Give brief first-aid advice such as*
  - *Continue with normal activities.*
  - *Look after physical well-being (eating, resting, not using intoxicants).*
  - *Allow time to pass and when symptoms might be pathological, seek help.*

It is important to remember the majority of research around trauma, including the introduction of post-traumatic stress disorder in 1980, was in relation to adults experiencing environmental disasters and discrete events such as wars. Not all traumatic events fit this profile and many clinicians suggest that we should consider two types of trauma, with interpersonal traumas more likely to have more profound effects than impersonal ones (Table 18.2).

What are Adverse Childhood Experiences (ACEs)?

The extent of childhood trauma and its long-term impact was clearly noted by Dr Felitti in the Adverse Childhood Experiences study [6]. While running an obesity clinic he heard about patients' experience of difficult childhoods and developed 10 questions.

In an American private health facility, 25,000 consecutive patients, mostly white and middle class, were given these questions and over 70% responded. Our prejudice may lead us to consider this a low-risk population but only a third reported no ACE. Felitti found ACEs are co-dependant; people don't live in a family where their mother is regularly beaten but life is otherwise fine. Felitti was able to access patients' full health notes and noted correlations between ACEs and pathology. Those with an ACE score of 6 or above had a 15% or greater chance than those with ACE scores of zero of currently suffering from any of the ten leading causes of death in the United States including chronic obstructive pulmonary disease (COPD), ischaemic heart disease (IHD) and liver disease. They were twice as likely to suffer from cancer and four times as likely to have emphysema.

Data from 4,000 people in Manchester [7] suggest that similar exposure to ACEs takes place in the UK and some worldwide consistency is beginning to appear. Given this large number, and considering that most people live healthy lives, it would be sensible to assume that the majority of people experiencing ACEs will have successful coping strategies and lead healthy fulfilling lives.

Mind and Body Response to ACEs

Threatening childhood events, whether single and impersonal (such as the Manchester bombing) or multiple random and interpersonal (such as witnessing domestic abuse), will be processed and stored differently to adulthood events. Piaget's model of children's psychological development explains why a child may not have the narrative language to describe events. Bowlby's attachment theory explains why there will be a profound trauma when someone who is deemed to be a caregiver is also a source of threat.

In terms of formal diagnosis, many people consider how mental illness after type 2 trauma

Table 18.2 Two Types of Trauma

Type 1 Trauma	Type 2 or Complex Trauma
Sudden and unexpected events, which are experienced as isolated incidents such as road traffic accidents, rapes or terrorist attacks. This can happen in childhood or adulthood.	This term refers to traumatic events which are repeated, interpersonal and often (although not always) occurring in childhood. This includes all forms of childhood abuse which are chronic and cumulative such as childhood sexual abuse, physical abuse, witnessing domestic abuse and neglect. Domestic abuse is the most common experience of complex trauma in adulthood.

warrants an alternative diagnostic label such as developmental trauma disorder. As this is not currently accepted, patients may accrue a variety of best fit diagnostic labels, including the following although this list is not exclusive: generalised anxiety disorder, substance misuse, depression, anorexia nervosa and personality disorder. In the ACE study, prevalence of chronic depression in people with an ACE score >4 was shown to be 66% in women and 35% in men. For those whose ACE score was 0, prevalence of chronic depression was 12%. The majority of psychiatric inpatients have been found to have histories of severe trauma, usually intrafamilial and at least 15% meet diagnostic criteria for PTSD. Herman and Van de Kolk concurred that many psychiatric patients had histories of trauma but that those suffering from borderline personality disorder stood out by having the most severe abuse histories. More than half had abuse starting before the age of 6 and 81% had histories of trauma in childhood [8].

When people recall intense negative emotion, brain scanning shows activity in gut, muscle and skin areas of basic bodily function. In his book, *The Feeling of What Happens* Demasio [9] explores how sense of self and sensory self are entwined. Many people express emotions using the language of the body: 'I'm heartbroken', 'I was all choked up'. People experiencing adrenaline release have many physical symptoms, beneficial if fight-or-flight is needed, but less helpful in daily life. They may then present these physical symptoms to clinicians who may investigate, e and provide temporary symptomatic relief but fail to address the underlying issues. Symptoms for which no clear physical basis is found are common in children and adults who have experienced trauma and can include chronic back and neck pain, headaches, digestive problems and chronic fatigue.

Coping with Difficult Emotions Caused by ACE

Many behaviours, such as use of intoxicants, eating leading to obesity and self-harm may provide short-term relief to someone coping with complex emotions. Clinicians see these behaviours as a problem and struggle to consider that although they confer long-term health risks, for the person these might be beneficial adaptations. In 1986,

Putman and Tickett [10] started a prospective study recruiting 84 girls referred to social services for family sexual abuse. The average age at recruitment was 11 years old and they were age-matched with follow up until the age of 25 with 96% remaining with the study. The results were unambiguous. Sexually abused girls show a wide range of negative effects including depression, high rates of obesity and self-mutilation.

Self-harm is a behaviour that baffles many clinicians. As early as 1978, Green [11] reported 41% of children who had been abused engaged in self-harming behaviours. Over the years, many terms have been used such as parasuicide, suicide attempt and deliberate self-harm. All of these assume we, as clinicians, can make accurate inferences as to people's intentionality, which is not possible. Though people who engage in self-harming behaviour are more at risk for suicide, we cannot assume each self-harming event was a suicide attempt. In fact, clinicians can become very frustrated when patients who have self-harmed are unable to give a clear narrative account of their actions. Considering much self-harm is in response to complex emotions whose base is in childhood trauma, maybe we are asking too much.

More information from scans helps us consider why people might self-harm. Dr Ruth Lannius asked 16 control people and 18 patients with severe chronic childhood abuse to be scanned while thinking about nothing [12]. The control patients' brain scans showed activation of a part of the brain called the default state network (DSN), the 'mohawk of self-awareness', which integrates sensations of physical relation in space with emotional and visceral perceptions from the body to create an ongoing sense of self. In the other group there was almost no activation in the DSN self-sensing brain, suggesting that, in an effort to shut off difficult sensations they had deadened their capacity to feel fully alive. It has been suggested self-harm might be an attempt to feel and restores the feeling of being alive. This loss of the ability to identify specific emotions, or alexithymia, was first noted by Henry Krystal [13] who worked with 1,000 Holocaust survivors. While often able to function well in daily life, they struggled to maintain intimate relations. The PET scans Frewen carried out showed that people with a diagnosis of PTSD who had most alexithymia also had least self-sensing. As one patient described, 'I don't know what I feel, it's like my head and body aren't connected…having a bubble bath and being burned or being raped is the same feeling. My brain doesn't feel'.

Long-term Sequelae of ACE

Rather than consider individual responses to trauma, it may be useful to consider public health data of some key areas of concern to our society. The LankellyChase Foundation's Hard Edges study [14] of severe and multiple disadvantage (SMD) reviewed three national data sets: people who are homeless; people in contact with the criminal justice system and those who have sought help for misuse of intoxicants. Of the people with all three markers of SMD, only 15% reported no traumatic or adverse events in childhood. Similarly, in a retrospective study of 30 homeless people asked to complete ACE questionnaires, just over 50% had ACE 3 and 90% had ACE 4. This suggests that many people within the complex homeless system and criminal justice system may also be the people least able to navigate these systems due to cognitive, physiological and behaviour patterns established in childhood due to trauma.

SUGGESTIONS FOR PRACTICE

- *Consider looking through a patient's history*
- *Be aware that people who may have had traumatic childhoods are at risk for the following:*
  - *Ill health (personality disorder, persistent physical symptoms).*
  - *Harmful coping strategies (self-harm, substance misuse, eating disorders).*
  - *Difficult living situations (homeless, domestic abuse, sex worker, in contact with the criminal justice system).*

Why Clinicians Should be Aware if Individuals Have A History of Trauma

UNDERSTANDING COGNITIVE DIFFICULTIES

Patients with alexithymia may struggle to answer simple clinical questions such as 'Where do you feel the pain?' or 'What does the pain feel like?'. When someone is experiencing flashbacks and responding with their emotional brain then higher-order cognitive functioning is never allowed to engage. A simple task, to the clinician, such as remembering an appointment or turning up on time may be difficult to complete. Patients may lack agency, which is a sense of being in charge of their life. Many patients who have a history of trauma lack agency and may struggle with decision-making questions such as 'Do you want to be referred for counselling?'

UNDERSTANDING EMOTIONAL (AFFECT) REGULATION

Though patients may not be able to verbalise the sensations related to arousal, clinicians can observe someone pacing the waiting room or the beads of sweat when sitting in the consulting room. For some patients the change from a normal, calm state to arousal and emotional dysregulation can be swift. Subtle signals picked up by the patient from the clinician may signal safety and trust and not heighten the arousal. Equally the clinician may be able to identify worsening triggers, such as seeing a male clinician, and mitigate this.

SUGGESTIONS FOR PRACTICE

- *Consider your posture, tone of voice, eye contact.*
- *Consider how to help people learn skills to regulate emotion such as*
  - *Controlled breathing.*
  - *Cooling themselves by opening a window, holding a cold item (bag of ice cubes in rubber glove) or holding a hand under a running tap.*
  - *Progressive muscle relaxation.*
  - *Counting down from 100 in sevens or 30 in twos.*
- *Practise modulating your own breathing with a colleague, using phrases such as 'I can see you are distressed', 'Can we breathe slowly together? First empty your lungs and then breathe slowly in and hold if you can, then breath slowly out'. Match your breathing to theirs and try to slow down.*

Do No Harm

Many clinicians have been complicit in replicating prior trauma. A very obvious example would be restraining patients who have been previously violently assaulted. Other forms of accidental complicity with the abuser may be less obvious, such as use of the common phrase, 'that's unbelievable' after disclosure of traumatic episode. There may also be some difficulty in fully accepting an incident took place and sometimes clinicians have been involved in difficult debates about repressed memories. As Ronald Summit wrote in 'The Child Sexual Abuse Accommodation Syndrome', '...initiation, intimidation, stigmatisation, isolation, helplessness and self-blame depend on a terrifying reality of child sexual abuse. Any attempts by the child to divulge the secret will be countered by an adult conspiracy of silence and disbelief" [15].

The failure of clinicians to consider developmental trauma disorder as a diagnosis in own right leads to patients accumulating many diagnoses of which emotionally unstable personality disorder is one. We then search for interventions, such as patient admissions, medications including antipsychotics and therapies like CBT with potentially little therapeutic benefit and which may actually perpetuate harm.

Encouraging Activities

There are many activities that are beneficial to patients with a history of trauma which are happening in local communities: yoga, pilates, mindfulness, singing in choirs, amateur dramatics, gardening and dog-walking. As clinicians we can learn where these activities take place in our locality, we can encourage people with historic trauma to continue such helpful activities and facilitate future participation.

SUGGESTIONS FOR PRACTICE

- *Find out where some local classes are, what time, how much they cost and whether they need to be booked.*
- *Consider having a 'mental well-being' list of activities to give to patients.*
- *Attend a yoga, meditation or mindfulness session so you can explain to people what to expect.*

Encouraging Team Involvement

There are many resources for health centres, GP practices or wards wanting to be more aware of how their behaviour can help people with historic trauma. These include everything from short videos all staff can watch, to larger documents with many steps. There are several key terms in use at present, including 'trauma-informed care' and 'psychologically informed environments' which should be understood. Health Education Scotland has a comprehensive tool that clinicians might use to be trauma or psychologically informed in practice.

SUGGESTIONS FOR PRACTICE

- *At the place where you work, encourage all the team to watch https://vimeo.com/274703693*

How Would I Ask About Historic Trauma?

As a clinician you may worry you lack the skills to deliver a comprehensive trauma-informed recovery plan for a patient. You may not want to know in detail about the trauma, but a person's presentation may make you consider trauma as a possible issue. People can worry about triggering a complex and uncontainable emotional response in asking about trauma and so it is good to have time and some skills to help people regulate emotions. Often it is not necessary to know specifics, but even asking about difficult situations helps patients know you are aware that abuse happens, and you are willing to hear about it. In asking the question there is also an implication that you have knowledge of pathways to recovery so you need, at least, to know what is available locally.

SUGGESTIONS FOR PRACTICE

- *Consider questions that might elicit difficult memories of childhood:*
  - *Can you remember a time when you were happy and well?*
  - *What was life like at home when you were growing up?*

What Will Help People in their Journey to Recovery?

Even if trauma is not recognized or acknowledged by the patient, the clinician can still know about steps involved in recovery as many do not require overt trauma focus. They also do not necessarily happen in a linear fashion. Judith Herman talks about establishing safety – both internal and external – grieving and reconnecting [16].

Establishing Internal Safety

Patients can establish control of body and mind by learning to recognise an ANS response and developing skills to regulate this response, thus feeling safe in body. The challenge, when working with people whose survival response is triggered too readily, is finding ways to reset their physiology so these mechanisms stop working against them. They then must use these skills when triggered by images, sensations, flashbacks or nightmares. This might happen in daily life or maybe during a therapy session. Some would call this being therapy-ready as people need to have skills to be able to cope with triggers to be able to talk to therapist or undertake eye movement desensitisation and reprocessing (EMDR).

SUGGESTIONS FOR PRACTICE

- *Know what services are offered in your area and what the referral routes are.*
- *Consider watching a YouTube clip about EMDR so that you are aware of basic principles and could explain briefly to a patient what to expect.*

Grieving (Restructuring the Personal Schema)

We all hold a narrative of who we are and where we have come from and for some this comes to be dominated by trauma. When someone is continually viscerally revisiting trauma a therapist may emphasise, 'That was then, this is now', encouraging hope for change. One particular narrative is, 'I was to blame' and a skilled therapist will challenge this belief, as all children deserve nurturing caregivers and a secure and happy childhood.

Reconnecting

This is where clinicians can encourage patients to engage with people around, develop social links and, over time, help establish secure social contacts.

REFERENCES

1. Van der Kolk BA. *The Body Keeps the Score: Brain, Mind and Body in the Healing of Trauma.* New York: Viking; 2014.
2. Porges SW. *The Polyvagal Theory: Neurophysiological Foundations of Emotion, Attachment, Communication and Self-Regulation, Norton Series on Interpersonal Neurobiology.* New York: WW Norton and Company; 2011.
3. McFarlane AC (1988) The longitudinal course of post traumatic morbidity. *Journal of Anxiety Disorders.* 1988; 1: 105–116.
4. Kulka RA et al. *Trauma and the Vietnam War Generation: Report of Findings from the National Vietnam Veterans Readjustment Study.* New York: Brunner/Mazel; 1990.
5. Lee KA et al. A 50-year prospective study of psychological sequelae of WW2 combat. *American Journal of Psychiatry.* 1995; 152 (4): 516–22.
6. Felitti VJ et al. Relationship of childhood abuse and household dysfunction to many of the leading causes of death in adults: The Adverse Childhood Experiences (ACE) study. *American Journal of Preventive Medicine.* 1998; 14(4): 245–58.
7. Manchester Council. Manchester Joint Service Needs Assessment: Adults and Older People: Adults with Complex Lives. Available from: https://www.manchester.gov.uk/downloads/download/6809/adults_and_older_peoples_jsna_-_adults_with_complex_lives [Accessed 25th May 2019].
8. Van der Kolk BA. The body keeps the score: Memory and the evolving psychobiology of post-traumatic stress. *Harvard Review of Psychiatry.* 1994; 1(5): 253–265.
9. Damosio AR et al. Subcortical and cortical brain activity during feelings of self-generated emotions. *Nature Neuroscience.* 2000; 3(10): 1049–1056.
10. Trickett PK, Noll JG, Putman FW. The impact of sexual abuse on female development: Lessons from a multigenerational longitudinal research study. *Development and Psychopathology.* 2011; 23: 453–476.

11. Simpson CA, Porter GI. Self-mutilation in children and adolescents. *Bulletin of the Menninger Clinic*. 1981; 45: 428–438.

12. Bluhm RL et al. Alterations in default network connectivity in posttraumatic stress disorder related to early-life trauma. *Journal of Psychiatry and Neuroscience*. 2009; 34(3): 187.

13. Krystal H, Krystal JH. *Integration and Self-Healing: Affect, Trauma, Alexithymia*. New York: Analytic Press; 1988.

14. Bramley G, Fitzpatrick S, Edwards J, Ford D, Johnsen S, Sosenko F, Watkins D. *Hard Edges: Mapping Severe and Multiple Disadvantage in England*. London: Lankelly Chase; 2015.

15. Summit RC. The child sexual abuse accommodation syndrome. 1983; *Child Abuse and Neglect*, 7, 177–193.

16. Herman J. Recovery from psychological trauma. *Psychiatry and Clinical Neurosciences*. 2002; 51(1), 98–103.

19

Building Resilience Through Self-care

CATHY CULLEN, MING RAWAT

To put it simply: you must take care of yourself in order to be able to take care of your patients.

As GPs with more than 20 years' experience, we believe passionately in the value of primary care for the health and well-being of our patients. We have both been involved in GP education for most of our careers and are involved in an educational programme which trains GPs to work in areas of deprivation and with marginalised groups.

One of the most important lessons we teach is this:

> Particularly when working in areas of deprivation or with marginalised groups, it is critical that, in addition to caring for their patients, physicians also practise self-care.

We call this, 'putting your own oxygen mask on first'. This safety principle, pronounced at the beginning of every flight, has just as much relevance to primary care as it does to airline travel. When passengers put on their own oxygen masks first, it enables them to breathe well enough to help others.

The same principle holds true for all clinicians. Particularly when working with vulnerable populations of patients, who often fail to value their health, clinicians must maintain their own physical and mental well-being in order to be effective.

To put it simply: you must take care of yourself in order to be able to take care of your patients.

HOW DO WE DEFINE RESILIENCE?

In our practices, resilience involves the art of equanimity. This means maintaining balance and composure during the peaks and troughs of primary care: the cool diagnoses, as well as the effective interventions; the surprising and rewarding positive patient outcomes as well as the unexpected deaths; nearly missed pathologies and failures despite our best efforts to improve patient health.

If you work long enough and see enough patients, there will be occasional negative outcomes. How you manage those outcomes, learn from them and carry on despite them will be a function of your own resilience.

WHY DOES RESILIENCE MATTER?

> The paradox at the heart of the health service is that we are damaging and killing the very people who are committing their working lives to caring for the health and wellbeing of other people. We are actually creating more customers for our system. It's a deeply disturbing paradox.[1]

Working in primary care is well recognised as being stressful [2–14]. A 2005 UK survey of 23,521 GPs found that 21% estimated the stress to be excessive and 55% felt it impinged excessively on their quality of life [15]. Another study estimated that 28% of GPs experienced significant stress, compared with around 18% in the general working population [16, 17].

Stress is a precursor to burnout, a condition long recognised as affecting clinicians of all age groups and genders. Prolonged stress can lead to maladaptive behaviours, which have a deleterious effect upon health. Doctors have long been known to have a higher rate of mortality from alcoholic cirrhosis and suicide (Proportional Mortality Ratios 162 and 193 for male and female doctors respectively) [20].

The relative risk of suicide among clinicians (in particular GPs), has been found to be between 1.1 to 3.4 times higher for male doctors and 2.5 to 5.7 times for female doctors when compared to general populations [21, 22].

Sadly, it is not only clinicians who suffer from this stress; their spouses also have higher suicidal rates than those in the general population. An early study by Sakinhofsky revealed that the wives of GPs were four times more likely to commit suicide than other women [23].

In the late 1980s, Cooper and others found that the four most important predictors of job stress were work-home interface, demands of the job, patients' expectations and practice administration [3]. For female doctors, the interference of the job with family life was the most significant predictor of stress, for male it was the joint stressors of practice administration and job demands [3].

Many of the main stressors for clinicians appear to be created or perpetuated by their own policies, including:

- Overbooking patients.
- Starting surgeries late.
- Accepting commitments too soon after surgeries are due to finish.
- Making insufficient allowances for extra emergency patients.
- Allowing inappropriate telephone calls or other interruptions [24].

When it comes to reducing the build-up of pressure, and the stress which results, partnership and practice arrangements [24, 25] appear to be more important factors than the length of time allotted for consultations. One study suggested practices which had equitable and inclusive partner and practice relationships managed workloads better than practices which were a collection of disparate individuals.

Protected time between consultations to tackle problems proactively as a partnership was identified as very important [26].

The same clinicians who considered that job stress was responsible for causing them psychological symptoms of ill health also reported being particularly stressed about the effects of work on their home and social lives [25]. Worrying about patients' complaints was a key stressor, as was the feeling that an increasingly hostile media was creating a culture of blame when it came to clinicians [25, 27, 28]. This last finding seems to be at odds with the enduring remarkably high levels of general public satisfaction with GP services [29].

Clinicians also frequently cited both imposed changes from NHS management and perceived loss of autonomy (greater accountability) as having a negative impact on morale [30, 31].

A stressed clinician is a poorly functioning one, also often displaying a lack of cooperation, irritability, aggressiveness, withdrawal behaviour and resentment. They have an increased tendency to make mistakes, a propensity to take shortcuts, are resistant to change [32–34] and are more likely to have poor concentration, bad timekeeping, impaired productivity and slow comprehension of new procedures.

Grol has demonstrated poor clinical performance in those doctors with negative feelings of tension, lack of time and frustration, as evidenced by a high prescription rate, in conjunction with offering little explanation to patients [35].

Research has shown a link between poor physician health and medical practices in areas of deprivation, in which increased patient demand and poorer outcomes adversely affect the ability of clinicians to manage the emotional burden of their work [36–38].

Like their patients, clinicians working long term in areas of deprivation are vulnerable to burnout, which can be defined as:

- Emotional exhaustion,
- Depersonalisation or disengagement,
- Reduced personal accomplishment, caused by chronic occupational stress.

PROTECTION AGAINST BURNOUT

When clinicians practice self-care they build resilience, which protects them from burnout.

At the core of self-care is maintaining a clinician's emotional and mental well-being. It is important you, as a clinician, assemble your own toolkit of self-care strategies. Be aware you will need different tools at different times in your life and career. The more you know about the tools available, the better you will be able to fine-tune and maintain your emotional and physical well-being. This also means knowing when you need to seek assistance.

CASE STUDY

How Self-Care Works for Me as a GP

Growing up in a family in which feelings were openly discussed, and in which we did a monthly written dialogue about feelings has meant that I have always been open to supportive work. In addition to my medical studies, I completed a diploma in cognitive behavioural therapy. I also became a Balint leader; as such, I meet with other doctors and facilitate a de-brief through confidential discussions about patients. Recently I completed a mindfulness-based self-compassion course.

Skills and strategies from all these sources have become part of my toolkit for self-care. In my general practice, being self-aware and allowing space for any realisations that occur during times of self-awareness are my keys to remaining balanced.

I know where I am on the stress curve, almost instinctively. If I find myself sighing or getting annoyed when people outside the consultation room look for support, I can tell that I am heading towards overload. When that happens, I will attempt to adjust things, or just try to be kinder to myself. That might be as simple as forgiving myself for being short with someone who usually didn't deserve it.

I feel that practising self-care, as with most other aspects of life, is a journey. I try to be mindful that what worked well at one time in my life may be less effective at another time. Practised well and often, self-care leads to a more satisfying work and home life.

Wholehearted Living

In teaching other clinicians about self-care, we have found it useful to draw upon the terms and language first used by researcher Brené Brown, the author of *Daring Greatly: How the Courage to Be Vulnerable Transforms the Way We Live, Love, Parent, and Lead.*

Brown emphasises the importance of wholehearted living.

People who live wholeheartedly are people you find admirable, not because of what they do professionally, but because of who they are.

- They are connected, joyful and compassionate.
- They know that love and belonging give a sense of purpose to their lives and they believe that they are worthy of that love and belonging.
- They aim to have lives defined by the courage to be imperfect.
- They are compassionate to others and to themselves.
- They are able to connect with others because of their authenticity.
- They are willing to be vulnerable.
- Inevitably, people who live wholeheartedly are people who self-care.

When we work with clinicians, we focus on the following areas to help them live more wholehearted lives. As a group, clinicians are often people pleasers. We want our patients to like us. We get a buzz when someone thinks we are a great doctor/nurse/practitioner but it is critical you remain authentic and stay true to who you are.

When clinicians feel under pressure to make patients like them, they are more likely to do things to please them, such as give them prescriptions they do not need and which may be harmful. Succumbing to this pressure leaves clinicians feeling dissatisfied and in the long run, disillusioned.

This can be best summarized by the following phrase: 'Be who you are and say what you feel, because the people who mind don't matter, and the people who matter don't mind' [39].

SUGGESTIONS FOR PRACTICE

- *Having the support of a solid group of peers, with whom you can do honest peer review, can aid you in becoming the clinician you want to be.*

As clinicians, we often advise others to take time out, to accept their frailties, and to allow themselves to make mistakes. However, we fail to give ourselves the same beneficial advice.

It is important that you learn to offer yourself the same kindness you extend to others.

Clinicians are often high achieving, high scoring people with perfectionistic tendencies. Society expects us to be superhuman and is unforgiving when we make errors. The fact of the matter is that clinicians will make mistakes. We can put in all the systems we like, but there will always be errors. As a wise man once said, 'The only one who doesn't make mistakes is God. If you think you are God, we really have a problem'.

SUGGESTIONS FOR PRACTICE

- *Always do your best but be kind to yourself when, despite your best, something goes wrong.*
- *Before there is a crisis, look for support from organisations, such as Health in Practice, when you feel you need extra care.*

We are hardwired to respond to negative experiences, because they are the ones that may endanger us, and we are programmed to try to survive. Research has shown that to counteract each single negative experience, we need five positive experiences.

So be aware of the ordinary things that spark joy: a bright sunny day, a colourful umbrella on a wet day, the smile of a friend. As a child, Cathy said goodnight prayers in which her family listed things for which they were grateful. A gratitude journal (another version of this practice) can play a similar role by reminding you of the little things that make an ordinary day into a good one.

In this world, in which we are always 'on', it is common to be plagued with a sense of scarcity: the fear of not having, or not being, enough. Many of us wake up in a panic, thinking, 'I didn't get enough sleep' or 'I don't have enough time to get through all my tasks today', or even 'If I get too busy I won't be able to switch off and then I will get overloaded'.

As a clinician who practices self-care, it is important to accept that even during times in which you are too busy, moments of joy can be found, for example in finally completing a chapter you promised to write ages ago!

Part of life and being connected to people is that bad things occasionally happen. Research into adverse childhood events has shown resilience is key in overcoming this negative start to life.

However, if an individual has just one person who believes that he or she is worthy of being loved, that can be enough to help that individual begin to develop resilience. For some patients, the one person who believes in their worth is their GP.

Even when you accept that occasional negative events are inevitable, sometimes it can seem as if you are sinking beneath an all-consuming wave of negativity. Try to remember this too will pass.

Avoidance of negative emotions is also known as numbing. Common forms of numbing include alcohol, drugs, overeating, and in the case of many professionals, being too busy. The problem is that these practices numb everything, not only the overwhelming negative emotions, but also the good experiences as well, such as the daily moments of joy.

So, when you reach for that third glass of wine or take on an extra task when you are already busy, ask yourself are you trying to numb or distract yourself because something is making you unhappy?

If you are authentic and honest with yourself, you will find it easier to make decisions. When something feels right, it usually is.

However, if you find that you are constantly checking with others and second-guessing yourself, you may not be trusting your inner self.

As a clinician it is important that you reflect upon your actions and check in with peers and check recognised sources of information. But often you need to trust yourself and the relationship you have built with your patient in order to achieve the best outcome for that patient at that time.

The good news is that time is often on your side. One of the great aspects of primary care is the length of the patient relationship. You don't need to fix everything at once. You and your patient are on a journey to better health together.

Creativity is good for self-care. However, most clinicians are high achievers, at least in the academic world. It can be hard for them to take pleasure in being creative simply for its own sake if they are used to constantly comparing themselves to their peers and jostling to be at the top of the class.

As it says in 'Desiderata', 'If you compare yourself with others, you may become vain and bitter; for always there will be greater and lesser persons than yourself'.

Find the part of you that is creative and don't be afraid to nurture it.

SUGGESTIONS FOR PRACTICE

- *Creative pursuits, such as drawing or playing music, can renew you and help you relax, particularly when you no longer have the competition of classmates.*
- *Even the simplest forms of creativity, such as the current trend for mindful colouring, can become tools for unwinding after stressful days.*

There is definite pleasure in a job well done, but there is much more to you than the job you do. Nurture and cherish the part of you that is not defined by your profession, to ensure your longevity as a wholehearted healthy person.

If you find you feel that being exhausted is a form of status symbol or feel that how productive you are defines your self-worth, it's time to take stock; this is not a sustainable pattern.

CASE STUDY

How Self-care Works for Me as a GP

Growing up in a family where sport was actively encouraged, we developed our own flow in different sporting activities. I was attracted to explore yoga as a way towards physical fitness but discovered the rich world of mind, body and breath connection. I benefitted from the contemplative practices of yoga where I was able to have a calmer mind and stronger physical core which I bring to my work as a GP. This led to a teacher training course in yoga, following which I then offered yoga classes to our GP trainees.

I continued to explore contemplative practices for my own well-being and I also completed a mindfulness teacher training course. This helped me to manage stress in my GP work where I was now experiencing the same workload, but with the new skills of awareness and the ability to self soothe. Skills and strategies from these sources have become part of my toolkit of self-care. Being mindful takes some training and with practice becomes a way of being

in life – in work and at home. This way of being brings a non-judgemental, grounded and trusting approach to my life and work. Self-care is a dynamic skill and at different stages calls for different strategies, but I feel the first skill is developing self-awareness – learning to read my own internal weather pattern and paying attention to those needs.

The fact that the modern world is always 'on' can cause anxiety. This is the reason that practising mindfulness has become so popular. As you assemble your own self-care toolkit, be sure to create a space when your mind can be calm and still. This space does not necessarily mean sitting and meditating. For some of us, the space for mindfulness can be walking the dog, without earphones, just being alone.

SUGGESTIONS FOR PRACTICE

- *Set boundaries: switch off phones, ignore emails at weekends, avoid diagnosing friends and family.*
- *Ensure that others respect those boundaries, as well as respecting them yourself.*

Society values us, and our role. If motivation is a mixture of mastery, autonomy and a sense of purpose, then primary care is a job area providing all those ingredients. This job gives you that.

Any job can be done better when it is done with joy. Encourage your patients. Praise them when they do well, whether it means being the parent who cares enough to present with their children, or being the teenager who values himself enough to lose weight, etc.

Self-awareness

To become more aware of your own state of mind, it can be helpful to use a stress curve, in which green indicates little or no stress while red indicates highly stressed (Figure 19.1).

As you develop awareness of your own feelings, take a moment to stop and observe where you fall on the stress curve.

There will be times, such as in a triage room in the Emergency Department, where being in the red zone of the stress curve is appropriate.

Observe where you fall on the stress curve during the rest of your day. Try to find your pattern of behaviour. And do not hesitate to get outside help, which could be a friend, a mentor, a Balint group or

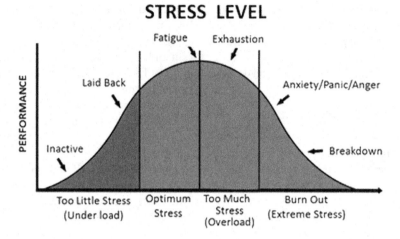

Figure 19.1 Stress levels.

psychological support. All of these resources can help you learn more about yourself and provide tools to help you manage stress better.

General Practice: The Best Medicine

As firm believers that general practice is a good thing, we know that far more than the handing over of a script occurs in a consultation. If we could ban the phrase, 'physician, heal thyself', we would.

SUGGESTIONS FOR PRACTICE

- *Treat yourself to a GP. Having a good GP, whose opinion you respect, is the best first step you can take in caring for, and about yourself. Go on: register today!*

There will always be more patients to be seen, and often they present with what appear to be greater needs than our own.

But to become the best clinician you can be, you need to sustain yourself. Come to know yourself and learn your limits. Recognise the signs of overload.

Remember that what worked to keep you on track when you were single might not work when you become a new parent, or when you are in financial difficulty. Don't be afraid to explore new solutions.

Find out what helps you unwind. Link in with colleagues and share your stresses. Seek out and use professional external help earlier rather than later.

Aim to live a wholehearted life. That really is the best you can do for your patients, for your family and for yourself.

REFERENCES

1. Dr Blanaid Hayes, Occupational Health Physician, quoting Michael West of Thought Leadership at the King's fund 2016.
2. Branthwaite A, Ross A. Satisfaction and job stress in general practice. *Fam Pract* 1988; 5 (2): 83–93.
3. Cooper CL, Rout U, Faragher B. Mental health, job satisfaction, and job stress among general practitioners. *BMJ* 1989; 298: 366–70.
4. Richards C. *The Health of Doctors.* King's Fund, London. 1989.
5. Howie J, Porter A, Heaney D, Hopton J. Long to short consultation ratio: A proxy measure of quality of care for general practice. *Br J Gen Pract* 1991; 41: 48–54.
6. Howie JG, Hopton JL, Heaney DJ, Porter AMD. Attitudes to medical care, the organisation of work, and stress among general practitioners. *Br J Gen Pract* 1992; 42: 181–5.
7. Sutherland VJ, Cooper C. Identifying distress among general practitioners: Predictors psychological ill health and job dissatisfaction. *Soc Sci Med* 1993; 37(5): 575–81.

8. Chambers R. Health and lifestyle of general practitioners and teachers. *Occup Med* 1992; 42: 69–78.

9. Caplan RP. Stress, anxiety and depression in hospital consultants, general practitioner and senior health service managers. *BMJ* 1994; 309: 1261–3.

10. Kirwan M, Armstrong D. Investigation of burnout in a sample of British general practitioners. *Br J Gen Pract* 1995; 45: 259–60.

11. Spurgeon P, Barwell F, Maxwell R. Types of work stress and implications for the role of general practitioners. *Health Services Management Research* 1995; 8(3): 186–97.

12. Chambers R, Campbell I. Anxiety and depression in general practitioners: Associations with type of practice, fund-holding, gender and other personal characteristics. *Fam Pract* 1996; 13 (2): 170–3.

13. Williams S, Michie S, Pattani S. *Improving the health of the NHS workforce*. Report of the partnership on the health of the NHS workforce. Nuffield Trust, London. 1998.

14. Chambers R, George V, McNeill A, Campbell I. Health at work in the general practice. *Br J Gen Pract* 1998; 48: 1501–4.

15. Stress and General Practice 2005 RCGP Information Sheet No 22.

16. Firth-Cozens J. Doctors, their wellbeing, and their stress. *BMJ* 2003; 326: 670–1.

17. Appleton K, House A, Dowell A. A survey of job satisfaction, sources of stress and psychological symptoms among general practitioners in Leeds. *Br J Gen Pract* 1998; 48: 1059–63.

18. Kirwan M, Armstrong D. Investigation of burnout in a sample of British general practitioners. *Br J Gen Pract* 1995; 45: 259–60.

19. Forsythe M, Calnan M, Wall B. Doctors as patients: Postal survey examining consultants and general practitioners adherence to guidelines. *BMJ* 1999; 319: 605–8.

20. Office of Population Censuses and Surveys. *Occupational Health Decennial Supplement for England and Wales*. HMSO, London 1995.

21. Lindeman S, Laara E, Hakko H, Lonnqvist J. A systematic review on gender-specific suicide mortality in medical doctors. *Br J Psych* 1996; 168: 274–9.

22. Hawton K, Clements A, Sakarovitch C, Simkin S, Deeks JJ. Suicide in doctors: A study of risk according to gender, seniority and specialty in medical practitioners in England and Wales, 1979–1995. *Journal of Epidemiol Community Health* 2001; 55: 296–300.

23. Sakinhofsky I. Suicide in doctors and their wives. *BMJ* 1980; 281: 386–7.

24. Howie J, Porter A, Heaney D, Hopton J. Long to short consultation ratio: A proxy measure of quality of care for general practice. *Br J Gen Pract* 1991; 41: 48–54.

25. McManus IC, Winder BC, Gordon D. The causal links between stress and burnout in a longitudinal study of UK doctors. *Lancet* 2002; 359: 2089–90.

26. Huby G, Gerry M, McKinstry B, Porter M, Shaw J, Wrate R. Morale among general practitioners: Qualitative study exploring relations between partnership arrangements, personal style, and workload. *BMJ* 2002; 325:140–4.

27. Spurgeon P, Barwell F, Maxwell R. Types of work stress and implications for the role of general practitioners. *Health Serv Manag Res* 1995; 8(3): 186–97.

28. Hayter P, Peckham S, Robinson R. *Morale in General Practice*. University of Southampton: Institute for Health Policy Studies 1996.

29. Edwards N, Kornacki MJ, Silversin J. Unhappy doctors: What are the causes and what can be done? *BMJ* 2002; 324: 835–8.

30. Cabinet Office. *Monitoring Satisfaction: Trends from 1998–2002*. Cabinet Office, London 2002.

31. Edwards N, Kornacki MJ, Silversin J. Unhappy doctors: What are the causes and what can be done? *BMJ* 2002; 324: 835–8.

32. Chambers R, Davies M. *What Stress in Primary Care!* Royal College of General Practitioners, London, 1999.

33. Cox T. *Stress research and stress management: Putting theory to work*. HSE Contract Research Report No 61/1993. Suffolk: Health and Safety Executive, 1993.

34. Mechanic D. Practice orientations among general medical practitioners in England and Wales. *Med Care* 1970; 8: 15–25.

35. Grol R, Mokkink H, Smits A, Van Eijk J, Beek M, Mesker P, Mesker-Niesten J. Work satisfaction of general practitioners and the quality of patient care. *Fam Pract* 1985; 2(3): 128–35.

36. Firth Cozens J. Predicting stress in general practitioners: 10 year follow-up postal survey. *BMJ* 1997; 315: 34–5.

37. Stirling AM, Wilson P, McConnachie A. Deprivation, psychological distress, and consultation length in general practice. *Br J Gener Pract* 2001; 51(467): 456–60.

38. Mercer SW, Watt GC. The inverse care law: Clinical primary care encounters in deprived and affluent areas of Scotland. *Ann Fam Med* 2007; 5(6): 503–10.

39. Unknown author.

20

Medical Advocacy: The Duty of Physicians as Advocates

JESSICA LEE

We are pushed towards a creeping sense of inevitability and assumed hopelessness.

The role of a physician is not easily defined. Certainly, we may readily list key elements: we diagnose, we prescribe, we aim to reduce suffering. Or we may appeal to values we ascribe to ourselves, such as professionalism, integrity, and empathy. However, such elements and values are not unique to our trade; they pertain to many other professions, both in health and otherwise.

Perhaps the simplest way for UK medics to outline our responsibilities is to turn to the duties expected of us by the General Medical Council. Although we are encouraged to neatly fit their mould, the duties have breadth in their brush-strokes. They leave room for a variety of personal motivations and health perspectives, provided we keep the care of our patients as our first concern; we take action wherever this is compromised, and we promote and protect health [1]. These duties ask us to be our patients' advocate and fulfil the social contract which exists between society and medicine, with society expecting from us the services of a healer. The WHO states that medical training has an obligation to,

'direct education, research and service activities towards addressing the priority health concerns of the community, region and/or nation that they have a mandate to serve'. [2]

Somewhere between our outlined responsibilities and daily practice this social contract of medicine gets lost. The slow unravelling begins early on. Medicine's mainstream curriculum teaches us what pills to prescribe and procedures to perform, whilst its hidden curriculum encourages us to value hierarchy, refrain from social or institutional critique and to avoid taking action on social determinants of health [3, 4]. It is well known that poverty causes ill health, and yet socioeconomic inequities tend to be overlooked throughout our training [5]. We learn to focus narrowly on treatment as medical management, rather than develop a wider, interrogative vista of the treatment of our patients by society. It is not surprising that collectively we then fail to recognise that the narrative of illness is far from a tale of behavioural and biological inevitability, but rather a symptom of a pathological system [6]. And so, we tend to focus on trying to change personal behaviour, rather than social circumstance, thereby artificially limiting our role.

The result is a physician poorly prepared for the complexity they face on the front line of medicine, where we find what is emphasised to us through single-best-answer scenarios in training leaves us firefighting in practice. In the face of this nihilism, time tends to push practitioners towards a creeping sense of inevitability and assumed hopelessness [7].

Learned helplessness in the face of poverty and its associated scarcity may be contagious, but it is a luxury that *we* can afford. The scarcity is not for ourselves, but for others. However, we *can* choose to reject it, by recognising the way we view sickness and its determinants is itself socially determined, and thus *may* be changed [8]. When we remember medicine's social contract, we recall that our professional duty to treat the sick, and promote and protect health, naturally includes *all* sick. To be poor does not mean to be less worthy of opportunity or good health. In our care of patients and their illnesses it therefore clearly falls within our role to identify, explore, and challenge the inequities which contribute to this sickness burden.

To advocate for a patient simply means to speak up for them. Advocacy prevents social passivity, curtails those feelings of helplessness and influences decision-making. It recognises that we create our culture and set our norms. We *can* influence resource allocation, and it is certainly within our competence and expertise to recognise, highlight and act upon health injustices. In fact, as physicians, we are uniquely placed to bear witness and facilitate a response. The Irish Medical Organisation identifies advocacy as one of the most important duties of a physician: not only to provide the best possible care, but also to do whatever one can for patients in the interests of their health [9]. Advocacy for equity is the perfect outlet for a frustrated physician, who, armed only with ten minutes and a potion packet, must hold back a tide of social sorrows.

Advocacy works. It has successfully ensured vaccination programmes, motor-vehicle safety, safer workplaces, control of infectious diseases, declines in deaths from coronary heart disease and stroke, safer and healthier foods, healthier mothers and babies, family planning, abortion, fluoridation of drinking water and recognition of tobacco use as a health hazard [10]. Considering the magnitude of issues tackled, it does not seem unreasonable to think that through advocacy real progress can be made for patients who are proportionally disadvantaged.

We know actions of advocacy do not need to be large. They might involve helping patients to better

access services or representing them in their dealings with other agencies (local housing authorities, the justice system, loan companies, financial institutions) [9]. Or it might mean creating a collective voice to raise a larger clamour and evoke widespread system change, such as the Deep End movement. Whatever the size of the action, perhaps the most important focus for change should be medical education and the knowledge that what we are teaching our students creates their perception of their role for the future.

Advocacy that articulates goals alone seldom attracts dissent. Contention arises when advocacy spells out strategies to achieve an end [11]; few people would publically disagree that early deaths for persons of lower income are tragic, but many may oppose potential solutions, such as the greater allocation of resources to these groups, or may wonder whether their plight is worthy of time in a medical curriculum. Understanding the unfortunate hypocrisy in this hostility should help us better confront it. The inevitable hostility at the start of real change may be unsettling, but it should be endured nevertheless.

It is worth remembering, despite a recent trend towards widening inequities, that it is less than 100 years since the National Health Service was created through advocacy and receptive leadership to ensure that everyone, regardless of their means, had access to health care. Those involved faced significant opposition from many groups, including the British Medical Association and several wealthy hospitals. Yet they were successful – with clear goals, sound arguments, and collective power, change may be achieved.

SUGGESTIONS FOR PRACTICE

- *A general practitioner, at the end of a long consultation about a patient's deteriorating mental health and feelings of hopelessness, may call the housing authority to stop the patient and their family from being evicted. This involvement is warranted if, as is so often the case, the eviction notice had come as a result of their late rent payments, which were caused by a delay in their universal credits payments, which they had been dependent on since the patient became unwell.*
- *A hospital doctor may contact and follow up with, various community services to ensure a regular attendee, who is homeless, is not*

discharged to the street, and gets access to the holistic care he/she requires. The doctor could then work to create local pathways to allow these actions to be replicated.

- A GP surgery could employ practitioners (e.g. focused care practitioners) to help with patients' unmet social needs, which is often something GPs struggle to address during consultations.
- Practitioners supporting medical education initiatives, such as elective components to the curriculum, medical societies, lectures, and research, which allow students exposure to the wider role of a physician.
- Health professionals engaging with third-sector and political organisations to promote wider system change and act upon social determinants of health.
- Physicians undertaking translational, cross-sectoral research that looks to highlight examples of structural violence, and to offer evidence-based solutions.
- Clinicians engaging with policy and resource allocation at every level whilst being conscious of their social contract.

REFERENCES

1. The General Medical Council. *Duties of a doctor* [Internet]. Good Medical Practice. 2019 [cited 2019 May 19]. Available from: https://www.gmc-uk.org/ethical-guidance/ethical-guidance-for-doctors/good-medical-practice/duties-of-a-doctor
2. Division of Development of Human Resources for Health. *Defining and Measuring the Social Accountability of Medical Schools*. Geneva, Switzerland; 1995.
3. Hafferty FW. Beyond curriculum reform: confronting medicine's hidden curriculum. *Acad Med*. 1998;73(4):403–7.
4. DasGupta S, Fornari A, Geer K, Hahn L, Kumar V, Lee HJ et al. Medical education for social justice: Paulo Freire revisited. *J Med Humanit*. 2006;27(4):245–51.
5. Marmot M. Health in an unequal world: Social circumstances, biology and disease. *Lancet*. 2006:2081–94.
6. De Pallok K, Maio F, Ansell DA. Structural racism — A 60-year-old black woman with breast cancer. *N Engl J Med*. 2019;380(16):1489–93.
7. Tomlinson J. Medical advocacy [Internet]. A Better NHS. 2012. Available from: https://abetternhs.wordpress.com/2012/08/18/medical-advocacy/
8. Powell A. Harvard's Paul Farmer on traveling the world to fight inequality in health – Harvard Gazette [Internet]. *Harvard Gazette*. 2018 [cited 2019 May 19]. Available from: https://news.harvard.edu/gazette/story/2018/05/harvards-paul-farmer-on-traveling-the-world-to-fight-inequality-in-health/
9. Irish Medical Organisation. *The Doctor as Advocate*. Irish Medical Organisation: Dublin; 2013.
10. CDC. Ten Great Public Health Achievements – United States, 1900–1999 [Internet]. *Morbidity and Mortality Weekly Report*. 1999 [cited 2019 May 19]. Available from: https://www.cdc.gov/mmwr/preview/mmwrhtml/00056796.htm
11. Chapman S. When is advocacy for change justified? *Int J Epidemiol*. 2001;30:1226–32.

PART 3

Populations and Groups

21

Child Health

JESSICA KEEBLE

A person's a person, no matter how small [1].

'Disadvantage starts before birth and accumulates through life...action to reduce health inequalities must start before birth and be followed through the life of the child. Giving every child the best start in life...is our highest priority recommendation' [2].

Child health is important not only for a child's current situation, but also for their long-term health and life outcome. The rate of child poverty in the UK in 2016 was 12% [3]. The need to address this was recognised by the UK government, who published the Every Child Matters green paper in 2003 [4]. This outlined plans to help every child have the support they need to achieve five key outcomes: be healthy, stay safe, enjoy and achieve, make a positive contribution and achieve economic well-being.

HOW IS CHILD HEALTH AND INEQUALITY MEASURED?

Measures of child health begin before birth, as the health and well-being of the mother is critical to the development of the child [2].

Teenage pregnancy rates are higher in deprived areas. Teenage pregnancies increase the risk of smoking during pregnancy, low birth weight, infant mortality, impaired maternal education and consequent further socioeconomic disadvantages [5].

Low birthweight at full term of pregnancy is an important public health measure as it indicates whether the baby was able to grow as expected while in the uterus and is a predictor of poorer long-term health and educational outcomes [6]. Between 2014 and 2016, 3.9% of live births in the most deprived areas were classified as low birthweight, compared to 2.0% in the least deprived areas [5].

Neonatal and infant mortality are also important markers of child health. The UN sustainable development goals include a target to end preventable deaths of newborns by 2030, with neonatal mortality (deaths under 28 days) at least as low as 12 per 1,000 live births [7]. In England and Wales, the 2016 infant mortality rate (deaths under 1 year) was 3.8 deaths per 1,000 births, and the neonatal mortality was 2.7 deaths per 1,000 births. Whilst this is well within the UN sustainable development goal, it hides inequality linked to deprivation. The most deprived areas of England had an infant mortality rate over twice that of the least deprived areas [8].

School readiness, measured between reception and year 1, can be seen as a rounded assessment of early physical, behavioural, cognitive and social development, as well as a social determinant of future health, as children who are ready for school are able to maximise their learning opportunities. Again, the data indicates this varies with deprivation. In 2016–2017, only 56% of children eligible for free school meals (due to low household income) were found to be ready for school, compared to 73% of children not eligible for free school meals [9].

Morbidity is also increased by socioeconomic deprivation, as illustrated by a study looking at data from the UK *Millennium Cohort Study*. Poor mental well-being, being overweight, long-standing illness, unintentional injuries and asthma, all increase with decreasing income [10].

CAUSES, CONSEQUENCES AND POTENTIAL SOLUTIONS FOR CHILD HEALTH INEQUALITY

The Marmot review found evidence that the conditions in which people find themselves, particularly in early childhood, are responsible for health inequalities [2]. The clear association between deprivation and child health means it is important to understand the environment in which the child is living. A method for understanding this is through the social determinants of child health [10]. This places the child at the centre, encompassed most closely by parenting and model healthy behaviour, then the physical, mental health and behaviours of parents and carers, household resources, community characteristics, living and working conditions and finally the socioeconomic, cultural, commercial, political and physical climate.

Deprivation is an unequal variation in the social determinants of child health. Changing child health outcomes requires an understanding of why this variation in the social determinants of child health exists. This may involve material, behavioural and psychosocial factors, but is often ultimately dependent on structural social determinants of health.

MATERIAL CAUSES

As an example, childhood obesity is associated with deprivation. Children who were overweight or obese in reception year (aged 4 to 5 years) were more likely to be overweight or obese in year 6 (aged 10 to 11 years) and then again more likely to go on to be overweight or obese adults, increasing mortality and morbidity in adulthood [5].

Low household income prevents parents from being able to provide a healthy diet. There is evidence for this. The government has published guidance about a healthy diet, known as the *Eat Well Guide* [11]. The poorest would have to spend 42% of their disposable income after housing to meet the costs. Initiatives such as the Healthy Start programme (for pregnant women and children under four) and free school meals are not universal, creating problems for those just above the threshold [12]. Children who do benefit from free school meals do not benefit from them during school holidays, and government measures to address this rely on third sector organisations, where reach may be haphazard [13].

BEHAVIOURAL CAUSES

An intervention which contributed to reduced child obesity rates in Leeds is the HENRY Approach. This works with 0–5-year-old children and their families, and focuses on parenting, family lifestyle habits, nutrition, activity and emotional well-being. It teaches authoritative parenting rather than authoritarian or permissive parenting [14].

The importance of parenting behaviour on child health is illustrated by the success of this. Other aspects of parental behaviour can have very significant effects on child health, from smoking in pregnancy [5] to child abuse. Analysis of serious case reviews highlight that in combination domestic violence, substance misuse and parental mental health problems are particularly toxic [15].

This links with research into adverse childhood experiences (ACEs): stressful events occurring in childhood have been shown to adversely affect adult health. The definition of ACE is varied and has expanded from the original research to include elements of socioeconomic deprivation as well as threats such as witnessing or experiencing abuse [16]. It is thought that threat and deprivation result in differing neurodevelopmental pathways [17]. Whilst early identification and appropriate intervention for ACEs is vital [18], modifiable socioeconomic inequalities should not be overlooked [19].

PSYCHOSOCIAL CAUSES

The attribution of health inequalities to behavioural factors risks absolving all but the disadvantaged themselves. It also falls short of addressing what might be underlying health behaviours. Feelings of inferiority caused by inequality, and the consequent lack of control have been shown to change physical and mental health. In addition to this, the stressors associated with disadvantage influence health behaviours. Overcoming this requires robust social support systems [10].

CASE STUDY

Shahida

Shahida, a mother of two, came to England in 2018 to escape her abusive husband. Together they had sought asylum in another European country, where she and her children experienced bullying, racism and discrimination.

On arriving in Bradford with her children, she felt 'very depressed, anxious, lost and alone'. She registered with a GP, who completed full medical health checks. 'The GP was very considerate and kind, it was like talking to a friend you can trust'. She was referred for counselling and to the well-being centre attached to the surgery where she saw the social prescriber. Her financial difficulties were addressed by an application to a local crisis fund, she has been supported in her asylum application and she was invited to participate in a recovery group for women survivors of abuse. 'I have no words for how much the Butterfly Project has helped me. It is not just about art, it has helped me become a better human and to stand on my own feet. It has made me a strong tree that is giving shelter and safety to my children. Before I was like a weak plant that was struggling to survive'.

Shahida confirmed that her mental health, confidence and self-esteem have improved significantly since arriving in Bradford. She identified that she is able to concentrate more, make better decisions and voice her opinions. She feels stronger, is worrying less and learning to live in the present. Her relationship with her children has improved and she feels she is a better mother and her children better children now. 'Bevan Wellbeing Centre has held us, made us feel safe and whole again. We were not complete when we arrived here, they have treated us with humanity and respect. Their sincerity, purity of heart and how much they want to help you can be seen in their eyes, it radiates from them and is contagious. They are perfect role models for what a human can be. They fill us up with so much hope for tomorrow'.

STRUCTURAL CAUSES

The structural social determinants of child health include the socioeconomic, political, cultural and community factors which determine access to employment, health services, education, housing and welfare. As the most powerful determinants of health inequality, it is important for clinicians to understand their impact, even though they may be more challenging to change.

Research into data from the *Millennium Cohort Study* looked at events which moved children into or out of poverty. The most important of these is gain or loss of household employment. Key factors made this harder, such as lone parenthood, larger numbers of children, disability of an adult and lower parental education [20].

A 2006 review commissioned by Shelter [21] thoroughly explores the impact of homelessness on child health. It explores the impact of homelessness (families placed in temporary accommodation by local authorities), overcrowding (e.g. when bedrooms are shared by different sex children over 10, by parents and children or by more than two children, and when living rooms or kitchens are used as bedrooms) and poor conditions or unfitness (needing substantial repairs, lacking in modern facilities or damp, cold and infested).

The review found evidence of how the 5 key outcomes stated in Every Child Matters are all impaired by homelessness [21]:

1. **Be Healthy**: Homeless children are 3–4 times more likely to have mental health problems. Overcrowding increases the risk of childhood meningitis, and poor home conditions (damp and mould) triple the risk of cough and wheeze.
2. **Stay Safe**: Almost half of all accidents involving children are related to physical conditions in and around the home. Families living in poor conditions are more likely to experience a domestic fire and less likely to own a smoke alarm.
3. **Enjoy and Achieve**: Homeless children are 2–3 times more likely to be absent from school, may change schools frequently and have lower levels of academic achievement. Overcrowding and poor-quality housing also affect school attendance.

4. **Make a Positive Contribution**: Aggression, hyperactivity and impulsivity are more common in homeless children and a significant proportion of young offenders have experienced homelessness.

5. **Achieve Economic Well-being**: Poor education and health outcomes associated with homelessness disadvantage future employment opportunities.

LIFE COURSE APPROACH

The many causes and consequences of health inequalities are not isolated but linked in complex cycles. Structural social determinants of health result in social stratification, which determine the socioeconomic circumstances of an individual. This results in differential exposure to material, psychosocial and behavioural health risk factors. These factors and the differential vulnerability caused by poor socioeconomic circumstances, influence child health directly and indirectly via parental health. This leads to social consequences and can be amplified by differential consequences. These consequences contribute to structural determinants.

For instance, a woman and child who entered the UK on a marriage visa but sought asylum because of domestic abuse from her partner are likely to be placed in poor-quality overcrowded housing with minimal benefits. The mother may already be psychosocially disempowered by the abuse from her partner and have a limited understanding and capability of how to access health or well-being services. The poor housing may put her child at risk of increased respiratory morbidity, increased risk of accidents and increased mental health and behavioural difficulties. The ability of the mother to cope with this may be limited by her pre-existing challenges and make it more difficult for her to access services on offer such as language lessons. She may therefore find it harder to access employment when and if her refugee status is granted.

Health inequalities can be reduced by modification of the effect of social stratification, through means such as employment, education and welfare systems. Modification of differential exposure includes universal programmes such as screening and immunisation, and the Healthy Child programme (free healthcare for children aged 0–19 through health visitors and school nurses).

Children's centres have been developed to modify differential vulnerability. Modification of the differential consequences of ill health occurs through welfare systems and parental workers rights [10].

The principle of proportionate universalism [2] recognises the value in providing services for all with a scale and intensity that is proportionate to the level of disadvantage. Health visiting and school nursing services are designed to focus on high impact aspects, such as transition to parenthood and the early weeks of pregnancy, maternal mental health, healthy weight and nutrition, resilience and emotional well-being and keeping safe. These are particularly relevant to deprived populations, and seek to directly address the causes of health inequality. Local government funded public health services have, however, recently been adversely affected by austerity measures [22].

More recently, children's centres were introduced to support the most deprived.

A government report published in 2015 found that these improved child, mother and household health outcomes, especially in centres that were maintaining or increasing services rather than experiencing cuts and restructuring [23]. Sadly, the number of children's centres has reduced since 2010 [24], in greater quantities than the government has admitted [25].

WHAT CAN BE DONE IN PRACTICE?

Pearce et al [10] suggest three ways that clinicians can impact child health inequality:

1. Understand the material, psychosocial or behavioural barriers to health that parents and children may be facing and consider possible solutions.

SUGGESTIONS FOR PRACTICE

Consider the following questions:

- *Do you know where to signpost people for benefits advice?*
- *Is there a food bank that your patients might be able to use?*
- *What parenting programmes are available locally?*
- *What services are offered by the local children's centre?*

- *What is the best way of helping this person access psychological support?*
- *How can I help my colleagues, students and trainees to understand this better?*
    2. Generate evidence of good practice and effectiveness. The NHS Long Term Plan requires proposed health programmes to state how they reduce health inequality and advocate within the NHS and wider government sectors [26].

SUGGESTIONS FOR PRACTICE

Consider the following:

- *Could you involve 'experts by experience' in service planning and evaluation?*
- *What data could you collect to investigate child health inequalities in your area?*
- *How could you disseminate examples of your good practice?*
    3. Advocate for child health equality within the NHS and in other government sectors [27].

SUGGESTIONS FOR PRACTICE

- *Consider where you have influence.*
- *Consider where you could have influence.*

CASE STUDY

Parveen

Parveen presented in a state of crisis. Her husband had recently left her to marry another woman and she'd just discovered that he had not been paying the rent on their home. Her landlord told her that she had to leave the property in a few days' time, which would result in Parveen and her three young children being made homeless.

She'd also been a victim of domestic abuse. As well as being hit physically by her husband over many years, he had complete control of the finances and had just given Parveen a small weekly allowance for food. This resulted in Parveen having no knowledge or skills with which to manage finances.

Her immediate issue of facing homelessness was addressed by professionals who advocated on her behalf with the landlord. This resulted in her eviction notice being revoked. Parveen was then signposted to a Benefits Adviser who supported her in applying for welfare benefits and explained the basics of managing finance, including the bills she would have to pay. It quickly became evident that her ex-husband had failed to pay the rent for a significant period of time, resulting in many months of arrears. A local faith-based crisis fund was able to meet this cost, setting Parveen free from debt.

In terms of Parveen's emotional needs and the impact the abuse had inevitably had on her, she was referred to local domestic abuse services for further support. She also participated in a creative recovery group for women survivors of abuse. Parveen is a very different woman now to the one who presented to us in crisis. Her smile is contagious, she is managing her home and family well and is providing a safe, secure and happy environment for her children to grow.

REFERENCES

1. Dr. Seuss. *Horton Hears a Who*. London: Harper Collins; 2012 (Original work published 1954).
2. Strategic Review of Health Inequalities in England post-2010. *Fair society, healthier lives: The Marmot review*. 2010. Available from: http://www.instituteofhealthequity.org/resources-reports/fair-society-healthy-lives-the-marmot-review/fair-society-healthy-lives-the-marmot-review-full-report.pdf [Accessed 12th May 2019].
3. Organisation for Economic Co-operation and Development. Compare your country: Income distribution and poverty: poverty by age. Available from: https://www1.compareyourcountry.org/inequality/en/1/316/default [Accessed 25th May 2019].
4. HM Treasury. Every child matters. 2003. Available from: https://assets.publishing.service.gov.uk/government/uploads/system/uploads/attachment_data/file/272064/5860.pdf [Accessed 13th May 019].
5. Public Health England. Health of children in the early years. *Health profile for England: 2018*. Available from: https://www.gov.uk/government/publications/

health-profile-for-england-2018/chapter-4-health-of-children-in-the-early-years [Accessed 3rd April 2019].

6. Jefferis B, Power C, Hertzman C. Birth weight, childhood socioeconomic environment, and cognitive development in the 1958 British birth cohort study. *BMJ*. 2002;325(7359): 305–305.

7. United Nations. Sustainable development goals. Available from: https://www.un.org/sustainabledevelopment/health [Accessed 13th May 2019].

8. Office for National Statistics. *Child and infant mortality in England and Wales: 2016*. Available from: https://www.ons.gov.uk/peoplepopulationandcommunity/birthsdeathsandmarriages/deaths/bulletins/childhoodinfantandperinatalmortality-inenglandandwales/2016 [Accessed 24th May 2019].

9. Public Health England. Wider determinants of health. *Health profile for England: 2018*. Available from: https://www.gov.uk/government/publications/health-profile-for-england-2018/chapter-6-wider-determinants-of-health [Accessed 3rd April 2019].

10. Pearce A, Dundas R, Whitehead M, Taylor- Robinson D. Pathways to inequalities in child health. *Archives of Disease in Childhood* [Preprint] 2019. Available from: doi: 10.1136/archdischild-2018-314808 [Accessed 8th April 2019].

11. Public Health England. *The Eatwell Guide*. 2016. Available from: https://www.gov.uk/government/publications/the-eatwell-guide [Accessed 13th May 2019].

12. Scott C, Sutherland J, Taylor A. Affordability of the UK's Eatwell Guide. Available from: https://foodfoundation.org.uk/wp-content/uploads/2018/09/Affordability-of-the-Eatwell-Guide_Final_Web-Version.pdf [Accessed 5th April 2019].

13. Henshaw C. DfE to expand programme targeting holiday hunger. Available from: https://www.tes.com/news/dfe-expand-programme-targeting-holiday-hunger [Accessed 13th May 2019].

14. Thornton J. What's behind reduced child obesity in Leeds? *BMJ*. 2019;365:l2045. Available from: doi: 10.1136/bmj.l2045 [Accessed 27th May 2019].

15. Brandon M, Bailey S, Belderson P. Building on the learning from serious case reviews: A two-year analysis of child protection database. Department for Education. 2007. Available from: https://www.gov.uk/government/publications/building-on-the-learning-from-serious-case-reviews-a-2-year-analysis-of-child-protection-database-notifications-2007-to-2009 [Accessed 2nd April 2019].

16. Taylor-Robinson D, Straatmann V, Whitehead M. Adverse childhood experiences or adverse childhood socioeconomic conditions? *The Lancet Public Health*. 2018:3(6):e262–e263.

17. McLaughlin K, Sheridan M, Lambert H. Childhood adversity and neural development: Deprivation and threat as distinct dimensions of early experience. *Neuroscience and Biobehavioral Reviews*. 2014;47:578–91. Available from: doi: 10.1016/j.neubiorev.2014.10.012

18. Paranjothy S, Evans A, Bandyopadhyay A, Fone D, Schofield B, John A, Bellis M, Lyons R, Farewell D, Long S. Risk of emergency hospital admission in children associated with mental disorders and alcohol misuse in the household: an electronic birth cohort study. *The Lancet Public Health*. 2018:3(6): e279–e288.

19. Straatmann V, Whitehead M, Taylor-Robinson D. RF31 Adverse childhood experiences or adverse socio-economic conditions? Assessing impacts on adolescent mental health in the UK Millennium Cohort Study. *BMJ*. 2018: A57.1–A57.

20. Barnes, M., Lord, C. and Chanfreau, J. *Child poverty transitions: Exploring the routes into and out of poverty 2009 to 2012*. UK: Department for Work and Pensions. 2015. Available from: http://openaccess.city.ac.uk/14349/1/Barnes%20et%20al%20%282015%29%20rr900%20child%20poverty%20transitions.pdf [Accessed 20th May 2019].

21. Harker L. Chance of a lifetime: The impact of housing on children's lives. *Shelter*. 2006. Available from: http://england.shelter.org.uk/professional_resources/policy_library/ policy_library_folder/chance_of_a_ lifetime_-_the_impact_of_bad_housing_on_childrens_lives.

https://england.shelter.org.uk/__data/assets/pdf_file/0016/39202/Chance_of_a_Lifetime.pdf [Accessed 13th May 2019].

22. Buck D. Local government spending on public health: death by a thousand cuts. Available from: https://www.kingsfund.org.uk/blog/2018/01/local-government-spending-public-health-cuts [Accessed 4th April 2019].

23. Sammoons P, Hall J, Smees R, Goff J, Sylva K, Smith T, Evangelou M, Eisenstadt N, Smith G. The impact of children's centres: studying the effects of children's centres in promoting better outcomes for young children and their families. Department for Education. 2015. Available from: https://assets.publishing.service.gov.uk/government/uploads/system/uploads/attachment_data/file/485347/DFE-RB495_Evaluation_of_children_s_centres_in_England__the_impact_of_children_s_centres_brief.pdf [Accessed 7th April 2019].

24. Department for Education. Number of children's centres by local authority. Available from: https://www.gov.uk/government/news/number-of-childrens-centres-by-local-authority [Accessed 7th April 2019].

25. Smith G, Sylva K, Sammons P, Smith T, Omonigho A. Stop Start: Survival, decline or closure? Children's Centres in England, 2018. The Sutton Trust. 2018. Available from: https://www.suttontrust.com/wp-content/uploads/2018/04/StopStart-FINAL.pdf [Accessed 7th April 2019].

26. NHS England. *The NHS Long Term Plan*. 2019. Available from: https://www.longterm-plan.nhs.uk/wp-content/uploads/2019/01/nhs-long-term-plan.pdf [Accessed 20th May 2019].

27. Weil L, Lemer C, Webb E, Hargreaves D. The voices of children and young people in health: Where are we now? *Archives of Disease in Childhood*. 2015;100(10):915–917.

22

Tackling Health Inequalities in Adolescence

MARIAN DAVIS

Despite the potential added difficulties, adolescents have, on average, two minutes less per consultation than adults.

Adolescence is a relatively modern construct. Traditionally, childhood was the period before puberty, before fertility. Children as young as 12 were expected to work as adults; this is still the case in many parts of the world. Over the last hundred years in the UK and other developed countries, societal changes and new regulations about education and employment have led to a different view. The median age for onset of puberty, marking the start of adolescence, is getting earlier. At the same time, there has been a blurring of the measures by which the end of adolescence and entry into adulthood is marked. Increasing access to further education and a delay in achieving financial independence has led to a widening gap between physical maturity and full independence. Adolescence can be thought of as the years from 10–18 and young adulthood as 19–24.

In recent years there has been an increase in understanding about the distinct characteristics of this age group physiologically, developmentally and societally.

Advances in knowledge about brain development have revealed that the brain continues to change during adolescence and young adulthood [1]. The prefrontal cortex, responsible for the development of abstract thinking, the ability to consider alternative views and the consequences of actions, develops up until the age of 25. In contrast, the limbic system, responsible for pleasure-seeking behaviours with immediate reward, peaks at age 16–18. This may go some way to explain adolescent risk-taking behaviours and the impact of peer pressure.

During adolescence, young people start to make independent decisions about music, fashion, friendships, employment or study and health behaviours. It is a crucial period for education and life chances; not participating fully in classes or having time off school with illness can have a long-term impact on those chances. Health behaviours adopted now, including smoking, use of alcohol, dietary choice and sexual behaviours are likely to continue into adulthood and can be a significant factor in the development of conditions such as type II diabetes, cardiovascular disease and cancer.

Western society frequently has a confused approach to these years. This is typified by some of the anomalies in the law: a young person can have consensual sex and join the army at 16 but is unable to vote, buy alcohol or cigarettes, or get married without parental consent until they are eighteen. Yet the age of criminal responsibility is

10 years in England, Wales and Northern Ireland, and 12 in Scotland.

These factors have brought about a change in approach. The years between 10 and 25, adolescence and young adulthood, are now recognised as a unique period, between being dependent on others to being an autonomous, fully mature adult. This has informed policy-making at a national level with an increasing focus on this age group in the NHS 10-year plan [2].

HEALTH INEQUALITIES IN ADOLESCENCE

Some of these differences are biological in origin or are a matter of choice; others arise as a result of external factors – social determinants [3].

Adolescence/young adulthood is a vital developmental stage, involving physical, psychological and behavioural changes. Health inequalities therefore impact heavily on this age group, particularly in terms of money and resources, living conditions, family, peers and social groups, education and worklessness [4]. There is a particular vulnerability associated with transitions such as leaving home.

Income inequality is a key structural social determinant which particularly impacts on this age group. Young people are disproportionately represented in the poorest households and the situation is getting worse. The percentage of young people living in households with less than 60% of the UK's median income increased from 19% to 25 % between 2008 and 2015 [5].

Nearly all health outcomes are worse for young people living in the most deprived areas compared with the least deprived. Obesity rates amongst 10- and 11-year-olds are twice as high, (Figure 22.1), 10- to 14-year-old pedestrians are 3.7 times more likely to be killed or seriously injured on the roads,15-year-olds are twice as likely to be regular smokers, and the under-18 conception rate is twice as high [5].

A similar picture is seen with mental health. Figure 22.2 shows the percentage of 11-year-olds with severe mental health problems by quintile of income [5]. This disparity is confirmed by a 2017 survey; young people aged 11–16 living in households in receipt of welfare benefits were twice as likely to have a diagnosable mental health disorder [6]. This has long-term implications because 50% of long-term adult mental health problems have presented by the age of 14 and 75% by the age of 25 [7].

In addition to socioeconomic deprivation, other factors are associated with poorer outcomes. Young people at particular risk include those who are LGBTQ, young carers, black and ethnic minorities, refugees, those who are in the justice system or not in education or training and those who live in care.

It is well documented that looked-after children and young people have poor health while they are in care and poor outcomes when they leave care [8]:

- 50% of young people in care have a diagnosable mental health disorder compared with 1 in 10 of their peers.
- When they leave care, they are five times more likely to commit suicide than others.

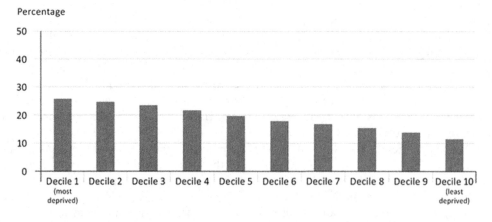

Figure 22.1 Percentage of 10–11-year-olds who are obese shown by decile of income.

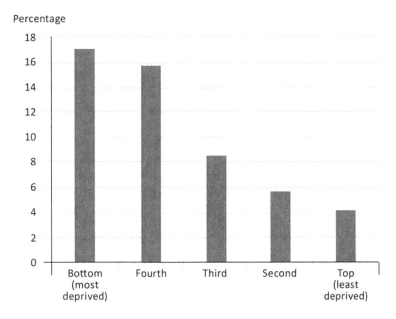

Figure 22.2 Percentage of 11-year-olds with severe mental health problems by quintile of income.

- 23% of all adults in prison and 40% of prisoners under 21 have been in care.
- 33% of care-leavers experience homelessness at some point within 2 years of leaving care.
- 25% of young women become teenage parents or pregnant within 1 year of leaving care, almost 50% within 2 years. (Of course, for some this may be a positive).
- Young people interviewed a year after leaving care are almost twice as likely to have problems with drugs or alcohol.

Young people often face multiple inequalities; the effect of combining these is both complex and additive. This is illustrated by looking at attendance in primary care. Attendance rates of 11–15-year-olds are significantly lower amongst those from the most deprived families (77%) compared with the least deprived (84%) and satisfaction rates are lower; with young people less likely to feel respected, to feel at ease or to be able to discuss personal matters [9]. Contributing factors include availability and accessibility of general practices in deprived areas, the young person and their family's ability to negotiate access to the healthcare system and higher rates of mental illness and psychological distress [10].

Health inequalities in this agegroup cannot be viewed in isolation but as part of a wider picture that includes education/employment, life chances, family relationships, influence of peers and long-term conditions. Indeed, young people themselves do not consider the various aspects of their lives in isolation. Their sense of health and well-being is derived from a multitude of factors including their relationships, mood, home situation and financial security. Living conditions, including type of neighbourhood and geographical location, are also important, e.g. injuries due to knife crime in some urban areas and difficulty of access to services in rural areas.

Health and well-being influence life chances including education, employment and relationships. In turn, life chances and choices affect health outcomes. This is illustrated by the wide-ranging consequences of living in care. It is only by a holistic approach addressing all these inequalities in our adolescents and young adults that the best health outcomes will be achieved.

The importance of highlighting the range of health inequalities that occur during these years is that many of the factors are amenable to change. Although adolescence is a period of vulnerability it also represents an opportunity to influence long-term health outcomes in a positive way, and the remainder of this chapter will focus on what we can do in primary care to achieve this.

CHANGING THE TRAJECTORY

Individual members of the primary care team have a limited ability to reduce inequalities at societal or even community level by improving employment and housing, or by sharing the nation's wealth more equitably. Clinicians, however, can make a difference to the lives of individuals by improving the quality of care offered to all our young patients and by helping them to make healthy choices.

This will involve action both within the individual consultation and at a practice level. Members of the primary healthcare team can also link with the community at various levels.

WITHIN THE CONSULTATION

Young people use primary care services more than is realised; 50% of 12–18-year-olds have visited their GP in the last 3 months. In the midst of a busy surgery, with many complex older patients with multiple morbidities, these are often the catch-up consultations –a young person presenting with a physical symptom and without the language to articulate the hidden agenda. Despite the potential added difficulty, adolescents have, on average, 2 minutes less per consultation than adults [11].

CASE STUDY

Archie

Archie, an 11-year-old boy attended the surgery in the company of his mum with an exacerbation of his asthma. The doctor spoke to him, with Mum chipping in where necessary. She showed him how to use the spacer and checked his understanding. At his review appointment a few weeks later, Archie took the lead in the consultation, reporting improvement in his symptoms. This fosters the development of skills necessary for self-management.

The foundation stone of primary care is the doctor/patient relationship. The GP or healthcare professional (HCP) has the potential to be a significant adult in the lives of some adolescents and young adults. They can start to develop a relationship from a very young age by addressing the child directly rather than talking over their heads to the parent. If the child is unable to describe their symptoms, the adult can answer. When developmentally appropriate, the child can speak for themselves.

SUGGESTIONS FOR PRACTICE

Practice Level

- *Include young people's opinions in practice surveys.*
- *Consider a patient information leaflet or web page specifically for young people.*
- *Train staff in dealing with young people.*
- *Consider use of technology and apps.*
- *Have a policy for transfer of patient records from parent to the young person.*
- *Provide internet access in waiting rooms with links to youth-friendly health websites.*
- *Consider providing outreach services – link with schools or local youth services.*
- *Advertise confidential services for all ages.*
- *Facilitate continuity of care with the same clinician.*
- *Take young people into consideration when planning waiting room design.*
- *Develop systems for seeking out hard-to-reach young people (e.g. young carers).*

Consultation Level

- *Encourage young people to start contributing to the consultation from a young age.*
- *Offer solo consultations, or part of consultation, to promote autonomy.*
- *Explain confidentiality (and its limitations) to parents and young people.*
- *Use the HEEADSSSSS assessment method to explore the psychosocial history.*
- *Give adequate time – don't cut it short.*
- *Facilitate return visits when needed.*
- *Ensure contact details are up to date to enable follow-up.*
- *Record vulnerabilities in the patient record.*
- *Develop rapport and trust over time.*
- *Facilitate transitions in healthcare.*

As the child gets older, say 12–14 years old, the GP can build into the routine consultation a couple of minutes at the end where the parent or carer leaves. This allows both parent and adolescent to get used to them consulting alone. Numerous studies have reported that confidentiality is the main concern for young people when they attend health services [12]. An explanation of what confidentiality means, together with its limitations, should be given before the parent leaves. Sometimes, the adolescent may have a concern that they wish to explore. This concern may be totally different to that of their parent. If there is nothing that they wish to discuss, the time can be used for health prevention topics or for giving information about what sort of problems, queries or concerns they can bring to the practice. This begins the process of the adolescent developing their own autonomous relationship with a clinician.

When an adolescent is seen alone, it is helpful to gain a picture of what their life is like. This can be done by having a conversation based around HEEADSSSSS [13]. This tool provides the headings for a psychosocial assessment of an adolescent or young adult – facilitating a conversation about

- Home
- Education
- Eating
- Activities
- Drugs
- Sexuality
- Sleep
- Screen use
- Safety
- Self-harm

It is always important to reinforce an assurance of confidentiality and its limitations at the start of every consultation. If this tool uncovers areas of concern such as inappropriate use of alcohol, give appropriate advice and arrange follow-up. A question about sleep is easy to ask and to answer but may lead to a conversation about anxiety or low mood or bullying. It might take a number of visits before the young person trusts the clinician enough to talk about the underlying problem. There is a need to be vigilant about safeguarding and act if there are concerns – ideally discussing the issue with the young person first.

CASE STUDY

Sarah

Sarah, aged 14, came to the surgery with her mother who was concerned that she might have anorexia. The GP saw Sarah by herself and having screened for an eating disorder arranged to review her in 2 weeks. At the second visit, Sarah was seen alone and told the doctor that she was struggling at school, not sleeping very well and feeling sad. The doctor assessed her safety and arranged further follow-up. At the third visit, Sarah told the doctor that a family friend had been behaving inappropriately and making her feel uncomfortable. The doctor explained to Sarah that this information needed to be shared and brought Mum in from the waiting room. Social services became involved. The problem was addressed and Sarah's depression resolved.

This illustrates the importance of seeing young people alone, in order to hear their story and understand that it can take time to gain trust.

Primary care has an important role in facilitating transitions – from the young person consulting in the company of parents or carers to consulting alone, to self-managing their long-term conditions such as asthma and diabetes, from paediatric to adult services and for young people entering employment and leaving home. In these and other situations, the clinician can be an advocate for adolescents or young adults.

CASE STUDY

Jake

Jake, a 17-year-old, came to the surgery with his father. He had been fired from his job as an apprentice the day before. His dad explained that Jake had ADHD but had stopped his medication a few months previously and disengaged from CAMHS. At first, Jake did not look out from under his cap – legs outstretched and arms firmly folded. The doctor suggested restarting his medication and re-referring him back to CAMHS and he agreed. She then offered to talk to the factory. They gave him his job back and he completed his apprenticeship.

This case study illustrates how a single intervention can be life-changing for a young person.

At Practice Level

Small-scale local studies about health services have identified that young care-leavers value supportive and friendly health professionals, would like to keep the same GP if possible and like the idea of young people's clinics [14]. Continuity of care is something that most patients will value. Yet changes in GP working practices and the increasing role of nurse practitioners, physician associates and paramedics mean that continuity of care can be harder to achieve [15]. The practice can develop systems to mitigate against this.

SUGGESTIONS FOR PRACTICE

- *Manage the transition from allowing parental access, to notes, to giving adolescents appropriate control. This should happen at an age which anticipates the need for privacy.*
- *Coding for vulnerabilities can ensure whichever HCP in the practice sees an adolescent or young adult there will be an alert to any concern or previous adverse childhood event.*
- *Deal with DNAs for both hospital and practice appointments and frequent attendance at A&E and out-of-hours services. These can be a red flag for adolescents and young adults with long-term conditions.*
- *Monitor repeat prescriptions in those who have long-term conditions – for example a high number of reliever versus preventer inhalers in patients with asthma.*
- *Record contact details for adolescent and young adult patients including mobile phone numbers and email. This will enable communication without involving parents.*
- *Seek out the hard-to-reach such as young carers.*
- *Train all practice staff in being youth-friendly and in confidentiality.*
- *Involve young people in the patient participation group and patient surveys.*
- *Communicate with the new GP when a young person with a long-term condition leaves home.*

In addition, a practice might establish services such as running a dedicated young person clinic or sending leaflets to young people and their parents on a particular birthday. They might develop the use of apps and other technology such as QR code access to the internet in the waiting room to communicate health information [16].

Adolescents and young adults require a holistic approach in order to achieve the best outcome. Health cannot be separated easily from other aspects of a young person's life such as education, family and housing. Ideally, healthcare provision will involve a team around the young person,

including school staff, social workers and parents working to the young person's agenda.

More generally, clinicians might go into local schools to deliver health education messages and to teach young people how to use primary care services appropriately. In some areas where access to the surgery is difficult, primary care clinics can be established within the school.

Health inequalities impact heavily on adolescents and young adults. They are frequent users of primary care and so the practice team has a vital role in reducing these inequalities, by taking action within the community, at practice level and within the consultation. They are a rewarding patient group to work with and clinicians have a vital role in facilitating the transition to consulting alone, promoting healthy behaviours, improving health literacy and fostering self-management of long-term conditions. There is enormous potential in primary care for changing the trajectory and consequences of health inequalities and optimising outcomes. Remember that a healthcare professional can be a significant adult in the life of a vulnerable young person and sometimes a single intervention can have life-changing consequences.

For further reading and resources, please see the RCGP Adolescent Health Group's webpage: https://www.rcgp.org.uk/clinical-and-research/resources/a-to-z-clinical-resources/youth-mental-health/the-rcgp-adolescent-health-group.aspx

REFERENCES

1. Blakemore S-J (2018) *Inventing Ourselves: The Secret Life of the Teenage Brain.* London: Doubleday.
2. NHS 10 year plan 2018 https://www.long-termplan.nhs.uk/
3. WHO Health Impact Assessment: Glossary https://www.who.int/hia/about/glos/en/index1.html
4. Hagell A, Shah R, Viner R, Hargreaves D, Varnes L, Heys M (2018) The Social Determinants of Young People's Health: Identifying the Key Issues and Assessing How Young People Are Doing in the 2010s. The Health Foundation.
5. Hagell A, Shah R, Coleman J (2017) *Key Data on Young People 2017.* London: Association for Young People's Health.

6. NHS Digital. Mental Health of Children and Young People 2017: Predictors of mental disorders https://files.digital.nhs.uk/85/7FFC57/MHCYP%202017%20Predictors.pdf

7. Kessler RC, Berglund P, Demler O, Jin R, Merikangas KR, Walters EE (2005) Lifetime prevalence and age of onset distributions of DSM-IV disorders in the National Co-morbidity Survey Replication. *Arch Gen Psych* 62(6):593–602.

8. Statutory Guidance on Promoting the Health and Well-being of Looked After Children. 2009 DCSF and DOH.

9. Yassaee AA, Hargreaves DS, Chester K et al. (2016) Experience of primary care services among early adolescents in England and association with health outcomes. *J Adolesc Health* 60:388–394.

10. Churchill RD (2017) Young people: Understanding the links between satisfaction with services and their health outcomes in primary care. *J Adolesc Health* 60:358–359.

11. Jacobson L, Wilkinson C, Owen P (1994). Is the potential of teenage consultations being missed?: a study of consultation times in primary care. *Fam Pract* 11:296–299. 10.1093/fampra/11.3.296.

12. Churchill RD, Allen J, Denman S et al. (2000) Do the attitudes and beliefs of young teenagers towards general practice influence actual consultation behaviour? *Br J Gen Pract* 50:953–957.

13. HEEADSSS http://m.appbuild.io/heeadsss

14. National Children's Bureau (2008) Promoting the health of young people leaving care. Healthy Care Briefing. www.ncb.org.uk/healthycare

15. Davis M (2018) Coding for Vulnerabilities in Adolescents. *Practice Management Magazine* September 2018.

16. Bright Idea Winner (2018) RCGP https://www.rcgp.org.uk/clinical-and-research/resources/bright-ideas/qr-info-pods.aspx

23

Understanding and Responding to Complexity in Young People

PHIL HARRIS

Young people begin to confront the challenge of formulating a coherent self-identity as parental influence wanes and critical age-related transitions loom on the horizon.

Complex needs in young people can embrace a diverse range of co-occurring problems including substance misuse, mental health, offending, early sexual involvement and educational disadvantage. This is a formidable battery of presenting needs for health care professionals who often have limited time and resources to impact on entrenched difficulties. This can be further compounded by the emotional labour of working with young lives, where it can seem that there is so much at stake.

ADOLESCENT DEVELOPMENT

Adolescence marks a period of rapid transition from a constrained social world to establishing an autonomous adult life that determines its own social context. It is a time of accelerated development at the physiological, psychological, relational and societal level.

A primary driver is developmental task achievement proposed by Havinghurst [1]. As we enter into adolescence higher levels of autonomy and more complex demands are expected of youth. This ranges from increased self-care, household and personal hygiene, self-regulation, the ability to manage peer relationships, romantic relationships and increased self-governance. This also requires the accomplishment of formal milestones such as selecting school options, passing exams, moving through the educational system and determining future life choices.

Biological drivers are significantly influenced by these social and cultural demands. For example, improved diet and nutrition has seen the onset of puberty now occur 5 years earlier than 100 years ago. Puberty itself is not restricted to sexual maturation but also triggers considerable changes to muscle mass, bone density, respiration and importantly neurological development, when 50% of the brain will undergo significant structural change. Critical neurological changes significantly increase the processing power of the brain, giving rise to more complex ways of understanding the world, particularly in terms of the development of empathy and the capacity to think about how we are thinking.

This gives rise to a deeper and nuanced self-awareness. Young people begin to confront the challenge of formulating a coherent self-identity as parental influence wanes and critical age-related transitions, like leaving school, loom on the horizon.

Research suggests that on average age 14 is a critical developmental point. Below the age of 14, young people are conservative about adult life. At age 14 young people emotionally separate from parents and become interested and even impatient for adult life, turning to peers to offer the developmental guidance that family once provided.

EVOLUTION OF SUBSTANCE MISUSE

Adolescent substance use does not just happen but aligns itself with these key developmental forces. For example, young people are quick to adopt socially novel drinking and drug practices and swiftly vector these behaviours into highly receptive peer networks of like-minded others. However, the rates of progression from experimentation to addiction are low. Research suggests that 76% of those who experiment with heroin do not go on to develop dependency [2].

From this variance we must conclude that young people do not have problems with substances, but certain young people have problems with a particular substance. For example, even though access routes and the range of substances have increased dramatically in recent years with the rise of new psychoactive substances, this has not created new groups of the population seeking treatment. Likewise, follow-up studies in North American states that decriminalized cannabis have revealed problematic consumption patterns in young people who were already high consumers prior to changes in the law [3]. Personality difficulties precede problem use rather than emerge from it [4].

Whilst risk and protective factors operate on a spectrum, protective factors are less significant in the lives of low-risk youth but incredibly important to high-risk youth. Furthermore, risk profiles are not fixed but accumulative. Young people are born with a background of

vulnerability factors, such as genetics, in-utero experience, socioeconomic status and family patterns of use. In childhood there can be risk factors such as the experience of a wide range of abuse, neglect, witnessing trauma and exposure to dysfunctional parental coping. Once young people move into early adolescence, innate suspicion of alcohol and drugs reduces. Peer belonging, lack of alternative sources of satisfaction, thrill seeking or emotional sedation result in continued use. As young people move into increasingly active substance using networks, new norms and wider availability is established and this creates greater access to a wider range of substances [5, 6].

Gateway drug theory suggests that the earlier the age of initiation the longer the subsequent substance-using career becomes. The Montreal Longitudinal and Experimental study of over 1,000 males in impoverished neighbourhoods in Canada examined drug and alcohol use at ages 17, 20 and 28 [7]. The results confirmed that the younger they started smoking cannabis, the more likely they were to have a drug problem later. Those who started before the age of 15 were at higher risk of problematic use – regardless of how often they consumed drugs [8, 9]. The typical sequence of substance involvement tends to follow a nicotine–alcohol–cannabis pattern of cheap and accessible drugs [10]. Even cannabis tends to be socially traded amongst young people no more than 2 years older [11]. Sequences which move into higher profile street drugs, like cocaine, indicate the young person is accessing drugs from an adult distribution network and could indicate risk of child sexual exploitation.

SUGGESTIONS FOR PRACTICE

• *Be aware of the age of initiation and the associated vulnerabilities with differing drug groups. Attempt to establish if young people are being bullied or exploited and what the motivating reasons for drug use are.*

TRAJECTORIES

Young people's natural conservatism towards adult behaviours under the age of 14 suggests that involvement in substance use prior to this time is strongly indicative of underlying complexity. This follows highly predictive patterns as vulnerability factors cluster together to form clear pathways into drug and alcohol involvement.

YOUTH WITH EXTERNALIZED DISORDERS; SMOKING BEGINS AGES 10–12

These young people grow up in areas of high deprivation with family histories of trans-generational poverty. They exhibit a high rate of externalized, impulse control disorders such as ADHD or oppositional defiance disorder/conduct disorder. There is strong evidence that poor impulse control is genetic but symptom severity is predicted by environments. When raised in stable, warm environments with clear boundaries, poor impulses tend to dissipate across adolescence. Where socially deprived parents lack the emotional, financial and social resources to provide this structure, it can lead to under-parenting that increases the impulsivity. Low-resourced parents with high-need offspring often leads to neglect, which for young people has more damaging long-term consequences than neglect in childhood that is identified and addressed [13]. These individuals are liable to be exposed to a wide range of abuse issues as children, move into early truancy and offending behaviour and are more likely to be diagnosed as adults with personality disorders.

YOUTH WITH INTERNALIZED DISORDERS; SMOKING BEGINS AGES 13–14

Profound neurological transitions, new emergent psychological processes and an increasingly demanding social environment place new pressures on young people, especially those with pre-existing vulnerabilities such as trauma, marginalization or abuse. This creates a dramatic spike in internalized mental illness including depression, anxiety, self-harm, eating disorders and anxiety. Astonishingly, 50% of all mental health diagnosis is made on 14-year-olds, whilst 75% of diagnosis is made by the age of 20 [14].

The anxiety-related disorders can be protective of young people's involvement in substance use due to the fretful nature of these disorders. However, if their experimentation with drugs and alcohol alleviates negative symptoms then their use can escalate dramatically.

NORMATIVE YOUTH; DRUG AND ALCOHOL USE BEGINS AGES 14–16

This is the period of peak peer influence. These young people hail from stable family backgrounds, attain reasonable educational achievements and have no underlying prior complexity. Young male use tends to be influenced by their peers whilst female use tends to be influenced by partners at this time. This places young women with a partner who is 2 or more years older at exposure and risk for substance use beyond their developmental capacity.

FLING YOUTH; AGES 16–21

These are high flyers in college settings who spend more money on beer than books. Research shows that these users are the highest consumers of drugs and alcohol of all four cohorts but in an intense, short bout of consumption. This is not without consequence for them. Up to 40% of college and university dropouts are drug- and alcohol-related and these are not evenly spread throughout the demographic groups attending university [15]. Instead they tend to occur in students from poorer or rural backgrounds who attend institutes of higher education. Poorer young peoples' identities tend to be forged by geographic belonging as opposed to highly portable academic credentials. Whilst drug and alcohol serve as bonding tools for many students, they also operate as coping strategies for those who work hard to escape their previous environments but find themselves in a new world where it is hard to belong. Combined with the transformative pressure of a rapidly changing sense of self, these young adults have increased rates of substance use, mental health and suicide. Young people are happier where they are socially connected to long-standing geographic peer groups [16].

UPSTREAM IMPACTS OF COMPLEXITY

Adverse childhood experience (ACE) research has charted the long-term negative health outcomes of negative experiences in childhood. Whilst ACEs have gained considerable traction in US and UK health policy, it should be noted that the items of the questionnaire which determines ACE are restricted to family experience, and do not consider external risk factors such as bullying or neighbourhood violence [17, 18]. Furthermore, whilst the ACE questionnaire is being widely promoted across primary and secondary health care services, there is no direct treatment or policy response to high-scoring individuals.

Emergent research is suggesting the deterioration in health outcomes that stem from ACEs are largely caused by epigenetic factors [19] whereby trauma triggers an evolutionary process of rapid ageing at a cellular level [20]. Rapid maturity offers greater capacity for self-preservation in children but the price may be a foreshortened life as an adult. This process can even influence the earlier onset of puberty. This places the impact of trauma beyond current medical science and restricts the value of ACEs to a preventative rather than interventive function, highlighting the need for much earlier age-related routine screenings than occur in the wider population.

Besides the human costs, these upstream outcomes come at a heavy economic cost. The Dunedin Multidisciplinary Health and Development Study in New Zealand has followed over 1,000 people born in 1972. This study found that just 20% of the sample accounted for 81% of criminal convictions, 66% of welfare benefits, 78% of prescription fills and 40% of excess obese kilograms [21]. Clinical predictors of the high-cost group were growing up in socioeconomically deprived environments, experience of maltreatment and low childhood impulse control. This research project also found that any subsequent upward social mobility did not reduce the health outcomes of children growing up in social deprivation on reaching adulthood [22].

Scant attention is directed at the psychosocial impact of social exclusion of adolescent development. Heavy substance use disconnects young people from the social settings where critical life tasks are rehearsed and achieved. This results in profound levels of development delay proportionate to the age of onset [23]. Biological age, calendar age and development age separate quickly in these circumstances.

SCREENING FOR COMPLEXITY

Screening and identification of young people with complex needs is challenging. The majority of symptoms that young people experience from substance use tend to be related to interference in social functioning as opposed to physical withdrawal [24]. This can weaken the associations that young people make between the substance use and the increasing social complications that build in their lives [225, 26]. Young people may be reluctant to divulge illicit behaviours such as drug use, sexual behaviours, criminal involvement or deteriorating mental health for fear of embarrassment, further social consequences or sanctions. The assumptions primary health care practitioners may hold regarding the health of youths also appears to reduce contact time, with young people experiencing the shortest consultation periods as catch-up patients.

Young people who experience neglect are also unlikely to be encouraged or supported into primary care by disengaged parents. Neglected adolescents are often distinguished through high rates of long-standing, undiagnosed health problems and poor dentistry [27].

SUGGESTIONS FOR PRACTICE

- *The complexity index [28] is a simple screening tool developed in order to identify the young person's risk trajectory in everyday clinical settings. Arranged in subscales, it indexes the unique risk profiles of each substance involvement pathway (Figures 23.1–23.3).*

TREATMENT

Scoring ranges on the complexity index (revised) offer greater insight into appropriate treatment

A. Domain	Screen	B. If Yes...Follow Up Questions	Score
Age of first use?		1. Did they initiate regular drug or alcohol use before the age of 14?	
Since you were young, have you always found it difficult to do what people ask you to do or follow rules?	Yes / No	2. Did they have a history of offending prior to treatment entry?	
		3. Have they been diagnosed with ADHD, Defiance or Conduct Disorder, or were they statemented?	
		4. Have they had social work involvement prior to treatment?	
		5. Do they have, or report a history of low commitment to school through persistent truancy?	

Figure 23.1 The complexity index (revised). (Adapted from Harris 2013.)

responses. Late-onset, fling and normative youth tend to benefit from very brief interventions. McCambridge and Strang [29] demonstrated that one hour of motivational interviewing [30] could generate significant reduction in drug and alcohol consumption in student populations. All brief interventions operate on a self-mastery model, supporting clients to identify their own personal skills, resources and networks and apply these resources to their emergent problems. As such, they are reliant on the existence of developed life task achievements and pro-social supports.

Internalized disorders' strong relationship to cognitive biases such as rumination, catastrophizing and emotional thinking tend to operate well in formalized counselling settings.

Environmental stabilization and consistency feature heavily in the outcomes of externalized and complex youth. Non-pharmacological approaches include behavioural rewards systems, family therapy, parenting models and social skills training [31].

This conceptual framework offers a more nuanced understanding of young people's complexity and the needs of divergent cohorts. It has assisted in the reconfiguration of services for young people, recognizing the wide range of presentations that accompany adolescent drug and alcohol use. This has required that they offer a range of interventions that span the variant trajectories of need and offer practitioners greater clinical direction in appropriate treatment selection [32–34].

SUGGESTIONS FOR PRACTICE

Pharmacological interventions prove effective for only about 50% of mental health presentations and some presentations are resistant to talking therapies. This suggests there is a profound gulf between established diagnostic frameworks and treatment formulations [35–36]. This is because mental health syndromes share overlapping symptoms that are difficult to isolate based purely on the patient's verbal presentation (Figures 23.4–23.5).

Computer-based therapies are showing increasing promise. This is not just therapy online but the development of software games [37] designed to work and improve functioning in particular neural systems. These have shown promise for improving impulse control [38], cravings [39] and depression [40] amongst other disorders and have obvious appeal to screen literate youth.

Do you ever feel very unhappy or find you worry a lot?	Yes / No	6. Do they have, or report, a history of depression or anxiety?	
		7. Do they have, or report, a history of self-harm prior to treatment?	
		8. Do they have, or report, a history of feeling suicidal?	
Have you only just started using drugs and alcohol and only with friends?	Yes / No	9. Do they report that previous pro-social activities they once enjoyed are no longer interesting?	
		10. Do they report only using drugs or alcohol with peers or partners?	
Are you currently, or have recently, been studying at college or university?	Yes / No	11. Do you feel you struggled to adjust to college / university life?	

Figure 23.2 The complexity index (revised). (Adapted from Harris 2013.)

There are a limited number of long-term treatment follow-up studies of young people with complex needs, although current results demonstrate the most complex youth have poorer outcomes at a 3-year follow-up [41]. Research suggests that the likelihood of lifetime drug abuse and dependence among young drug users was reduced by 4% and 5% with each year drug use onset was delayed [42]. Hser et al [12] identified that a difference in age of initiation of just 6 months led to remission from opiates in the late 20s as opposed to lifelong involvement.

This gives confidence to the belief that pragmatic, well targeted and appropriately informed interventions can make a significant impact on the long-term outcomes of young people.

This young person does not fit any of these criteria	Yes / No	12. Not scored-this is a reliability measure to ensure all young people are captured or those that do not fit the criteria are identified.	
Are you currently using alcohol?	Yes / No	13. Do they use Alcohol?	
Are you currently, or have recently, been involved with any non-prescribed drugs?	Yes / No	14. Do they use Class C Drugs? (Benzos, GHB, Ketamine, etc.)	
	Yes / No	15. Do they use Class B Drugs? (Cannabis, Ecstasy, Amphetamine etc.)	
	Yes / No	16. Do they use Class A Drugs? (Heroin, Cocaine, Crack etc)	
	Yes / No	17. Do they use Steroids \ Solvents \ Other Non-Classified (New psychoactive substances, OTC, Prescriptions Drugs etc)	

Figure 23.3 The complexity index (revised). (Adapted from Harris 2013.)

	Presentation	Clinical Interventions	Adjunct Support
Normative	Experimental	• Brief Intervention • Assertiveness • Sexual Health • Volunteer Support	• Re-Establish Pro-Social Activity • Improve Personal Decision Making • Sustain Reduced Substance Use
Internalized	Low Mood	• Medication Compliance • Mapping Strengths • Coping Strategies • Peer Support	• Improve Family Communication • Symptom Control • Increase Resilience • Develop Self-Efficacy • Reduce Self-Destructive

Figure 23.4 Trajectory informed interventions.

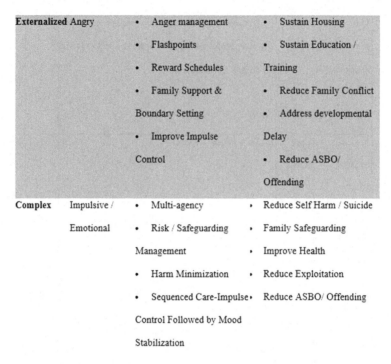

Figure 23.5 Trajectory informed interventions.

REFERENCES

1. Havighurst, R.J. *Developmental Tasks and Education.* New York, McKay, 1972.
2. Antony, J.C., Waner, L.A. & Kessler, R.C. Comparative epidemiology of dependence on tobacco, alcohol, controlled substances and inhalants: Basic findings for the National Co-morbidity Survey. *Experimental and Clinical Psychopharmacology.* 1994; 2 (3): 244–268.
3. Kerr, D.C.R., Bae, H., Phibbs, S. & Kern, A.C. Changes in undergraduates' marijuana, heavy alcohol, and cigarette use following legalization of recreational marijuana use in Oregon. *Addiction.* 2017; 112 (11):1992–2001.
4. Defoe, I.N., Khurana, A., Betancourt, L.M., Hurt, H. & Romer, D. Disentangling longitudinal relations between youth cannabis use, peer cannabis use, and conduct problems: Developmental cascading links to cannabis use disorder. *Addiction.* 2018; 114 (3): 485–491.
5. Newcomb, M.D., Maddahian, E., Skager, R. & Bentler, P.M. Substance abuse and psychosocial risk factors among teenagers: Associations with sex, age, ethnicity, and type of school. *The American Journal of Drug and Alcohol Abuse.* 1987; 13 (4): 413–433.
6. Martin, C.S., Langenbucher, J.W., Kaczynski, N.A. & Chung, T. Staging in the onset of DSM-IV alcohol symptoms in adolescents: Survival/hazard analyses. *Journal of Studies on Alcohol.* 1996; 57 (5): 549–558.
7. Tremblay, R.E, Vitaro, F., Nagin, D., Pagani, L. & Seguin, J.R. The Montreal longitudinal and experimental study rediscovering the power of descriptions. In Thornberry, T.P & Krohn, M.D. (eds) *Taking Stock of Delinquency: An Overview of Findings from Contemporary Longitudinal Studies.* New York, Kluwer, 2003, pp 205–254.
8. Kandel, D. & Yamaguchi, K. From beer to crack: Developmental patterns of drug involvement. *American Journal of Public Health.* 1993; 83 (6): 851–855.
9. Taylor, M., Collin, S.M., Munafò, M.R., MacLeod, J., Hickman, M. & Heron, J. Patterns of cannabis use during adolescence and their association with harmful substance use behaviour: Findings from a

UK birth cohort. *Journal of Epidemiology and Community Health.* 2017; 71 (8): 764–770.

10. Schulenberg, J., O'Malley, P.M., Bachman, J.G., Wadsworth, K.N. & Johnston, L.D. Getting drunk and growing up: Trajectories of frequent binge drinking during the transition to young adulthood. *Journal of Studies on Alcohol.* 1996; 57 (3): 289–304.

11. Hamil-Luker, J., Land, K.C. & Blau, J. Diverse trajectories of cocaine use through early adulthood among rebellious and social conforming youth. *Social Science Research.* 2004; 33 (2): 300–321.

12. Hser, Y.I., Chou, C.P. & Anglin, M.D. Trajectories of heroin addiction: Growth mixture modelling results based on a 33-year follow-up study. *Evaluation Review.* 2007; 31 (6): 548–563.

13. Smith, C.A., Ireland, T.O. & Thornberry, P. Adolescent maltreatment and its impact on young adult antisocial behavior. *Child Abuse & Neglect.* 2005; 29 (10): 1099–1119.

14. Kessler, R.C., Berglund, P., Demler, O., Jin, R., Merikangas, K.R. & Walters, E.E. Lifetime prevalence and age-of-onset distributions of DSM-IV disorders in the National Comorbidity Survey Replication. *Archives of General Psychiatry.* 2005; 62 (7): 593–603.

15. Kassenboehmer, S.C., Leung, F. & Schurer, S. University education and non-cognitive skill development. *Oxford Economic Papers.* 2018; 70 (2): 538–562.

16. Borschel, E., Zimmermann, J., Crocetti, E., Meeus, W., Noack, P. & Neyer, F.J. Me and you in a mobile world: The development of regional identity and personal relationships in young adulthood. *Developmental Psychology.* 2019; Advance online publication. http://dx.doi.org/10.1037/dev0000677.

17. World Health Organization. Adverse Childhood Experiences International Questionnaire. In *Adverse Childhood Experiences International Questionnaire (ACE-IQ).* Geneva, WHO, 2018 [website]: https://www.who.int/violence_injury_prevention/violence/activities/adverse_childhood_experiences/en/

18. Felitti, V.J., Anda, R.F., Nordenberg, D., Williamson, D.F., Spitz, A.M., Edwards, V., Koss, M.P. & Marks, J.S. Relationship of childhood abuse and household dysfunction to many of the leading causes of death in adults: The Adverse Childhood Experiences (ACE) Study. *The American Journal of Preventative Medicine.* 1998; 14 (4): 245–258.

19. Sumner, J.A., Colich, N.L., Uddin, M., Armstrong, D. & McLaughlin, K.A. Early experiences of threat, but not deprivation, are associated with accelerated biological aging in children and adolescents. *Biological Psychiatry.* 2019; 85 (3): 268–278.

20. Vinkers, C.H., Kalafateli, A.L., Rutten, B.P., Kas, M.J., Kaminsky, Z., Turner, J.D. & Boks, M.P. Traumatic stress and human DNA methylation: A critical review. *Epigenomics.* 2015; 7 (4): 593–608.

21. Caspi, A., Houts, R.M., Belsky, D.W., Harrington, H., Hogan, S., Ramrakham, S., Poulton, R. & Moffitt, T.E. Childhood forecasting of a small segment of the population with large economic burden. *Nature Human Behavior.* 2016; 1(article 0005). doi:10.1038/s41562-016-0005

22. Poutlon, R., Caspi, A., Milne, B.J., Thomson, M., Taylor, A., Sears, R. & Moffitt, T.E. Association between children's experience of socioeconomic disadvantage and adult health: A life-course study. *The Lancet.* 2002; 360 (9346): 1640–1645.

23. Melrose, M., Turner, P., Pitts, J. & Barrett, D. *The Impact of Heavy Cannabis Use on Young People Vulnerability and Youth Transitions.* York, The Joseph Rowntree Foundation, 2007.

24. Storbjork, J. & Room, R. The two worlds of alcohol problems: Who is in treatment and who is not?' *Addiction Research and Theory.* 2008; 16 (1): 67–84.

25. White, W.L. & McLellan, A.T. (2008). Addiction as a chronic disease: Key messages for clients, families and referral sources. *Counselor.* 2008; 9 (3): 24–33.

26. Scott, C., White, W. & Dennis, M.L. Chronic addiction and recovery management: Implications for clinical practice. *Counselor.* 2007; 8 (2): 22–27.

27. Raws, P. *Understanding Adolescent Neglect: Troubled Teens A Study of the Links Between Parenting and Adolescent Neglect.* The Children's Society, 2016.

28. Harris, P. *Youthoria: Adolescent Substance Misuse-Problems, Prevention and Treatment*. Lyme Regis, Russell House Publishing, 2013.

29. McCambridge, J. & Strang, J. The efficacy of single-session motivational interviewing in reducing drug consumption and perceptions of drug-related risk and harm among young people: Results from a multi-site cluster randomized trial. *Addiction*. 2004; 99 (1): 39–52.

30. Miller, W.R. & Rollnick, S. *Motivational Interviewing: Helping People Change*. New York, Guilford Press, 2012.

31. Weisz, J.R., Kristin, M., Hawley, K.M. & Doss, A.J. Empirically tested psychotherapies for youth internalizing and externalizing problems and disorders. *Child and Adolescent Psychiatric Clinics of North America*. 2004; 13 (4): 729–815.

32. Cummings, J.R., Bornovalova, M.A., Ojanen, T., Hunt, E., MacPherson, L. & Lejuez, C. Time doesn't change everything: The longitudinal course of distress. *Journal of Abnormal Child Psychology*. 2013; 41 (5): 735–748.

33. Weisz, J., Kuppens, S., Ng, M.Y., Vaughn-Coaxum, R.A., Ugueto, A., Eckshtain, D. & Corteselli, K. Are psychotherapies for young people growing stronger? Tracking trends over time for youth anxiety, depression, attention-deficit/hyperactivity disorder, and conduct problems. *Perspectives on Psychological Science*. 2019; 14 (2): 216–237.

34. www.nimh.nih.gov/research/research-funded-by-nimh/rdoc/index.shtml

35. Miller, S.D., Duncan, B.L., Brown, J., Sorrell, R. & Chalk, M.B. Using formal client feedback to improve retention and outcome: Making ongoing, real-time assessment feasible. *Journal of Brief Therapy*. 2006; 5 (1): 5–22.

36. Lambert, M.J., Whipple, J.L., Smart, D.W., Vermeersch, D.A., Nielsen, S.L. & Hawkins, E.J. The effects of providing therapists with feedback on patient progress during psychotherapy: Are outcomes enhanced? *Psychotherapy Research*. 2001; 11 (1): 49–68.

37. Fleming, T., Bavin, L.M., Stasiak, K., Hermansson-Webb, E., Merry, S.N., Cheek, C., Lucassen, M.F.G., Lau, H.M., Pollmuller, B. & Hetrick, S.E. Serious games and gamification for mental health: Current status and promising directions. *Frontiers in Psychiatry*. 2017; 7, Article I.D. 215. http://dx.doi.org/10.3389/fpst.2016.00215.

38. Brooks, S.J, Wiemerslage, L., Burch, K.H., Maiorana, S.A., Cocolas, E., Schiöth, H.B., Kamaloodien, K. & Stein, D.J. The impact of cognitive training in substance use disorder: The effect of working memory training on impulse control in methamphetamine users. *Psychopharmocology*. 2017; 234 (12): 1911–192.

39. Skorka-Brown, J., Andrade, J. & May, J. Playing 'Tetris' reduces the strength, frequency and vividness of naturally occurring cravings. *Appetite*. 2014; 76: 161–165.

40. Elgamal, S., McKinnion, M.C., Ramakrishnan, K., Joffe, R.T. & MacQueen, G. Successful computer-assisted cognitive remediation therapy in patients with unipolar depression: A proof of principle study. *Psychological Medicine*. 2007; 37 (9): 1229–1238.

41. Chung, T., Martin, C.S., Grella, C.F., Winters, K.C. & Abrantes, A.M. Course of alcohol problems in treated adolescents. *Alcoholism: Clinical and Experimental Research*. 2003; 27 (2): 253–261.

42. Grant, B.F. & Dawson, D.A. Age of onset of drug use and its association with DSM-IV drug abuse and dependence: Results from the national longitudinal alcohol epidemiologic survey. *Journal of Substance Abuse*. 1998; 10 (2): 163–173.

24

Addressing the Health and Well-being of Young Carers

HANNAH THOMPSON

Hear the young person's voice – and ensure it is neither missed nor given less credence as a result of the strength of the voices of adults around them.

Young carers are children and young people who provide care to another family member. The level of care they provide is wide-ranging, from nursing and personal intimate care to domestic and financial care. The roles young carers are required to carry out are usually those undertaken by an adult and as a result of this they take on a level of responsibility that is inappropriate to their age and development. This is likely to have a significant impact on their childhood experiences.

IMPACTS OF CARING

Caring responsibilities can be difficult and stressful at any age. Taking on the physical and emotional demands of supporting a family member or friend with a long-term sickness, disability, mental ill health or addiction is a lot for young minds to deal with. For many young people, particularly those who go unidentified, caring can lead to a significant and long-term negative impact on their physical and mental health and well-being. [1]

Young carers often talk about feeling tired and under pressure. Many experience traumatic life changes such as bereavement, family break-up, losing income or housing, and seeing the effects of an illness or addiction on the person they care for. All these things, alongside the pressures of school or college and the social isolation experienced by many, can lead to stress, anxiety and depression. Research by Carers Trust and the University of Nottingham found that almost a third of young carers reported that their own physical health was 'just OK' and 38% reported having a mental health problem.

Young carers' physical health may also suffer. Financial pressures, time pressures, exhaustion as a result of interrupted sleep and physical injuries can be acquired from repeatedly having to support or move someone with poor mobility.

The health of young carers may be affected for a variety of reasons and might not be addressed if their health appointments are being missed, not prioritised or if there is a distrust of health services. The 2011 census found that young carers providing between 20 and 49 hours are over three times more likely to report their health as not being good compared to those without caring responsibilities.

IDENTIFICATION OF CARERS

Before young carers can be supported, they must be identified. In March 2018 the Greater Manchester Combined Authority (GMCA) conducted a review of young carer provisions across the 10 local authorities [2]. Whilst responses indicated 2.3% of the North West population of young people identified themselves as carers, evidence suggests this figure is closer to 8%.

As there is no standardised recording or capturing tool, the true numbers of young carers within the population is increasingly difficult to estimate. With most referrals for support coming from schools or via social workers, health professionals can play a key role in identifying young carers and offering support.

SUGGESTIONS FOR PRACTICE

- *When in consultation with families where there might be young carers, consider asking the following questions [3]*
    - *Who helps to care for the person at home?*
    - *What effect does their condition and personal care needs have on the family?*
    - *Is there a child/young person in the family who helps to provide care?*
    - *How does this affect the child/young person physically, emotionally or educationally?*
    - *Is there any direct help that would support the young carer?*
    - *Does the parent need support in their parenting role?*
    - *What can be offered to help the whole family?*
    - *When prescribing medication for your client, consider whether a young carer may be administering it. Is this appropriate? Do they need support?*
- *Offer training to primary care staff in identification and recognition of young carers. (Some young carers services offer this.)*

When establishing that there could be a young carer in the family, it is best to adopt the whole family approach which considers the impact of an individual's additional needs on the rest of their family and addresses the child's needs within the context of their family, instead of in isolation [4].

The Carers Trust details different components of the whole family approach:

- Whole family assessments.
- Support for adults and other family members within the family, such as parenting support; provision of practical and emotional support.
- Building support networks including engaging the wider family through, for example, family group conferences.
- Relationship building within the family, such as support with building roles, routines and responsibilities and engaging families in positive activities [4].

It is important to honestly discuss what the options might be for all the individuals in question. It's wise to explore preferences from an early stage, to ensure a dialogue that suits the adult, young person and the family. You would need to check with your local authority to see who to refer to for assessment. If you have an established young carers service in your area, it would be beneficial to liaise with them on a regular basis for support, information and advice. They may be able to provide material to go on your practice website and noticeboards.

When considering how to standardise identification, the Carers Trust and Children's Society, in their pilot scheme, *Making a Step Change for Young Carers and their Families*, described 'what good looks like', and highlighted 8 key considerations:

1. A collaborative approach and joint responsibility for identification of young carers across children's and adults' services, including health and education.
2. Include young carers in Joint Strategic Needs Assessment.
3. Secure support for young carers from senior health stakeholders.
4. Joint ownership of pathways for the identification and assessment of young carers across agencies.
5. Local authorities should encourage young carers to self-refer and develop a clear and transparent offer of support to young carers and their families.

6. Schools should be supported to identify young carers and encouraged to participate in the Young Carers in Schools programme.
7. Every school should have a young carers champion.
8. Local authorities should promote and support the young carer champion role within health services, particularly within GP practice.

SUPPORTING YOUNG CARERS

Dedicated support for young carers can help to protect their health and well-being. Being a young carer impacts negatively on school attendance, punctuality and academic achievement. Additionally, isolation, low mood, low aspiration, bullying, lack of leisure time and poverty are identified as frequent concerns amongst young carers [2].

Having someone to talk to, to share their concerns with, such as a young carers' support worker, is hugely important.

Young carers say that peer support online or within a young carers' service for example, where they can relax, be themselves and take part in activities is vital. For others, dedicated emotional support from specialist services may be appropriate.

Respite activities and sports may also be important opportunities where young carers can simply be young people and have fun. The role of all health professionals involved in their identification and care is to reduce social isolation and protect their health and well-being.

SUGGESTIONS FOR PRACTICE

- *Research the local young carers support in your area, make contact, keep up-to-date and understand their referral criteria.*
- *Can you create an accessible resource or information pack for young carers which can signpost them to online support or local activities? (remember looking at youth centres, sports, activity groups such as cadets and scouts and opportunities for creative expression where young people are able to be separate from duties and responsibilities).*

LEARNING FROM SERIOUS CASE REVIEWS [5]

Case Study

ANNIE

Annie was a 37-year-old mother of two who died from sepsis relating to pressure ulcers as a complication of malnourishment and self-neglect. It was not clearly understood why she had stopped eating. She had a history of alcohol misuse as well as mental health needs. She had previously been a victim of domestic abuse and experienced a decline in self-care when she lost her job following an accident, causing damage to herself.

She had also been diagnosed with breast cancer. She had two sons who had previously been on child protection plans who had gone to live with maternal grandparents. The younger son Stanley, aged 15, moved back to care for Annie when his grandparents became unwell themselves. The second son, aged 18, moved out of the family home to live with his girlfriend.

Annie had self-discharged from hospital 6 months before her death. Professionals dealing with her did not always seem to understand the complexity of her social circumstances. There was a tendency to accept at face value what she was saying. Sometimes people involved in her care demonstrated a lack of professional curiosity and as a result did not really understand the true situation. For example, although it was recognised that she was not eating, it was not clear why she was not eating. She would sometimes not engage with health services and would often not allow services to access her home.

At this point, a safeguarding concern could have been raised and a holistic assessment completed to address the needs of both mother and her youngest son.

FINDINGS [6]

- Annie was an independent person who was reluctant to accept help or support.
- She had experienced difficulties with her physical and mental health needs and these were exacerbated by the use of alcohol.
- Agencies involved with Annie did not complete a capacity assessment.

- Services assumed Annie had capacity and that she chose to make unwise decisions around eating and drinking.
- As Annie's physical health deteriorated and her self-neglecting behaviour increased, there was evidence to suggest agencies did not work together to reassess the family's needs.
- Annie's bedroom was unkempt and evidence of her poor condition.
- Annie's tenancy was compromised due to rent arrears (despite the fact that she had been offered and accepted support for help to set up the new family home).
- Concerns were raised by the school suggesting that the boys were unkempt and malnourished.
- Consent for CAF was not given.
- There was a lack of understanding of Stanley's needs, particularly in relation to caring for his mother rather than seeing him as a child in need of protection.
- School supported Stanley to cope with home situation and focused on his needs.

LEARNING AND SUGGESTIONS FOR PRACTICE

Communication

- *Some services did attempt to offer support although when support was refused persistence and professional curiosity could have been explored. Schools have an important role to offer and often care deeply about their students yet feel they do not know how and where to link up support. Be aware that they offer their own pastoral teams and often have counsellors that a young person may not have had access to if staff are not aware of extended family health needs.*
- *Frank and open conversations with service users about their choices and the impact on others is to be supported, particularly when related to children and adults at risk. Training and supervision to facilitate such conversations must take place to ensure positive outcomes are achieved.*
- *If a person raises concerns and doesn't want to work alongside professionals, question why and try to find a way to change this.*
- *If high-risk cases are recognised early, then collaboration with partner agencies is vital*

to ensure joint risk assessment and planning is in place. This approach would allow early and effective identification of risk, improved information sharing, joint decision-making and coordinated action.

Understanding Carer's Needs

- *Consider the impact on a child being a carer to a parent and involving support organisations for carers from all ages and backgrounds. Some communities will not consider that caring for an older relative is an increased burden and therefore conversation with a professional from a similar background may be more productive in explaining the risks of being a young carer and why support might be beneficial.*
- *Consider whether it is appropriate to use a childcarer to convey information to and from a possible adult at risk. Remember community advocates and identify a trusted adult support figure for information sharing. Use of family members for translation is rarely appropriate, so consider getting an interpreter involved from the offset.*
- *Practitioners working with children and young people are reminded of the importance of hearing the young person's voice, and ensuring it is neither missed nor given less credence as a result of the strength of the voices of adults around them.*

Multi-agency Working

- *Practitioners are urged to seek support and supervision early (and with management oversight) when involved in such complex circumstances, so that time and resources are available to support this.*
- *Consider involvement from all agencies, especially local mental health services, as seeking that support in safeguarding children is vital. Navigating the local availability and waiting lists is a challenge as services may be linked to postcodes or funding may have been withdrawn so previously known providers will no longer be available. But they are there. Look especially into schools and youth*

centres as they include caring individuals passionate about young people's well-being and provide ongoing continuity to monitor and communicate back new concerns or changes in behaviour.

- Safeguarding issues span across generations – the think family approach is a significant area of focus, particularly with services working across boundaries and in partnership within adult and children's services. [7]

Young carers are a hugely underrepresented and unidentified group within our population. They often see their duties as normal and don't consider asking for help as they already have a family member who is 'suffering'. The incremental impact over the years is a growing and unnoticed concern by both themselves and clinicians, so our duty is to identify carers early in order to reduce the sequence of deteriorating physical and mental health. Knowledge of your localities' available services is crucial, as the biggest factor identified in improving well-being is access to a continued support network in order to enhance opportunities for expression and conversation. These individuals deserve time to develop their own interests and personalities and this in itself is the key to a lifetime of improved outcomes.

REFERENCES

1. Carers Trust. Protecting the Health and Wellbeing of Young Carers. https://professionals.carers.org/protecting-health-and-wellbeing-young-carers (accessed).
2. Heeran C. Where Are We Now. GM LA Response Summary 2018 (accessed).
3. The Children's Society. A guide for supporting, identifying and signposting young carers in your practice. 2017 (accessed).
4. Carers Trust. Whole Family Approaches. https://professionals.carers.org/whole-family-approaches (accessed).
5. Mair R. Young Carers: Still Ignored or Do They Now Have Reason to Be Hopeful. Care Knowledge 2019 (accessed).
6. Mortimer E, Kingston P. Serious Case Review / Safeguarding Adults Review. Briefing Paper 2018. http://www.safeguardingadultsinstockport.org.uk/wp-content/uploads/2019/04/Briefing-paper-Annie-Stanley.pdf (accessed).
7. Stockport Council. The Stockport Council Plan 2018–2019. 2018. https://assets.ctfassets.net/ii3xdrqc6nfw/2X8eT6UA1aMOgWIEg2SU8Y/fc9f82d94912a34798115d-1b82a5c869/Stockport_Council_Plan_2018-19.pdf (accessed).

25

Women's Health and Health Inequality

RACHEL STEEN

The fear of being stigmatised means that many do not access such support.

There is a complex relationship between gender, deprivation, ethnicity and health inequalities. For this reason, we need to think about gender when considering ways to reduce health inequalities. Women face different health challenges to men due to biology and culture [1]. Michael Marmot encourages what he calls, 'proportionate universalism' [2]: targeting healthcare where it is needed most. Thinking about proportionate universalism for both gender and poverty is essential in tackling health inequality.

Despite steady increases in life expectancy for both sexes in the UK, rates of increase have stalled since the financial crisis in 2008, particularly when compared to the rest of Europe [3]. In the lowest deprivation deciles, there has been a fall in life expectancy for women (Figure 25.1) [4]. Beyond maternal health, women living in deprivation are more at risk of mental health problems, certain cancers, and are more likely to be victims of domestic violence.

Vulnerable groups, such as drug users and Travellers, are known to have poorer health, and women from these groups have worse health than their male counterparts [5, 6]. Tackling health inequalities for vulnerable groups poses multiple challenges without the added burden of gender and socioeconomic deprivation (Figure 25.1).

SPECIFIC HEALTH ISSUES FACING WOMEN IN THE CONTEXT OF DEPRIVATION

Maternal Health

With increasing knowledge and understanding of adverse childhood experience and the importance of early years, we know the pregnancy and well-being of a mother and her baby impacts throughout the course of child's life into adulthood. Maternal health can influence a child's subsequent educational achievement and economic status as well as lead to negative health outcomes such as obesity or mental health issues [7].

Access to maternal health services is particularly poor for women from low socioeconomic backgrounds. This in turn has significant consequences for both maternal and child health [8]. Women living in poverty are more at risk of unplanned pregnancy, late antenatal care booking and poor maternal/child outcomes in pregnancy [9]. Ethnicity also plays a part. Evidence suggests UK-born women have a lower rate of maternal mortality (7.87 per 100,000 women) than non-UK-born women (8.8 per 100,000 women) [1].

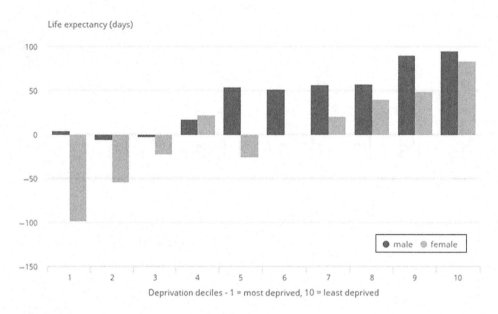

Figure 25.1 Change in life expectancy in days between 2012–2014 and 2015–2017.

SUGGESTIONS FOR PRACTICE

- *Provide support to families and be aware of local services that can provide additional help to women and mothers.*
  - *Examples of such support include the female parent support programmes like Wild Young Parents in Cornwall or MAMTA, the women's health support service in Coventry [1].*

SEXUAL HEALTH

Despite increasing efficiencies in sexual and reproductive health (SRH) services following the move of SRH funding from the NHS to local authorities (LA) in 2012, rates of STIs are increasing while SRH services are reducing [10]. LA spend on SRH services reduced by 3.5% yearly from 2015–2018 [11]. Clinics shut down, reduced their hours or moved to locations which are harder for patients to access. When clinics are geographically harder to access, women from deprived areas are impacted most, in particular women from marginalised groups [6].

Recent reductions in staffing in sexual health services means there is pressure to focus on diagnostics and treatment rather than a more holistic approach. A holistic approach may be needed, for example, to help meet the complex social, financial and psychological needs of a sex worker [12]. The voluntary sector covers some gaps by providing support to vulnerable groups, but these are often on short term and raise issues of sustainability [11]. Local and national variations in the availability of SRH services create 'cold spots' of access for the most vulnerable patients [13].

SUGGESTIONS FOR PRACTICE

- *Communicate, advocate and negotiate locally so it is clear where sexual health services are offered and the ongoing importance of securing funding on the basis of deterioration to long-term health outcomes for marginalised groups.*

MENTAL HEALTH

Women in areas of low socioeconomic deprivation are more likely to suffer from mental health problems than women living in affluent areas. With a higher number of comorbidities, these women have an increased disease burden making them more likely to suffer from mental health problems. Women from all backgrounds are more likely to present with symptoms of anxiety, depression and somatic complaints than men [14].

DEMENTIA

The UK has an ageing population, and it is important to recognise the intersectionality of age and gender for women's health services. Female pensioners have higher rates of poverty compared to male pensioners. Women are more likely to have dementia than men and this is also the leading cause of death for women. Women with dementia also have less contact with GPs than men [3]. It is essential therefore to understand the risks for women when caring for our ageing population.

DOMESTIC VIOLENCE

Women in areas of socioeconomic deprivation are particularly at risk of domestic violence [15]. Domestic violence has an impact on many aspects of a woman's health but particularly on mental health and long-term conditions [16, 17]. Health professionals often report a lack of confidence in asking about domestic violence and when a patient does disclose this information, they often feel they don't know what to do next [15].

SUGGESTIONS FOR PRACTICE

- *Support your team to routinely ask patients about domestic violence and abuse. Ask more than once if violence or abuse is suspected.*
- *Familiarise yourself and your team with the appropriate local referral and services. Lack of local services is not an excuse not to ask about domestic violence or abuse.*
- *Educate yourself and your team about the barriers that victims face. Support with this could be through services such as* The Change That Lasts: Ask Me *scheme.*

CANCER

In women, cervical cancer is most likely to be affected by levels of deprivation, in terms of both incidence and mortality [18]. Macmillan Cancer Support reports that 25% of people living with cervical cancer are from the most deprived group compared to 16% in the least deprived [19]. Most other cancers are also more common for women living in deprivation [18]. While the incidence of breast cancer is higher in more affluent areas (possibly due to increased screening in more affluent women), age-related mortality in breast cancer is higher for women living in deprivation [18].

Deprivation also has strong associations with the risk factors for female cancers such as the

association of human papillomavirus (HPV) with cervical cancer. HPV is known to be increased in patients that smoke, have sexual intercourse at an early age, and patients who have not been vaccinated. Studies have shown a link to deprivation for all of these factors [20, 21]. Cervical cancer screening aims to prevent cervical cancer by detecting HPV early or before invasive disease. Cervical cancer screening has been shown to have a lower uptake in more deprived areas [20] meaning women in these areas are more likely to present late when the disease is more advanced and less treatable [18].

In addition to the effect of deprivation on incidence and mortality in cancer, women living in deprived areas are more likely to be in financial difficulty. This means they are much more likely to be affected by the financial implications of living with cancer such as increased energy bills and fuel poverty [22].

SUGGESTIONS FOR PRACTICE

- *Be relentless in your pursuit of non-responders to screening invitations regarding women living in deprivation in your patient population.*
- *Work with local services to support patients with preventing cancer risk factors, examples being smoking cessation, reducing alcohol consumption and HPV prevention through vaccination uptake.*
- *Signpost and support patients with the financial challenges at the time of cancer diagnosis.*

VULNERABLE GROUPS

Women's health is particularly affected if they are in a vulnerable group, leaving them most at risk of maternal death [23]. The National Institute for Health and Care Excellence (NICE) recommends training in recognition and management of vulnerable high-risk groups taking into account social, religious and psychological factors that impact the patient [24]. Each factor does not exist in isolation. Domestic violence, for example, is present in many vulnerable groups but as an overriding feature we know this is particularly linked to poverty [15]. Evidence suggests that by thinking about how to tackle health inequalities in one specific vulnerable group we can have positive effects on other groups too [6].

DRUG USE IN WOMEN

Despite research showing men outnumber women in alcohol and drug use, when we consider the effect of substance use on women we find a complex web of issues affecting all aspects of women's health [25].

Women's drug use differs from men. Women use and need small amounts for a stronger effect. They get addicted quicker and find it more difficult to give up [12]. Women users are more likely to commit crimes in order to buy drugs and drug offences contribute to the majority of female prison sentences in the UK [26].

Women entering drug use services are also likely to have more complex psychological and social problems than men, including those associated with substance use. Women are more likely to drop out of support programmes than men due to childcare pressures and fear of having children taken into care [25]. Pregnancy, for example, highlights the challenges for this group of women. Pregnancy is a point when women drug users are often offered support with reducing or stopping drug use due to potential harm to their unborn child. However, the fear of being stigmatised means that many do not access such support [25].

SUGGESTIONS FOR PRACTICE

- *Consider a drug user's financial, psychological and social situation. Ask about*
  - *Children, and support with childcare,*
  - *Financial situation and crime,*
  - *Domestic violence and abuse.*
- *Maximise the opportunities of extra support and services around antenatal and pregnancy care with specialist midwifery, safeguarding health visitor teams and ongoing community input to support women with drug use.*

GYPSY AND TRAVELLER HEALTH

Gypsies and Travellers are among the worst affected vulnerable groups in the UK when it comes to health inequalities, with only 6% surpassing the age of 65 [27]. They have high rates of chronic disease, mental health problems and suicide [5]. Life expectancy of Gypsy and Traveller women is 12 years less than for non-Gypsy and Traveller women. They also face problems during pregnancy, with increased rates of miscarriage, stillbirth, neonatal and maternal deaths [28].

Gypsy and Traveller patients are likely to face discrimination and stigma accessing services, so it is important that practice staff are welcoming and understanding of their needs. Registration is often difficult with many reporting GP surgeries not allowing registration without a fixed address or identification. This is not an excuse for a surgery not to register a patient. It is also important that the low level of literacy of Gypsies and Travellers is taken into account (45% have low or no literacy) in the current roll-out of digital technology in primary care [5].

SUGGESTIONS FOR PRACTICE

- *Familiarise yourself with and work with local services that support Gypsies and Travellers.*
- *Consider the importance of attaching outreach services/identified liaison team members from your practice in order to improve communication and therefore understanding about how best to improve access and service uptake for this group of women.*

MIGRANT HEALTH

Women refugees and migrants often arrive from situations where they have faced extreme discrimination and barriers to accessing health services. This has significant effects on both their mental and physical health. Physical health problems range from acute infectious diseases to nutritional deficiencies and chronic disease [30]. Female genital mutilation can also contribute to poor reproductive health. Additionally, the challenges of arriving and starting a new life in a new country adds a further stressor on health [31]. Women refugees have often been exposed to physical, emotional and sexual abuse, speak little or no English, and/or may be victims of human trafficking [30].

SUGGESTIONS FOR PRACTICE

- *Be sensitive to cultural differences especially when it comes to sexual and reproductive health. It may be more appropriate to use a female interpreter for example.*

- *Think about whether a patient may be a victim of human trafficking and refer appropriately. More information is available at the Human Trafficking Centre.*

Healthcare professionals have the privileged position of being able to ask our patients about how they are impacted by their social, financial and psychological health. Creating an ethos of care and trust allows open conversations about specific problems women are facing.

Many of the solutions to practise discussed during this chapter have some overlap so these have been brought together and summarised below. We know that helping one group of vulnerable patients can have a positive impact on another group of vulnerable patients too [6]. By improving health for women living in deprivation we can also have an impact on the health of the whole family, including men and children living in deprivation. Keeping women's health in mind, we can help improve an individual's health as well as taking steps to tackle health inequalities in the population.

SUGGESTIONS FOR PRACTICE

- *Find out more about your local population*
  - *Identify the specific vulnerable groups and health needs of women in your patient population and what barriers these women face to accessing services.*
  - *Consider arranging some cultural awareness training for your team on the vulnerable groups of women specific to your patient population.*
- *Be open and supportive to vulnerable groups*
  - *Make time to smile and welcome your patient.*
  - *Challenge a culture of stigma around specific vulnerable groups. Examples being drug users or Gypsies and Travellers.*
  - *Think about ways that your team can support women accessing services. An example being supporting women with low literacy with registration.*
  - *If you are working in a GP practice, ensure your registration policy is correct. Proof of address or ID is not needed to register.*
  - *Find out about local groups or services in your area which support vulnerable groups of women. Work together with these services*

to support these patients. An example organisation is Pensioners Link: Leigh and Wigan.
  - *Include women from vulnerable groups in designing how you deliver and design healthcare in your area.*
  - *Act as ambassadors in your areas for the specific needs of women and women from vulnerable groups.*
- *Keep specifics to women's health in mind when seeing patients*
  - *Work closely with local maternity services and encourage women to book early for antenatal care.*
  - *Consider asking about social support, children crime and drug and alcohol use.*
- *Improve services for women in your area*
  - *Advocate for your patients and lobby local and national policies to include the specific needs for the health of women and those in vulnerable groups, not just for pregnancy.*
  - *Lobby for increased resources for services to support women's health. Examples of this include lobbying to prevent cuts to women's refuges or local sexual health services.*
  - *Work in partnership with services in your area.*

REFERENCES

1. BMA. Addressing unmet needs in health inequality. 2018 24.4.19. Available from: file:///C:/Users/rache/Downloads/Womens-health-full-report-aug2018.pdf.
2. Review TM. Fair society, healthy lives. Strategic review of health inequalities in England post 2010. 2010. Available from: http://www.instituteofhealthequity.org/resources-reports/fair-society-healthy-lives-the-marmot-review/fair-society-healthy-lives-full-report-pdf.pdf.
3. Equity Ulfh. Marmott indicators 2017-Health institute breifing 2017 24.4.19. Available from: http://www.instituteof-healthequity.org/resources-reports/marmot-indicators-2017-institute-of-health-equity-briefing/marmot-indicators-briefing-2017-updated.pdf.
4. Statistics OoN. Health state life expectancies by national deprivation deciles, England and Wales: 2015 to 2017. 2019.

5. Parry G, Van Cleemput P, Peters J, Moore J, Walters S, Thomas K et al. The health status of gypsies & travellers in England. 2004. Available from: https://www.sheffield.ac.uk/polopoly_fs/1.43714!/file/GT-final-report-for-web.pdf.

6. O'Donnell P, Tierney E, O'Carroll A, Nurse D, MacFarlane A. Exploring levers and barriers to accessing primary care for marginalised groups and identifying their priorities for primary care provision: A participatory learning and action research study. *International Journal for Equity in Health*. 2016;15:197.

7. Marmott M, Goldblatt P, J A et al. The Marmott Review: Fair society, healthy lives. Strategic review of health inequalities in England post 2010. Available from: http://www.instituteofhealthequity.org/resources-reports/fair-society-healthy-lives-the-marmot-review/fair-society-healthy-lives-full-report-pdf.pdf.

8. Haddrill RJG, Mitchell CA, Anumba DO. Understanding delayed access to antenatal care: A qualitative interview study. *BMC Pregnancy and Childbirth*. 2014;14(1):207.

9. Kapaya H, Mercer E, Boffey F, Jones G, Mitchell C, Anumba D. Deprivation and poor psychosocial support are key determinants of late antenatal presentation and poor fetal outcomes-a combined retrospective and prospective study. *BMC Pregnancy and Childbirth*. 2015;15(1):309.

10. Ministry of House CaLG. Local authority revenue expenditure and financing England: 2017 to 2018 individual local authority data - outturn 2019. Available from: https://www.gov.uk/government/statistics/local-authority-revenue-expenditure-and-financing-england-2017-to-2018-individual-local-authority-data-outturn.

11. Robertson R. What do cuts in sexual health services mean for patients? The Kings Fund; 2017.

12. Hamilton I. Breaking the silence on women and drug abuse. 2017. Available from: https://www.pharmaceutical-journal.com/opinion/comment/why-women-who-misuse-drugs-have-different-needs/20203081.article?firstPass=false.

13. Buck D. Prevention is better than cure – except when it comes to paying for it. 2018. Available from: https://www.kingsfund.org.uk/blog/2018/11/prevention-better-cure-except-when-it-comes-paying-it.

14. Gender disparities and mental health. Available from: https://www.who.int/mental_health/media/en/242.pdf?ua=1.

15. Scott S, Williams J, Mcnaughton Nicholls C, McManus S, Brown A, Harvey S et al. Violence, abuse and mental health in England. 2015. Available from: http://www.natcen.ac.uk/media/1057987/REVA_Brief-1_Population-patterns_FINAL_071015.pdf.

16. Goodway M. Domestic violence and abuse. 2019. Available from: https://www.fairhealth.org.uk/dva.

17. Change that lasts: ask me. Women's Aid Federation. Available from: https://www.womensaid.org.uk/our-approach-change-that-lasts/askme/.

18. O'Leary E, Cooper N, Peake M, Oehler C, Hounsome L, Elliss-Brookes L et al. Deprivation and cancer: In search of a common measure across England, Wales, Scotland, Northern Ireland and Ireland. London: Public Health England; 2016.

19. Support MC. 20 Year Cancer Prevalence, England. Available from: https://www.macmillan.org.uk/documents/aboutus/research/researchandevaluationreports/ourresearchpartners/20yrcancerprevalenceengland.pdf.

20. Hughes A, Mesher D, White J, Soldan K. Coverage of the English National human papillomavirus (HPV) Immunisation Programme among 12 to 17 year old females by area-level deprivation score, England, 2008 to 2011. *Euro Surveill*. 2014;19(2).

21. Parkin D. Tobacco-attributable cancer burden in the UK in 2010. *British Journal of Cancer*. 2011;105.

22. Support MC. Cancers hidden price tag: Revealing the cost behind the illness. Available from: https://www.macmillan.org.uk/_images/Cancers-Hidden-Price-Tag-report-England_tcm9-270862.pdf.

23. Askew I. Poorest and most marginalized women continue to be most at risk of maternal death. 2016. Available from: https://www.who.int/reproductivehealth/news/maternal-death/en/.

24. Excellence NIoC. Pregnancy and complex social factors: Service provision overview. 2019. Available from: https://www.nice.org.uk/guidance/CG110.

25. Abuse NIoD. Substance use in women. 2018. Available from: https://www.drugabuse.gov/publications/drugfacts/substance-use-in-women.

26. Drugscope. *Using Women*. London: Drugscope; 2005.

27. Statistics OoN. 2011 Census analysis: What does the 2011 Census tell us about the characteristics of Gypsy or Irish travellers in England and Wales? Office of National Statistics; 2014.

28. Worrell S. Gypsy and Traveller Healthcare. 2018. Available from: https://www.fairhealth.org.uk/learning/gypsytraveller.

29. LeedsGATE. LeedsGATE: Working to improve the quality of life for Gypsies and Travellers. Available from: http://leedsgate.co.uk/.

30. Costa D. Healthcare for refugee women. Reprinted from *Australian Family Physicians*; 2007.

31. England PH. Women's health: Migrant health guide: Advice and guidance on the health needs of migrant patients for healthcare practitioners. 2014. Available from: https://www.gov.uk/guidance/womens-health-migrant-health-guide.

26

Men's Health

PETER BAKER

Better men's health contributes to better health for women and children.

Defining men's health has not proved entirely straightforward for researchers, practitioners and advocates working in this field. In the 25 years or so that men's health has been identified and discussed as a discrete health issue, many definitions have been suggested [1]. One useful definition has been developed by the Men's Health Forum (MHF), a national UK charity. This asserts that a male health issue is one that fulfils either of the following conditions: it arises from physiological, psychological, social, cultural or environmental factors that have a specific impact on boys or men; and/or it necessitates male-specific actions to achieve improvements in health or well-being at either individual or population level [2].

The MHF's holistic definition is helpful in many ways. It suggests that any consideration of men's health should include the health of boys, mental as well as physical health, and both clinical and social issues, including (at least by implication) the role of male gender norms. It also highlights that improvements in male health may require more than uniform population-wide interventions; put simply, what works for women may not work for men.

THE SCALE OF THE PROBLEM

Men's health is in many significant ways poorer than women's. According to the World Health Organisation (WHO), global male average life expectancy at birth in 2016 was 69.8 years compared to 74.2 years for female life expectancy [3]. In the 53 countries of the WHO's European region, male life expectancy stood at 74.2 years and female at 80.8 years. Europe is the world region with the largest male-female gap: this is because of the very large differences between male and female life expectancy in several Eastern European states.

In the United Kingdom (UK) specifically, the respective figures for males and females were 79.2 years and 82.9 years for the period 2015–2017 [4]. Premature mortality also impacts significantly more men than women. In England and Wales in 2017, 19% of all male deaths were in age groups under 65 years and 38% were in age groups under 75 years [5]. The respective female figures were 12% and 25%.

There are marked local variations in male life expectancy within the UK. Glasgow city had the lowest male life expectancy in the UK in 2015–2017 at 73.3 years [6]. This contrasts with the much more affluent district of Hart in Hampshire which had the UK's highest male life expectancy (83.3 years). A similar difference in male life expectancy can be found when comparing data from small neighbourhoods across England. This shows that, in 2014–2016, life expectancy at birth among the most deprived males in England was

73.9 years, compared with 83.3 years among the least deprived [7].

There are some other specific groups of men who experience particularly poor health outcomes. Homeless men are very vulnerable; the mortality rates of homeless men in Dublin are 3–10 times higher than those of the general population [8] and prisoners have very high rates of mental health problems [9]. Mental health problems, suicide and self-harm are higher than average amongst gay men in the UK and these issues are associated with the challenges and stress experienced by men as a direct result of their sexual identity [10]. The use of illegal drugs before or during sex ('chemsex') has also been identified as a significant risk factor for gay men's health as it facilitates high-risk sexual behaviour.

The main causes of death in men vary depending on their life course. But overall in 2015 ischaemic heart disease was the leading cause of death in males, accounting for 14% of all deaths [11]. It was the cause of almost twice as many deaths as the second leading cause of death, dementia and Alzheimer's disease. Stroke was responsible for a further 6% of deaths. Four of the 10 leading causes of death were cancers and of these, lung cancer caused the most deaths. If deaths from all forms of cancer were grouped together, cancer deaths would account for 30% of all deaths in males.

THE CAUSES OF POOR MEN'S HEALTH

The main causes of men's poor health are men's risk-taking practices and, to a lesser extent, their sub-optimal use of health services. Underpinning both of these factors are the gender norms men have been socialized to follow as well as a lack of attention to men's health issues by health providers and policymakers. Male biology may play some role in determining their poorer health – it is the most likely explanation for the higher levels of perinatal, neonatal and post-neonatal mortality in males – but is not thought to be a major factor across a man's life, perhaps accounting for 1 or 2 years at most of men's shorter life expectancy [12].

The evidence is clear that male gender norms – expectations to be self-sufficient, to act tough, to be physically attractive, to be heterosexual, to have sexual prowess, and to use aggression to resolve conflict [13] – encourage men to take more risks

with their health than women [14]. Men are, for example, more likely to drink alcohol at levels hazardous to health, to eat red and processed meat and to drive dangerously. Men are less likely to eat fruit and vegetables. Historically, men have smoked tobacco at much higher levels than women and, although the difference is now much smaller, men who smoke cigarettes are still likely to smoke more per day than female smokers. Men are generally more physically active than women but, even so, only a minority are active at recommended levels. Men often combine several unhealthy practices; one study found that physical inactivity combined with a lack of fruit and vegetables was the most common combination [15].

Men's less healthy practices are reflected in data on the mortality rates for causes considered preventable: in the UK in 2017, the rate was 238 per 100,000 for males compared to 143 per 100,000 for females [16]. Almost 72,000 male deaths and about 47,000 female deaths were considered preventable.

Men generally under-use health services, particularly primary care services [17]. Men are particularly reluctant to seek help for mental health problems [18]. They are less likely to participate in free health checks designed to detect undiagnosed cardiovascular disease and diabetes or the risk factors for these conditions [19]. Men are also less likely to have an eye health check [20]. Despite being at greater risk of bowel cancer, they are less likely to take part in screening programmes [21]. Men's use of self-management support interventions for long-term conditions is also sub-optimal [22]. Infrequent use of and late presentation to health services have been associated with men experiencing higher levels of potentially preventable health problems and having reduced treatment options, possibly resulting in higher hospitalisation rates [23].

One explanation for men's problematic use of services is their lower health literacy. British men have been found to be twice as likely as women to have limited health literacy [24]. Men are less likely to recognize a number of common cancer symptoms [25]. The largest sex difference is for recognition of a change in the appearance of a mole; the odds of recognizing this symptom are 60% higher in women than men. Men are also more likely than women to misperceive their weight, less likely to consider their body weight a risk for their health and less likely to consider managing or be actively trying to manage their weight [26].

Men are not simply reluctant to use primary care services, they also often find them difficult to access for practical reasons [27]. Booking systems can be hard to use – many GP surgeries require patients to phone for an appointment at a time when men may be commuting or at work – and appointments themselves may not be available at convenient times or places, again because of work commitments [28]. The increasing number of men working in the insecure 'precariat' sector of the economy may well find it even harder to take time off work for medical appointments, and there may also be a loss of income for the time taken off work.

Despite men's poorer health outcomes, there has not been a strategic response in the UK. Even though the Equality Act 2010 and the Health and Social Care Act 2012 place a duty on health services to tackle gender health inequalities, as does the NHS constitution, the UK has not followed the lead of Australia, Brazil and Ireland and developed a national men's health policy. There have been no signs that the government plans to take any specific action to implement WHO Europe's men's health strategy, adopted by its 53 member states (including the UK) in 2018 [29]. National policy on promoting equality has not translated into systematic local action either. Gender generally, and men's health specifically, have been poorly addressed in the majority of Joint Strategic Needs Assessments (JSNAs), the key policy document used to determine and subsequently implement local health priorities and activities [30].

WHY MEN'S HEALTH SHOULD BE TACKLED

The case for committing resources to improving men's health is very clear. First and foremost, it is an ethical imperative. The WHO Constitution, adopted in 1946, speaks of 'the highest attainable standard of health as a fundamental right of every human being' [31]. This places an obligation on states to ensure access to timely, acceptable, and affordable healthcare of appropriate quality as well as to provide for the underlying determinants of health, such as safe and potable water, sanitation, food, housing, health-related information and education and gender equality.

Better men's health contributes to better health for women and children. The benefits for women are most obvious in the area of sexual and reproductive health where safer sex practices by men would clearly prevent the transmission of a wide range of infections and their consequences. Greater male involvement in contraception would also help to reduce the number of unplanned pregnancies. High morbidity and mortality rates in men impact on women in another way, especially in lower-income households: the loss or incapacity of the primary breadwinner, frequently a man, can have a hugely detrimental effect on partners and children [32]. They may have to take on caring responsibilities, limiting employment and educational opportunities and reducing current and future income.

Addressing men's mental health issues, including alcohol and drug misuse, could contribute to a reduction in male violence against women, children and other men. A WHO report suggested that, in the USA and in England and Wales, victims of domestic violence believed their partners to have been drinking prior to a physical assault in 55% and 32% of cases respectively [33].

Healthcare costs could fall. It has been calculated that relatively small annual improvements in four key risk factors – smoking, alcohol, weight and physical activity – in Canadian men would produce a cumulative cost saving of CAD 51 billion over about 20 years [34]. A separate analysis suggests that men's premature mortality and morbidity costs the US economy approximately USD 479 billion annually [35].

When making a case for men's health, it is essential not to imply that women's health does not also require greater attention (in many specific areas of health, women's outcomes are worse than men's) or that tackling men's health is more important than addressing women's health [36]. In reality, there is not a binary choice to be made nor is this a zero-sum game; investment is needed in gender-responsive approaches that improve the health of all.

Efforts to address men's health should not be avoided because of a belief that men are somehow to blame for their poor health as a result of their risk-taking or reluctance to seek help. Instead, it is necessary to understand the causes and consequences of men's health practices and to develop practical and non-judgemental responses [37]. Men are still brought up with an expectation that they will conform to male gender norms and it can be difficult for individual men to reject them, especially if they have limited agency because of their income, employment status or personal history. This does not mean, of course, that individual men should not be held accountable when they put others at risk or cause them actual harm, or that men should not support gender equality for women.

HOW MEN'S HEALTH CAN BE IMPROVED

Men's health has without doubt improved significantly since the early 1990s. Male life expectancy has increased as has male healthy life expectancy. Male cigarette smoking and cardiovascular disease and cancer mortality rates have steadily declined. Men can now access national screening programmes for bowel cancer, chlamydia and abdominal aortic aneurysms as well as NHS health checks which aim to detect the early signs of stroke, kidney disease, heart disease, diabetes and dementia. As a result of a vigorous 5-year campaign led by a coalition of professional and patient organisations, from 2019–20 adolescent boys will be covered by the national HPV vaccination programme (available to girls since 2008). There has also been a marked increase in national and local men's health interventions, including the annual Men's Health Week, launched by MHF in 2002.

The challenge is to accelerate these trends to ensure that more men, especially men in those groups with the worst outcomes, can enjoy the benefits of optimal health. There is certainly no longer any shortage of ideas about the steps that are needed.

SUGGESTIONS FOR PRACTICE

- *At a national strategic level: there should be an introduction of men's health policy and also for other health policies, whether on cancer, cardiovascular disease or obesity, to take explicit account of the specific needs of men [38].*
- *At the local level: data on men's health should be reflected in JSNAs and men's needs recognized in health and well-being strategies.*

More local authorities could follow the example of Leeds City Council which, in 2016 published a report on the state of men's health in its area and has taken account of its findings in service development [39].

A range of practical steps could improve men's use of primary care services, including general practice. For example, the greater availability of digital technologies for making appointments and for information, advice and even some consultations could make a difference, especially if combined with an extension of opening hours beyond the normal working day.

SUGGESTIONS FOR PRACTICE

- *Services could feel more male-friendly by having male-interest magazines in waiting rooms and displaying health information (posters, leaflets, etc.) targeted at men.*
- *Taking services, including NHS Health Checks, to where men are is an effective strategy; workplaces, faith and leisure venues (such as clubs, pubs and sports stadia) are settings where men can more easily be engaged.*
- *Practitioners should also consider how they can make every contact count with men, especially with those they may see rarely.*
- *Services could consider allocating responsibility for developing work on men's health to a specific member of staff.*

Training for health professionals on men's health issues is important, although it is currently very limited and not part of pre-qualification curricula. However, the Royal College of General Practitioners (RCGP) does offer occasional men's health training workshops for GPs and practice nurses; MHF has a training programme aimed mainly at public health practitioners; and the Centre for Pharmacy Postgraduate Education (CPPE) has developed a distance learning module on men's health for pharmacists and pharmacy technicians. Ireland's now well-established ENGAGE men's health training programme offers another way forward [40]. It aims to increase participants' understanding of best practice in engaging men with health programmes. Health practitioners from a variety of services are informed about evidence-based tools, connect with a network of supportive peers, and learn about harmful gender roles and norms that contribute to practices such as the under-utilization of health services. ENGAGE helps raise awareness about gender-responsive healthcare in order to improve the quality of care given to men and to generate positive and sensitive clinical engagements.

Practitioners require easily accessible and robust evidence and guidance about how to develop and deliver effective men's health interventions. Such information is increasingly available in a wide variety of journals and reports but is generally not provided in synthesized and user-friendly formats. However, MHF has published three useful 'how to' guides to engage men in self-management support, weight management and mental health [41–43]. Each guide summarizes key research, contains case studies and offers practitioners 10 top tips. The Queen's Nursing Institute (QNI) has also published information and guidance for nurses working with men in the community [44–45]. More such resources are required.

There are several macro-level steps that could be taken to improve men's health. Tougher controls on tobacco, alcohol, sugar and gambling would disproportionately benefit men's health and wellbeing. More egalitarian social and economic policies would also help because the social gradient in life expectancy is steeper for men than women, meaning that deprivation appears to have a bigger negative impact on men's health.

CASE STUDIES

Service providers can also learn from the increasing number of case studies which demonstrate good practice in engaging men through a gender-responsive approach.

Men's Health Forum

MHF pioneered the production of health information for men in the form of 'Man Manual' booklets which are non-didactic and contain easy-to-read non-medical text and humorous cartoons [46]. They are published and co-branded by Haynes, a publisher of car maintenance manuals which is well-known and trusted by many men. Written by health experts, the 'Man Manuals' cover a wide range of topics, including specific health problems (eg. diabetes, cancer, stress) as well as general health. Some are aimed at specific groups of men, such as farmers, gay men and transgender men. The booklets can be purchased by men via Amazon or in bulk by organizations. Some companies have commissioned booklets specifically for their male employees. Well over one million 'Man Manuals' have been distributed to date.

Premier League Health

Premier League Health was a national men's health programme delivered by 15 Premier League soccer clubs in England. It succeeded in reaching men with multiple health practices contributing to chronic conditions who were typically regarded as 'hard to contact or engage' (over one-third of the participating men reported that they did not consult their GP and over half never engaged with a health advice service) [47]. Despite having substantial health needs, these participants were unlikely to be exposed to conventional health promotion opportunities. Men taking part in the programme demonstrated significant increases in weekly physical activity and daily consumption of fruit and vegetables and significant decreases in daily sitting time, weekly alcohol consumption and body mass index. The evaluation confirmed that health interventions delivered in professional football clubs have a powerful reach with male supporters, but also with men not engaging with primary care and health information services.

Football Fans in Training

Football Fans in Training (FFIT) in Scotland provides another good example of a lifestyle programme – in this case, weight management – which uses sport to target men specifically. Based at top-flight football clubs, it has achieved significant participation and resulted in positive outcomes: men who took part in the programme lost almost 5kg more weight than men in the comparison group [48]. They also had lower waist size, lower percentage body fat and blood pressure, reported higher levels of physical activity, better diets and felt better about themselves. The FFIT approach is now being used more widely in Europe, where it is branded as EuroFIT [49] and also for hockey fans in Canada [50].

AHEAD

The nurse-led AHEAD project in the UK aimed to improve the uptake by men aged 40–65 of free health checks and respiratory, cardiovascular and diabetes chronic disease reviews in a GP surgery. Male patients who had already declined three previous invitations to attend either a health check or a chronic disease review were identified and targeted. They were invited for a blood test and posters, promotion banners and practice staff reinforced the message that men should attend. The value of health checks is debatable [51] but this initiative clearly demonstrates that it is possible to engage men in primary care services. The number who attended for health checks increased by over 250% year-on-year (to over 400 men a year) and over 50 new cases of chronic disease (hypertension, diabetes, asthma, COPD, mental health, coronary heart disease or stroke) were detected. The number of men on the pre-diabetic register more than doubled.

Men's health has improved significantly since men's health was identified as a discrete field of work about 25 years ago. But it remains unnecessarily poor, especially for men on low incomes or who belong to certain disadvantaged groups (e.g. men who are gay, homeless or in prison). Gender norms, which encourage men to take risks, act tough and avoid help-seeking, impact on men's health practices. They are more likely than women to smoke, drink alcohol and have a poor diet, for example. Men also use primary care services less effectively. Policymakers and practitioners have not yet responded to these problems systematically by developing male-targeted strategies and services which could more effectively engage men.

In the UK, there is a legal requirement, albeit currently largely overlooked by health policymakers and providers, to address gender inequalities in health. There is also a strong ethical argument for action to improve men's health and potentially major savings in healthcare expenditure as well as contributing to improved outcomes for women and children.

Outcomes could be improved if national and local men's health policies were introduced, services made more male-friendly (e.g. by using digital technologies and being delivered 'where men are', such as workplaces and sports stadia), staff properly trained and user-friendly guidance provided to practitioners. There are now many well-evaluated case studies of gender-responsive interventions which have effectively engaged men. Well-established platforms, such as Men's Health Week, also provide opportunities for practitioners to reach out to men.

The prospects for improving men's health are better than ever. What is now needed are greater levels of investment and, even more importantly, a new and vigorous commitment at all levels to tackle this still largely overlooked area of inequality.

REFERENCES

1. Bardehle D, Dinges M, White A. What is men's health? A definition. *Journal of Men's Health*. 2017 Oct 24;13(2):e40–52.
2. Wilkins D. *Untold Problems: A Review of the Essential Issues in the Mental Health of Men and Boys*. London, Men's Health Forum and National Mental Health Development Unit; 2010.
3. WHO. Global Health Observatory data repository. Life expectancy and Healthy life expectancy: Data by WHO region. http://apps.who.int/gho/data/view.main.SDG2016LEXREGv?lang=en (accessed 21 March 2019).
4. Office for National Statistics (2018). Health state life expectancies, UK: 2015 to 2017. https://www.ons.gov.uk/peoplepopulationandcommunity/healthandsocialcare/healthandlifeexpectancies/bulletins/healthstatelifeexpectanciesuk/2015to2017 (accessed 21 March 2018).
5. Office for National Statistics (2018). Death registrations summary tables - England and Wales. https://www.ons.gov.uk/peoplepopulationandcommunity/birthsdeathsandmarriages/deaths/datasets/deathregistrationssummarytablesenglandandwalesreferencetables (accessed 27 March 2019).
6. Office for National Statistics (2018). Life expectancy at birth and at age 65 years by local areas, UK. https://www.ons.gov.uk/peoplepopulationandcommunity/healthandsocialcare/healthandlifeexpectancies/datasets/lifeexpectancyatbirthandatage65bylocalareasuk (accessed 21 March 2019).
7. Office for National Statistics (2018). Health state life expectancies by national deprivation deciles, England and Wales: 2014 to 2016. https://www.ons.gov.uk/peoplepopulationandcommunity/healthandsocialcare/healthinequalities/bulletins/healthstatelifeexpectanciesbyindexofmultipledeprivationimd/englandandwales2014to2016 (accessed 21 March 2019).

8. Ivers JH, Zgaga L, O'Donoghue-Hynes B, Heary A, Gallwey B, Barry J. Five-year standardised mortality ratios in a cohort of homeless people in Dublin. *BMJ Open.* 2019 Jan 1;9(1):bmjopen-2018.

9. Tyler N, Miles HL, Karadag B, Rogers G. An updated picture of the mental health needs of male and female prisoners in the UK: Prevalence, comorbidity, and gender differences. *Social Psychiatry and Psychiatric Epidemiology.* 2019:1–0.

10. Davis S, Marwa W. Is being gay in the UK seriously bad for your health? A review of evidence. *Journal of Global Epidemiology and Environmental Health.* 2017 Dec 12.

11. Public Health England (2017). Health profile for England: 2017. https://www.gov.uk/government/publications/health-profile-for-england (accessed 21 March 2019).

12. Monasta L, Ronfani L, Gallus S, Beghi E, Giussani G, Bosetti C, Cortinovis M, Bikbov B, Perico N, Remuzzi G. Global, regional, and national age-sex-specific mortality and life expectancy, 1950–2017. *The Lancet.* 2018 Nov 10;392(10159):1684–735.

13. Heilman B, Barker G, Harrison A. The Man Box: A Study on Being a Young Man in the US, UK, and Mexico. Unilever Axe, Promundo; 2017.

14. Baker P. *Who Self-Cares Wins: A Global Perspective on Men and Self-care.* London, Global Action on Men's Health; 2019.

15. Zwolinsky S, Raine G, Robertson S. Prevalence, co-occurrence and clustering of lifestyle risk factors among UK men. *Journal of Men's Health.* 2016;12(2).

16. Office for National Statistics (2019). Avoidable mortality in the UK. https://www.ons.gov.uk/peoplepopulationandcommunity/healthandsocialcare/causesofdeath/datasets/avoidablemortalityintheuk (accessed 21 March 2019).

17. Baker P. Men's Health: An overlooked inequality. *British Journal of Nursing.* 2016 Oct 27;25(19):1054–7.

18. Lindinger-Sternart S. Help-seeking behaviors of men for mental health and the impact of diverse cultural backgrounds. *International Journal of Social Science Studies.* 2015;3:1.

19. Coghill N, Garside L, Montgomery AA, Feder G, Horwood J. NHS Health Checks: A cross-sectional, observational, quantitative study on equitability of uptake and selected outcomes. In South West Public Health Scientific Conference 2017. 2017 Apr 14.

20. Dickey H, Ikenwilo D, Norwood P, Watson V, Zangelidis A. Utilisation of eye-care services: The effect of Scotland's free eye examination policy. *Health Policy.* 2012 Dec 1;108(2–3):286–93.

21. Klabunde C, Blom J, Bulliard JL, Garcia M, Hagoel L, Mai V, Patnick J, Rozjabek H, Senore C, Törnberg S. Participation rates for organized colorectal cancer screening programmes: An international comparison. *Journal of Medical Screening.* 2015 Sep;22(3):119–26.

22. Galdas P, Darwin Z, Kidd L, Blickem C, McPherson K, Hunt K, Bower P, Gilbody S, Richardson G. The accessibility and acceptability of self-management support interventions for men with long term conditions: A systematic review and meta-synthesis of qualitative studies. *BMC Public Health.* 2014 Dec;14(1):1230.

23. Juel K, Christensen K. Are men seeking medical advice too late? Contacts to general practitioners and hospital admissions in Denmark 2005. *Journal of Public Health.* 2007 Nov 2;30(1):111–3.

24. von Wagner C, Knight K, Steptoe A, Wardle J. Functional health literacy and health-promoting behaviour in a national sample of British adults. *Journal of Epidemiology & Community Health.* 2007 Dec 1;61(12):1086–90.

25. Niksic M, Rachet B, Warburton FG, Wardle J, Ramirez AJ, Forbes LJ. Cancer symptom awareness and barriers to symptomatic presentation in England—are we clear on cancer? *British Journal of Cancer.* 2015 Jul;113(3):533.

26. Robertson C, Archibald D, Avenell A, Douglas F, Hoddinott P, Van Teijlingen E, Boyers D, Stewart F, Boachie C, Fioratou E, Wilkins D. Systematic reviews of and integrated report on the quantitative, qualitative and economic evidence base

for the management of obesity in men. *Health Technology Assessment (Winchester, England).* 2014 May;18(35):v.

27. Coles R, Watkins F, Swami V, Jones S, Woolf S, Stanistreet D. What men really want: A qualitative investigation of men's health needs from the Halton and St Helens Primary Care Trust men's health promotion project. *British Journal of Health Psychology.* 2010 Nov;15(4):921–39.

28. Lopes RC, Luiz FS, Barbosa AC, dos Santos Juliatti RP, dos Santos AS, da Costa Carbogim F. Sociodemographic profile of men users of primary care and health/Perfil sociodemográfico de homens usuários da atenção primária e cuidado à saúde/Perfil sociodemografico de hombres usuarios de la atención primaria y cuidado... *Revista de Enfermagem da UFPI.* 2018 Nov 25;7(3):29–34.

29. WHO Europe (2018). Strategy on the health and well-being of men in the WHO European Region. http://www.euro.who.int/__data/assets/pdf_file/0003/378165/68wd12e_MensHealthStrategy_180480.pdf?ua=1 (accessed 27 March 2019).

30. Centre for Public Scrutiny, MHF. Men Behaving Badly? Ten Questions Council Scrutiny Committees Can Ask About Men's Health. London, Centre for Public Scrutiny; 2015.

31. WHO. Human rights and health. https://www.who.int/news-room/fact-sheets/detail/human-rights-and-health (accessed 28 March 2019).

32. Edström J, Hassink A, Shahrokh T, Stern E (2015). Engendering Men: A collaborative review of evidence on men and boys in social change and gender equality. https://opendocs.ids.ac.uk/opendocs/bitstream/handle/123456789/7059/EMERGE.pdf?sequence=1 (accessed 28 March 2019).

33. WHO (2006). Intimate partner violence and alcohol. https://www.healthsystemsglobal.org/upload/resource/fs_intimate1.pdf (accessed 28 March 2019).

34. Krueger H, Goldenberg SL, Koot J, Andres E. Don't change much: The economic impact of modest health behavior changes in middle-aged men. *American Journal of Men's Health.* 2017 Mar;11(2):275–83.

35. Brott A, Dougherty A, Williams ST, Matope JH, Fadich A, Taddelle M. The economic burden shouldered by public and private entities as a consequence of health disparities between men and women. *American Journal of Men's Health.* 2011 Nov;5(6):528–39.

36. Baker P, Shand T. Men's health: Time for a new approach to policy and practice? *Journal of Global Health.* 2017 Jun;7(1).

37. Whitley R. Men's mental health: Beyond victim-blaming. *The Canadian Journal of Psychiatry.* 2018 Aug 24; 63(9):577–80.

38. Men's Health Forum (2014). Men's health manifesto. https://www.menshealthforum.org.uk/sites/default/files/pdf/mens_health_manifesto_lr.pdf (accessed 27 March 2019).

39. White A, Seims A, Newton R (2016). The state of men's health in Leeds: Main report. https://www.leeds.gov.uk/docs/The%20State%20of%20Mens%20Health%20in%20Leeds%20-%20Main%20Report.pdf (accessed 27 March 2019).

40. Osborne A, Carroll P, Richardson N, Doheny M, Brennan L, Lambe B. From training to practice: The impact of ENGAGE, Ireland's national men's health training programme. *Health Promotion International.* 2016 Dec 24;33(3):458–67.

41. Galdas P. *How to Engage Men in Self-management Support.* London, MHF; 2015.

42. Wilkins D. *How to Make Weight-Loss Services Work for Men.* London, MHF; 2014.

43. Wilkins D. *How to Make Mental Health Services Work for Men.* London, MHF; 2015.

44. Baker P. *Men's Health: Nurse-led Projects in the Community.* London, The Queen's Nursing Institute; 2018.

45. MHF. Man manuals. https://shop.menshealthforum.org.uk/collections/man-manuals (accessed 27 March 2019).

46. Pringle A, Zwolinsky S, McKenna J, Daly-Smith A, Robertson S, White A. Effect of a national programme of men's health delivered in English Premier League football clubs. *Public Health.* 2013 Jan 1;127(1):18–26.

47. Wyke S, Hunt K, Gray C, Fenwick E, Bunn C, Donnan P, Rauchhaus P, Mutrie N, Anderson A, Boyer N, Brady A. Football fans in

training (FFIT): A randomised controlled trial of a gender-sensitised weight loss and healthy living programme for men. *Public Health Research*. 2015.

48. Wyke S, Bunn C, Andersen E, Silva MN, Van Nassau F, McSkimming P, Kolovos S, Gill JM, Gray CM, Hunt K, Anderson AS. The effect of a programme to improve men's sedentary time and physical activity: The European Fans in Training (EuroFIT) randomised controlled trial. *PLoS Medicine*. 2019 Feb 5;16(2):e1002736.

49. Blunt W, Gill DP, Sibbald SL, Riggin B, Pulford RW, Scott R, Danylchuk K, Gray CM, Wyke S, Bunn C, Petrella RJ. Optimization of the Hockey Fans in Training (Hockey FIT) weight loss and healthy lifestyle program for male hockey fans. *BMC Public Health*. 2017 Dec;17(1):916.

50. Krogsbøll LT, Jørgensen K, Gøtzsche PC. General health checks in adults for reducing morbidity and mortality from disease: *Cochrane Database of Systematic Reviews*.

27

Ageing Unequally

LOUISE TOMKOW

Although life expectancy is increasing, people are not necessarily ageing well.

The UK population is ageing and inequalities in both health and wealth are growing. Those living in the most affluent areas live disability-free for 15 years longer than their poorest counterparts, thus health disparities are expressed most profoundly in later life [1]. Numerous studies demonstrate the association between social disadvantage and ill health. The contemporary political climate of economic austerity impacts health both through the rationalisation of health resources and cuts to public services, which worsen the socioeconomic determinants of health [2]. These structural inequalities are modifiable at a policy level. However governmental and media discourse frequently overlooks both these political dynamics, and the benefits of living longer, and instead construct the older population as a threat to the economic sustainability of health services [3].

Health inequalities in later life can be understood to reflect social advantage and disadvantage accumulated over the life course. Consequently, when looking to address health inequalities in older populations, practitioners often justifiably feel overwhelmed. Rather than proffering a one-size-fits-all approach, a focus on person-centred care for older people, which actively considers the cumulative and intersecting disadvantages experienced over the life course should be considered. Importantly, it is suggested that in order to close the gap in health in later life, health care professionals must be advocates beyond the clinic.

INTERSECTIONAL INEQUALITIES OVER THE LIFE COURSE

Although life expectancy is increasing, people are not necessarily ageing well. Significant and growing proportions of the population are living with multiple chronic diseases: 23% of those aged 50–64 in the UK have two or more long-term health conditions. This increases with age and is unequally distributed across the population [4]. Physical and mental health outcomes in later life are largely determined by socioeconomic position across the life course [5, 6]. As disadvantaged social groups are exposed to increased and prolonged episodes of adversarial environments, the toll on individuals' biopsychosocial systems accumulates unequally [7].

The association between poverty and morbidity is well described. In England, men older over the age of 50 in the poorest population quintile are three times more likely to have heart disease, twice as likely to have diabetes, and twice as likely to have arthritis, in comparison to their wealthiest counterparts [8]. Inequalities in wealth and health are also associated with functional deficiencies. Over 50s in the poorest quintile are four times more likely to struggle with activities of daily living (ADLs) than the richest [8].

Inequalities in health are also observed across additional social domains, including gender and ethnicity. Although women live longer than men, older women tend to be poorer than older men; in 2014 only 36% of women were eligible for full state pension [4]. Functional impairments also appear to be more pronounced for poorer older women than their poor male and wealthier female counterparts: 41% of women in the poorest quintile struggle with ADLs, compared with 34% of men in the same quintile, and 13% of women in the wealthiest quintile [8].

Older black and minority ethnic (BAME) groups tend to report significantly worse health than white British. Amongst 61–70-year-olds, 34% of white British report fair or bad health, compared to 63–69% of Indian, Pakistani and Caribbean, and 86% of Bangladeshi [8]. The households of ethnic minorities are some of the poorest in the UK [9], but ethnicity has implications for health in later life independent of socioeconomic factors. Although often underestimated, exposure to racism across the life course is associated with poor physical and mental health outcomes [10]. Migration to the UK is increasing, as is diversity amongst the older population, with a projected 11-fold increase in the number of BAME individuals over the age of 70 between 2018 and 2051 [11]. Marginalised social groups such as older asylum seekers and refugees face multiple social disadvantages. Here, poverty, violence, ethnicity, gender and immigration status place some older people in unique positions of disadvantage [12].

FRAILTY: AN EXPRESSION OF INEQUALITY

The concept of frailty has received increasing policy, media and academic attention over the past two decades. Frailty is defined as a 'medical syndrome with multiple causes and contributors, characterised by diminished strength, endurance, and reduced physiologic function that increases an individual's vulnerability for developing increased dependency and/or death' [13]. Frailty can be understood as a manifestation of inequality across the life course: poorer groups become frail at a younger age than wealthier groups and poverty is associated with a faster decline in frailty [14].

The concept of frailty is facing increasing resistance from health care providers and older people [15]. The lay perception of frailty is of a negative state of existence; frailty 'links with the negative social imaginary of a feared old age', and is connected with powerlessness, impairment, and loss of control which causes social devaluation [16]. Although many describe experiences of feeling frail, qualitative research suggests older people resist frailty as a diagnosis and an identity [17]. Furthermore, socioeconomic inequalities contribute to differential experiences of ageing and frailty. Poorer frail individuals have worse subjective well-being than their equally frail but wealthier counterparts [18]. The fact that poverty augments the negative psychological components of frailty draws attention to the pervasiveness of socioeconomic inequalities on multiple dimensions of health and well-being.

The approaches used to measure frailty are broadly divisable into the frailty phenotype and the deficit accumulation model. The phenotype understands frailty as an observable clinical syndrome with five characteristics: unintentional weight loss, exhaustion, weakness, slow walking speed and low physical activity [19]. The deficit accumulation model, operationalised though the frailty index (FI), conceptualises frailty as the accumulation of physical, psychological and social losses [20]. Both approaches attempt to quantify older individuals' complex needs and are independently predictive of often costly adverse outcomes such as unplanned hospitalisation, admission to long-term care facilities and death [21].

Likely as a result of this population-predictive tools, there is a governmental drive to identify frail older people. The routine diagnosis of frailty was written into the NHS GP contract in 2017 and encourages clinicians who identify frailty to 'take action' [22]. Physical activity regimes, particularly resistance training, have the most convincing evidence base for modifying the trajectory of frailty [23, 24]. However, these self-management strategies have been shown to have a lower uptake in poorer socioeconomic groups [25].

The gold standard management of frailty is a comprehensive geriatric assessment (CGA) (Figures 27.1 and 27.2). CGA is a multidimensional interdisciplinary process that identifies an older person's medical, psychological and functional capacity in order to coordinate a plan of treatment [26]. CGA has been shown to reduce death and disability in frail older people when delivered to the acutely unwell in the context of specialist inpatient secondary care [27–29] (Figures 27.1 and 27.2).

SUGGESTIONS FOR PRACTICE

- *Primary care physicians should deliver a CGA to their frail patients, with the support of geriatricians if needed.*

The medical review of frail older individuals, based on consensus guidance from the British Geriatrics Society [30], focuses on a holistic review and is shown in Figure 27.3.

The Role of the Healthcare Professional in Addressing Unequal Ageing

Many of the socioeconomic inequalities described in this chapter determine the health of older people in ways that clinicians may find difficult to challenge. However, understanding the multiple dimensions of disadvantage allows practitioners to consider the structural determinants of health inequalities, both in the management of older individuals and when implementing health policy. A three-pronged approach, focusing on prevention, mitigation and management can be taken when looking to address drivers and effects of unequal ageing.

Prevention

Preventing health inequalities in later life requires a life-course approach that works to avert disadvantage before it accumulates. Early-life interventions that target the prevention of key risk

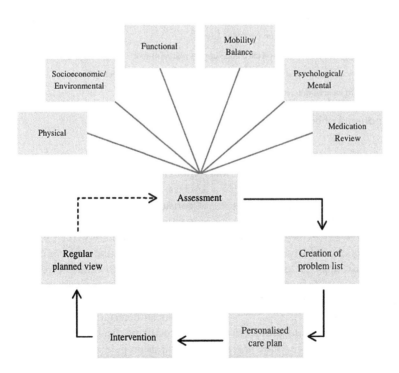

Figure 27.1 Components of a CGA, version 1.

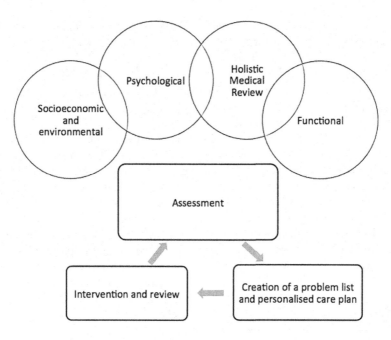

Figure 27.2 Components of a CGA, version 2.

- Diagnose and optimise the treatment of medical conditions.
- Utilise evidence-based medication reviews, such as STOPP/START criteria, alongside patients' personal priorities and degree of frailty.
- Discuss the significance of illness and impairment with older people and carers to define the impact this on everyday life.
- Design an individualised care and support plan collaboratively with the older person, outlining who takes responsibility for particular aspects of care and what to do in case of deterioration.

Figure 27.3 Components of holistic medical review for frail individuals.

factors and population groups can disrupt the links between socioeconomic disadvantage and health status [31].

SUGGESTIONS FOR PRACTICE

- *At a practice and policy level: organise local services in a way that supports disadvantaged populations of all ages, guided by the understanding that the drivers of inequality intersect across multiple domains*
- *At an individual patient level: adopt a person-centred approach at all ages is fundamental to identifying and addressing the particular social disadvantages that impact health*

Levels and conditions of education, employment, housing and welfare vary widely across social class, gender, race and migration status. Holistic consultations build practitioners' knowledge of the particular forms of disadvantage facing the local population and allow the provision of appropriate advocacy and support for individual patients.

In addition to clinical care, practitioners looking to address health inequalities should use their individual and collective voices to promote action on the social determinants of health. This can include restructuring health education towards a greater emphasis on public and social health. These sustainable measures should strive to shift perspectives away from an accusatory focus on the health behaviours of poorer individuals, towards a critical analysis of how unequal societies produce unequal health in later life. Using global health to illustrate examples of successful initiatives elsewhere, such education would draw attention to the structural barriers to good health and the modifiable and political nature of health inequalities. In addition, and as a result, health workers might feel more motivated and better equipped to lobby governments for redistributive measures to address gaps in health and wealth.

Mitigation

Mitigation of unequal ageing involves alleviating the disadvantage that has accumulated over the life course, thus it is a necessarily broad domain. Whilst the aforementioned person-centred approach can steer clinicians' specific mitigation strategies, research shows that social positioning is associated with particular modifiable determinants of health. One example is health care access. Recent research has demonstrated how particular groups, such as migrants, face barriers to accessing health care in the UK [32].

SUGGESTIONS FOR PRACTICE

- *Target user-friendly and accessible information at socially disadvantaged groups to support breaking down of barriers.*
- *Consider information sharing between practitioners, public health professionals and researchers on how to mitigate ingrained inequalities.*

Management

To manage the effects of unequal ageing it is recommended to adopt a person-centred, interdisciplinary approach, based around the principles of a CGA. However, whilst consulting with older people about their health needs, practitioners should consider the cumulative and intersecting dimensions of disadvantage faced by patients over their life course. As the chapter has highlighted, the unequal distribution of resources across the domains of gender, race and social class means that certain patients may react differentially to stigmatising diagnoses such as frailty. Moreover, particular management strategies may be seen as more or less acceptable by different social groups.

By being mindful of the multifaceted drivers of health inequalities, practitioners are more likely to reject a one-size-fits-all approach to health in later life. Instead, by centralising the older patient in decisions about their management, culturally sensitive and socially engaged care is provided. Such bespoke service provision requires resources.

SUGGESTIONS FOR PRACTICE

- *Service providers should prioritise the development of specialist geriatric services which embed the principles of an interdisciplinary CGA into an accessible service for older individuals.*

There is much that healthcare professionals can do to improve the lives of the most disadvantaged older people. This chapter has suggested that the prevention, mitigation and management of health inequalities in later life requires the rejection of a one-size fits all approach. Instead, emerging geriatric concepts such as frailty can be used as a tool through which practitioners explore, mitigate and manage the multiple and intersecting disadvantages impacting older people. A person-centred approach should strive to collaborate with the older population. Community practitioners can capitalise on the expertise of allied health care professionals and local specialist geriatric medicine services to address patients' priorities. Specific strategies, such as addressing barriers to health care for disadvantaged populations, should accompany individual patient advocacy.

Current demographic changes, such as increasing life expectancy, smaller family sizes, and economic policies that increase income disparity over the course of working life predict growing inequalities in later life for today's younger generation. Addressing the drivers of these inequalities should be priority. Much of the change required concerns the social determinants of health inequalities across the life course. Specifically, a policy focus on equitable access to quality education and improvement of the living and employment conditions for the most disadvantaged groups is needed. This social change requires political impetus and social policy reform, domains often assumed to be outside of the clinical realm. However, in order to address the human cost of increasing health inequalities on vulnerable older people, practitioners must take steps outside of their clinical encounters. Here, restructuring medical education, steering policy and research and capitalising on medical credentials to lobby politicians, are potential avenues though which health care professionals might influence and reform the social policy that drives inequality.

REFERENCES

1. Office for National Statistics. Living longer: How our population is changing and why it matters. [Internet]. 2018 [cited 11.4.19]. Available at: https://www.ons.gov.uk/peoplepopulationandcommunity/birthsdeathsandmarriages/ageing/articles/livinglongerhowourpopulationischangingandwhyitmatters/2018-08-13#how-is-the-uk-population-changing

2. Dorling D. The mother of underlying causes–economic ranking and health inequality. *Social Science & Medicine*. 2015 Mar 1;128:327–30.

3. Campbell D. NHS cannot cope with ageing population, warns top doctor. *The Guardian*. [Internet]. 2015 [cited 11.4.19]. Available at: https://www.theguardian.com/society/2015/jan/19/nhs-we-have-not-fit-for-future-warns-top-doctor-bruce-keogh

4. Department for Work and Pensions. Fuller Working Lives Evidence Base, using Annual Population Survey data July 2015–2016. [Internet]. 2017 [cited 11.4.19]. Available at: https://assets.publishing.service.gov.uk/government/uploads/system/uploads/attachment_data/file/648979/fuller-working-lives-evidence-base-2017.pdf

5. Singh-Manoux A, Ferrie JE, Chandola T, Marmot M. Socioeconomic trajectories across the life course and health outcomes in midlife: Evidence for the accumulation hypothesis? *International Journal of Epidemiology*. 2004 Jul 15;33(5):1072–9.

6. Otero-Rodríguez A, León-Muñoz LM, Banegas JR, Guallar-Castillón P, Rodríguez-Artalejo F, Regidor E. Life-course socioeconomic position and change in quality of life among older adults: Evidence for the role of a critical period, accumulation of exposure and social mobility. *Journal of Epidemiology and Community Health*. 2011 Nov 1;65(11):964–71.

7. Vanhoutte B, Nazroo J. Life course pathways to later life wellbeing: A comparative study of the role of socio-economic position in England and the US. *Journal of Population Ageing*. 2016 Jun 1;9(1–2):157–77.

8. Banks J, Batty D, Nazroo J, Oskala A, Steptoe A. The dynamics of ageing: Evidence from the English Longitudinal Study of ageing 2002–16 (Wave 8). [Internet]. 2017 [cited 11.4.19]. Available at: https://www.elsa-project.ac.uk/publicationDetails/id/13512

9. Department for Work and Pensions. Households below average income time series, 1994–95 to 2016/17. [Internet]. 2018 [cited 11.4.19]. Available at: https://www.gov.uk/government/statistics/households-below-average-income-199495-to-201617

10. Wallace S, Nazroo J, Bécares L. Cumulative effect of racial discrimination on the mental health of ethnic minorities in the United Kingdom. *American Journal of Public Health*. 2016 Jul;106(7):1294–300.

11. Runnymede and the Centre for Policy on Ageing. The future ageing of the ethnic minority population of England and Wales. London. [Internet]. 2010 [cited 11.4.19]. Available at: https://www.runnymedetrust.org/uploads/publications/pdfs/TheFutureAgeingOfTheEthnicMinorityPopulation-ForWebJuly2010.pdf

12. Tomkow L. Health in a hostile hospitality [PhD thesis] University of Manchester, 2019 Under Review.

13. Morley JE, Vellas B, Van Kan GA, Anker SD, Bauer JM, Bernabei R, Cesari M, Chumlea WC, Doehner W, Evans J, Fried LP. Frailty consensus: A call to action. *Journal of the American Medical Directors Association*. 2013 Jun 1;14(6):392–7.

14. Marshall A, Nazroo J, Tampubolon G, Vanhoutte B. Cohort differences in the levels and trajectories of frailty among older people in England. *Journal of Epidemiology and Community Health*. 2015 Apr 1;69(4):316–21.

15. Shaw RL, Gwyther H, Holland C, Bujnowska-Fedak MA, Kurpas D, Cano A, Marcucci M, Riva S, D'Avanzo BA. Understanding frailty: Meanings and beliefs about screening

and prevention across key stakeholder groups in Europe. *Ageing & Society.* 2018 Jun;38(6):1223–52.

16. Gilleard C, Higgs P. Frailty, disability and old age: A re-appraisal. *Health.* 2011 Sep;15(5):475–90.

17. Grenier A. The distinction between being and feeling frail: Exploring emotional experiences in health and social care. *Journal of Social Work Practice.* 2006 Nov 1;20(3):299–313.

18. Hubbard RE, Goodwin VA, Llewellyn DJ, Warmoth K, Lang IA. Frailty, financial resources and subjective well-being in later life. *Archives of Gerontology and Geriatrics.* 2014 May 1;58(3):364–9.

19. Fried LP, Tangen CM, Walston J, Newman AB, Hirsch C, Gottdiener J, Seeman T, Tracy R, Kop WJ, Burke G, McBurnie MA. Frailty in older adults: Evidence for a phenotype. *The Journals of Gerontology Series A: Biological Sciences and Medical Sciences.* 2001 Mar 1;56(3):M146–57.

20. Mitnitski AB, Mogilner AJ, Rockwood K. Accumulation of deficits as a proxy measure of aging. *The Scientific World Journal.* 2001;1:323–36.

21. Rockwood K, Andrew M, Mitnitski A. A comparison of two approaches to measuring frailty in elderly people. *The Journals of Gerontology Series A: Biological Sciences and Medical Sciences.* 2007 Jul 1;62(7):738–43.

22. Tomkow L. The emergence and utilisation of frailty in the United Kingdom: A contemporary biopolitical practice. *Ageing & Society.* 2018:1–8.

23. Theou O, Stathokostas L, Roland KP, Jakobi JM, Patterson C, Vandervoort AA, Jones GR. The effectiveness of exercise interventions for the management of frailty: A systematic review. *Journal of Aging Research.* 2011;2011.

24. Liu CJ, Latham NK. Progressive resistance strength training for improving physical function in older adults. *Cochrane Database of Systematic Reviews.* 2009(3).

25. Cramm JM, Twisk J, Nieboer AP. Self-management abilities and frailty are important for healthy aging among community-dwelling older people; a cross-sectional study. *BMC Geriatrics.* 2014 Dec;14(1):28.

26. Welsh TJ, Gordon AL, Gladman JR. Comprehensive geriatric assessment–a guide for the non-specialist. *International Journal of Clinical Practice.* 2014 Mar;68(3):290.

27. Ellis G, Whitehead MA, Robinson D, O'Neill D, Langhorne P. Comprehensive geriatric assessment for older adults admitted to hospital: Meta-analysis of randomised controlled trials. *BMJ.* 2011 Oct 27;343:d6553.

28. Briggs R, McDonough A, Ellis G, Bennett K, O'Neill D, Robinson D. Comprehensive Geriatric Assessment for community-dwelling, high-risk, frail, older people. *Cochrane Database of Systematic Reviews.* 2017(6).

29. Turner G, Clegg A. Best practice guidelines for the management of frailty: A British Geriatrics Society, Age UK and Royal College of General Practitioners report. *Age and Ageing.* 2014 Nov 1;43(6):744–7.

30. British Geriatrics Society. CGA in Primary Care Settings: The elements of the CGA process. [Internet]. 2019 [cited 11.4.19]. Available at: https://www.bgs.org.uk/resources/2-cga-in-primary-care-settings-the-elements-of-the-cga-process

31. OECD. *Preventing Ageing Unequally.* OECD Publishing. [Internet]. 2017 [cited 11.4.19]. Available at: https://dx.doi.org/10.1787/9789264279087-en

32. Kang C, Tomkow L, Farrington R. Access to primary health care for asylum seekers and refugees: A qualitative study of service user experiences in the UK. *British Journal of General Practice.* 2019 Feb 12:bjgp19X701309.

28

How Can We Improve Health and Healthcare Experiences of Black, Asian and Minority Ethnic (BAME) Communities?

ENAM-UL HAQUE, BUSHERA CHOUDRY AND RIYA E. GEORGE

At a young age, I learnt of the heartache my father suffered with the loss of his father and brother to hepatocellular carcinoma and liver cirrhosis, both caused by hepatitis; a condition that could now be managed effectively. My parents, like many Bangladeshi patients, also suffered with type II diabetes, and I have seen the consequences and complications of these conditions through them…

As authors, we have all experienced our family members suffer with hepatitis, diabetes or mental illness; conditions prevalent in BAME communities [1]. Whilst the health of the population as a whole in the United Kingdom may be improving, health inequalities remain stubbornly ubiquitous [2]. In most healthcare systems it is acknowledged that BAME populations experience poorer health and barriers to accessing services [3]. The sources of these ethnic disparities are complex and multifactorial and have been described as 'pervasive' (2003, 2004), 'prevalent' (2006), 'persistent' (2008) and worryingly 'not improving' (2010) and 'not changing' (2012, 2015).

Differences in health across ethnic groups has been reported internationally for a range of health outcomes. The relationship between ethnicity and health is multifaceted, with evidence suggesting much of this variation is associated with socioeconomic position [4]. Conventional indicators and measurements of ethnicity have statistically explained health differences between BAME and white populations. However, they do not tell the full story and must be interpreted with caution [5].

REMEMBERING THE 'ME' IN BAME

The UK is multicultural with a demographic that is frequently described as diverse: 86% of the UK population is reported as white and 14 % from BAME backgrounds. Within this 14%, 7.5% are from Asian ethnic groups, 3.3% are belonging to Black ethnic groups, 2.2% being mixed or multiple ethnic groups and 1% classed as other ethnic groups [6]. The acronyms BAME (Black, Asian and Minority Ethnic) and BME (Black and Minority Ethnic) are popular terms and these arguably simplistic abbreviations are used to describe richly heterogeneous and varied populations.

However, in reality the terms BAME and BME are vaguely defined, poorly understood and used interchangeably [7]. Various criticisms have been made over the disregard for the inherent complexity in these different populations, with authors stating terms such as BAME and BME are 'outdated', 'misleading' and 'simply code for not being White' [8]. Additionally, the binary division of the population into white and BAME (or non-white) categories discounts the heterogeneity within white populations. The UK census data from 2001 to 2011 showed the percentage of the population of England and Wales that was classed as 'White British' decreased from 87.4% to 80.5%, whilst the 'Other White' group saw the largest increase in their share of the population from 2.6% to 4.4% [6]. Some argue that black, Asian and minority ethnic groups are three discrete populations with distinct differences, and potentially specific ethnic groups among them. As authors, when asked to define our ethnicity our responses differed: second-generation Bangladeshi, first-generation British Pakistani and British Asian, South Indian; yet statistically we are all classed as BAME. By grouping diverse individuals into one category (that can be seen as homogenous populations), it may serve to mask the distinct experiences and disadvantages specific ethnic groups face [9].

Conventional routine population data such as the census has conflated the concepts of race (broadly meaning biological or physical differences between groups of people) and ethnicity (a broader concept describing shared cultural practices, perspectives and distinctions such as nationality, religion or language that set apart one group of people from another) as being the same and have divided the population into quantifiable categories to explore differences between ethnic groups [10]. These ethnic categories become crude surrogates for the experiences of individuals within these predefined groupings. This categorisation renders invisible additional factors that contribute to disparities in health such as discrimination, racism, language barriers and the stressors associated with migration. In the UK census data there are 18 ethnic group categories, which are grouped into five broad ethnic classifications; these are outlined in Table 28.1.

It appears that ethnicity has been indexed either by race, nationality or country of birth. This can become problematic for individuals whose nationality differs from their country of birth or whose nationality changes due to other life experiences such as marital status. Even within these 18 categories it is impossible to represent every ethnic group. The introduction of new pre-coded choices, such as 'mixed ethnicity' categories has resulted in marked changes in the relationship between different ethnic groups and health [11]. This demonstrates that the way in which methods of data collection construe ethnicity can alter how healthcare experiences are understood among different ethnic groups. Similarly, Table 28.2 outlines the ethnic group classifications for the United States and Canada.

Table 28.1 UK Census Data – Ethnicity Classifications

Ethnic Group Classifications
White
• English/Welsh/Scottish/Northern Irish/British
• Irish
• Gypsy or Irish Traveller
• Any other White background
Mixed/Multiple ethnic groups
• White and Black Caribbean
• White and Black African
• White and Asian
• Any other Mixed / Multiple ethnic background
Asian/Asian British
• Indian
• Pakistani
• Bangladeshi
• Chinese
• Any other Asian background
Black/African/Caribbean/Black British
• African
• Caribbean
• Any other Black / African / Caribbean background
Other ethnic group
• Arab
• Any other ethnic group

Table 28.2 US and Canadian Census Data

United States of America Census Data Racial and Ethnic Group Classifications	Canada Census Data Ethnic Group Classifications	
White A person having origins in any of the original peoples of Europe, the Middle East, or North Africa.	Canadian English Scottish French	Irish German Chinese Italian
Black or African American A person having origins in any of the black racial groups of Africa.	First Nations (North American Indians) East Indian Dutch	Ukrainian Polish
American Indian or Alaska Native A person having origins in any of the original peoples of North and South America (including Central America), and who maintains tribal affiliation or community attachment.	FilipinoM British Isles Origins Russian Metis	Portuguese Welsh Norwegian
Asian A person having origins in any of the original peoples of the Far East, Southeast Asia, or the Indian subcontinent including, for example, Cambodia, China, India, Japan, Korea, Malaysia, Pakistan, the Philippine Islands, Thailand, and Vietnam.		
Native Hawaiian or Other Pacific Islander A person having origins in any of the original peoples of Hawaii, Guam, Samoa, or other Pacific Islands.		
Hispanic or Latino A person of Cuban, Mexican, Puerto Rican, South or Central American, or other Spanish culture or origin, regardless of race. The term, "Spanish origin", can be used in addition to "Hispanic or Latino".		
Two or more races **Other races**		

Parallel to the UK census, it seems ethnicity has been indexed by race, nationality, country of birth and in some cases by language. Ethnicity and race are socially constructed concepts which are challenging to compartmentalise into specific categories [10]. The rapid growth of diverse ethnic communities, each with their own health profiles and cultural norms and practices, further departs from the appropriateness in using terms such as BAME and BME. In writing this chapter, it became apparent that using the term BAME is problematic as it begs the question who does this include and exclude? Throughout this chapter the exact details of how ethnicity is classified in different studies is made transparent, this is to ensure

the constructed nature of the categories is fully apparent. The illustrated examples of possible interventions are targeted broadly at specific ethnic minority populations in the UK (this includes white ethnic minority groups such as Gypsy and Travellers), which typically fall under the umbrella term BAME.

HEALTH CONDITIONS AND BARRIERS TO ACCESSING SERVICES FOR BAME COMMUNITIES

A multitude of research shows the differential risk of disease for specific ethnic minority communities. These patterns of ethnic variations in health are hugely diverse and interlinked with a variety of complex risk factors [12]. A summary of the differential risk of disease and variations in a few behavioural risk factors is shown in Table 28.3 and 28.4; this has been developed from the information presented in the 2018 National Institute of Clinical Excellence (NICE) briefing paper [13].

Echoing the information presented in Table 28.3, certain diseases are more prevalent in specific ethnic minority populations. For example, South Asian patients are six times more likely and black patients three times more likely to be diagnosed with type II diabetes compared to the general population (defined in this research as white) [14]. South Asians are also 1.5 times more likely to die from cardiovascular disease, such as coronary heart disease and stroke, than the general white population, with insulin resistance suggested as attributable to this disease [15]. However, other studies show South Asian patients are delayed in receiving appropriate care which is thought to be due to misunderstanding the presenting symptoms [16]. Interestingly, black patients have less cardiovascular risk compared to the general white population [15]. The Gypsy, Roma and Traveller (GRT) communities experience some of the worst health inequalities of any ethnic minority populations in the UK; life expectancy is 12 years lower in GRT compared to the general white population [17]. GRT women also experience higher rates of miscarriage, and stillbirths and infant mortality are three times higher in comparison to the general white population [18]. Ethnic populations also differ genetically, making certain diseases more prevalent, for example sickle cell disease and Creutzfeldt-Jakob in black ethnic groups [19].

The 'Adult Psychiatry Morbidity Survey: Survey of Mental Health and Wellbeing' showed black women were more likely to have common mental disorders (29.3% of black women compared to 20.9% in the white population) [20]. Black and Asian women were also more likely to experience panic disorders. Grey et al.'s systematic review exploring mental health inequalities facing UK minority ethnic populations found black Caribbean patients were two to eight times more likely to be diagnosed with severe mental health problems compared with the white population [21]. Irish populations have the highest suicide rates for female children in the European Union. The 2018 'Out of Silence' report outlined specific mental health needs of Irish women and girls [22].

The information above is merely a snapshot of the ethnic disparities in health outcomes between ethnic minority groups in comparison to the general population. These ethnic disparities represent a cumulative effect of a variety of risk factors. The issues highlighted in Table 28.4 are mostly associated with lifestyle factors, however other influences such as health beliefs and expectations, socioeconomic position and direct/ indirect discrimination contribute to the expression of health inequalities and warrants further research to understand the interrelationship between these attributable factors [23, 24]. Table 28.5 highlights a broad overview of responses from a survey carried out among doctors in north England who were asked to identity, from their clinical experiences, barriers to accessing services for BAME communities.

Table 28.3 Differential Risk of Disease for Different Population Subgroups

Disease	Highest Prevalence
Angina	Pakistani men of all ages and Indian women
Myocardial infarctions	Pakistani men and women over 55 years old
Cardiovascular disease	South Asian men are 50% more likely to have coronary heart disease than men in the general population. Bangladeshis have the highest rates (followed by Pakistanis, then Indians and other South Asians).
Hypertension	Black Caribbean groups
Diabetes	Bangladeshi, Pakistani, Indian, Black African and Chinese populations
Sexually transmitted diseases (including HIV)	Black ethnic groups

Table 28.4 Variations in Behavioural Risk Factors among Different Population Subgroups

Risk factors	
Smoking	Highest in Black, Asian, Black Caribbean and Bangladeshi men and Black Caribbean women.
Physical activity	Pakistani and Bangladeshi groups report low levels of physical activity.
Alcohol consumption	Alcohol consumption above the recommended level reported in men of Indian, Black Caribbean, Black African and Chinese populations.
Obesity or being overweight	Highest in Black and Asian populations.

CASE STUDY

AskDoc

AskDoc is an organisation that was set up in Manchester 2011 with the aim to educate, engage and empower local BAME populations. It has achieved this through a series of tailored public health interventions designed to raise awareness and knowledge and facilitate early access to screening and treatment for prevalent health conditions. AskDoc has worked collaboratively with a range of healthcare organisations over the past 8 years to slowly dismantle barriers to accessing healthcare services for BAME populations.

Raising Awareness and Early Access to Screening for Hepatitis C

A collaborative project between AskDoc and Public Health England's north-west centre was established to raise awareness and encourage uptake of screening for hepatitis C among the British Pakistani community. Third-sector organisations, such as the Hepatitis C Trust and local hepatologists, were also involved. The project involved two core stages; the first stage was centred on challenging common misconceptions. A series of ten workshops at local public areas such as mosques were facilitated to challenge patient perceptions of hepatitis C, covering aspects such as aetiology, clinical features and potential complications, see Figure 28.1.

The workshops were developed in English and Urdu, thus enabling an accurate understanding of the condition. Feedback from the workshops showed they were positively received by the audience, with an attendee commenting, 'It has really opened my eyes'. As authors, from our clinical experiences this was extremely positive to hear as many patients with hepatitis C are reluctant to discuss their condition due to the ongoing stigma surrounding it.

Table 28.5 Barriers to Accessing Services – Survey Responses

Socioeconomic position	Experiences of discrimination	Cultural health beliefs and expectations
• Poor health literacy resulting in misunderstandings/ misconceptions of modern medicine i.e. MMI, conditions and treatments • Funding for travel to healthcare services • Poor knowledge and engagement in health protective factors • Migrant status resulting in language barriers	• Experiences of individual or institutional racism in healthcare services • Domestic abuse among women • Coercion from family members or healthcare practitioners • Culturally insensitive language with healthcare practitioners	• Stigma concerning certain conditions i.e. mental health and hepatitis. • Communication issues between healthcare providers and patients/ lack of and limited training with interpreters/ translators • Under-representation of BAME healthcare professionals • Preference for alternative medicines and herbal treatments

Misconceptions	True or False
1. Hepatitis C is spread through **shaking hands** with an infected person	**False** We reassured the audience that spread did not occur this way. Spread is normally by blood to blood transmission, such as using contaminated medical equipment.
2. Hepatitis C is spread through **sharing food** with an infected person	**False** We reassured the audience that the infection was not spread through saliva but through blood
3. Hepatitis C was spread mainly by **unprotected sex** and so a person affected by this was stigmatised by the community	**Possible, but not primary route** Although sexual transmission was possible, the main cause of spread was through use of non-sterile medical equipment and used razors. This then challenged the stereotype and stigma accompanying Hepatitis C.

Figure 28.1 Misconceptions around hepatitis C.

The second stage of the project involved designing and delivering a screening programme for hepatitis C which was tailored to the British Pakistani community. This involved adapting conventional methods of screening, see Figure 28.2 as an example. Orasure hepatitis C screening methods were used which can detect the virus in saliva. Patients were tested by swabbing their buccal mucosa, with results being available within the hour. The risk of blood-borne transmission and needle-stick injuries was therefore avoided, and there was no distress for patients. Two screening events in 2015 and a further two events in 2016 were run. A total of 208 individuals were tested in 2015 with four individuals found to be positive, 237 individuals were tested in 2016 with five individuals found to be positive.

With the support of Public Health England, patients testing positive were referred back to their general practitioner for more detailed tests. Those who were not registered with a general practitioner were referred to a specialist hepatology clinic locally. Key challenges in this project were around obtaining funding and the required manpower to run the screening events. Fortunately, funds were provided by the Hepatitis C Trust and volunteer doctors and medical students involved in AskDoc assisted with the testing and counselling.

Health Awareness Workshops

Health awareness workshops are a primary method in equipping BAME communities with the necessary knowledge and information and provide an opportunity to challenge patient perceptions. The structure of the workshops, which compliment AskDoc's vision of educating, engaging and empowering BAME communities, involves formal presentations, small group discussions, question-and-answer panels, and feedback and evaluation.

Numerous workshops on a wide variety of topics such as cardiovascular health, obesity, mental health and type II diabetes have been delivered to a diverse array of ethnic minority communities in the Greater Manchester area, see Figure 28.3 as examples. This has enabled AskDoc to develop a reputation as experts in public health interventions tailored towards BAME communities, which has led to them speaking at a range of different healthcare conferences.

Figure 28.3 highlights the results of regular feedback evaluation that is conducted as part of the workshops; this illustrates immediate

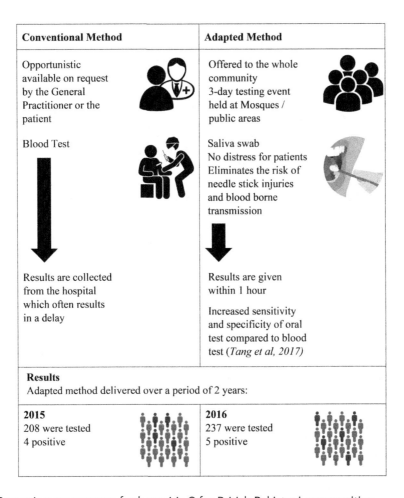

Conventional Method	Adapted Method
Opportunistic available on request by the General Practitioner or the patient	Offered to the whole community 3-day testing event held at Mosques / public areas
Blood Test	Saliva swab No distress for patients Eliminates the risk of needle stick injuries and blood borne transmission
Results are collected from the hospital which often results in a delay	Results are given within 1 hour Increased sensitivity and specificity of oral test compared to blood test (*Tang et al, 2017*)

Results
Adapted method delivered over a period of 2 years:

2015 208 were tested 4 positive	**2016** 237 were tested 5 positive

Figure 28.2 Screening programme for hepatitis C for British Pakistani communities.

improvements in knowledge after the workshops. Three key BAME health issues identified by recent NICE guidance have been the focus of the health awareness workshops, these include cardiovascular health, diabetes and mental health. A permanent base in Oldham has been established to deliver a programme of activities. This has been created in collaboration with a local charity which has ensured a regular menu of activities for the local British Pakistani community.

The greatest challenge AskDoc has experienced is capturing the quality of impact. Evaluation questionnaires were utilised to assess if the intervention was successful in improving knowledge and changes in attitudes on a short-term basis, but further evaluative methods are needed to assess the longer-term impact of the interventions. This will highlight whether these short interventions have made tangible improvements to the health of BAME communities.

Improving Health Outcomes for Patients with Poorly Controlled Diabetes

AskDoc was invited by a locality group in Manchester Clinical Commissioning Group to work with them in improving health outcomes for BAME patients with poorly controlled type 2 diabetes. It was identified that the locality had a large proportion of BAME patients with diabetes with poor health outcomes. A series of bespoke cultural diversity workshops on diabetes were delivered to the local community, with resources and support provided by Diabetes UK. The workshops focused on lifestyle factors such as diet and

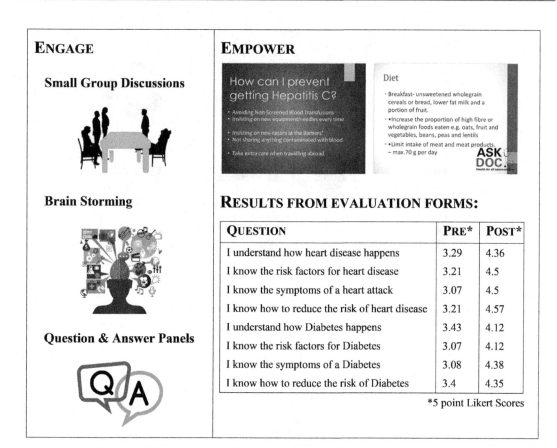

Figure 28.3 Methods to engage and empower BAME communities.

exercise, with coverage on recommended food choices in South Asian meals, thereby making the content meaningful and relatable, see Figure 28.4.

One of the presentation slides had a traditional South Asian breakfast and it was interesting to see members of the audience admitting to having *halwa puri* (high sugar and carbohydrate content) for breakfast. It gave the presenters an opportunity to explore alternative options with the community. Following the workshops, specialist interventions for patients with poorly controlled diabetes took place. Patients were invited to attend a workshop on diabetes which was accompanied by a tailored support plan with health trainers. The workshop was designed and delivered by a medical student as a part of a special study module, and evaluation data was obtained. The intervention focused on raising awareness of a healthy diet and the importance of exercise and weight reduction, ensuring the information was adapted to a typical South Asian lifestyle. Nine patients were recruited from GP surgeries in the locality. However, only three attended the training event. The impact of the workshop was

measured via a 5-point Likert score, ranging from strongly disagree [1] to strongly agree [5]. Patients scored an average of five for better understanding the importance of diabetic control and methods for improving their diabetic control. Similarly, to the challenges mentioned in other interventions, obtaining funding proved difficult and much of this work relied on the goodwill of volunteers.

Diversity has been recognised as an increasingly important component in the undergraduate medical curriculum [25]. Disparities in the experiences between BAME and white medical and dental students exists across the UK. BAME students are more likely to perform poorly in examinations and experience discrimination [26]. Tackling these issues, we believe, is also part of empowering BAME communities in healthcare as a whole and securing a culturally diverse workforce for an increasingly diverse patient population. Case examples 4 and 5 showcase some of the initiatives to empower BAME student/ healthcare provider communities within medicine and dentistry.

NHS Conventional Diabetes Diet Advice	Diet Advice tailored for South Asians
You can eat many types of foods There's nothing you can't eat if you have type 2 diabetes, but you'll have to limit certain foods. You should: • eat a wide range of foods – including fruit, vegetables and some starchy foods like pasta • keep sugar, fat and salt to a minimum • eat breakfast, lunch and dinner every day – don't skip meals If you need to change your diet, it might be easier to make small changes every week. Information about food can be found on these diabetes sites: • food for people with diabetes • tips on eating with your family and eating out • recipes for people with diabetes • food and nutrition message board	**Healthy Eating and Diet Tips for South Asians** Asians have a particularly high susceptibility to type 2 diabetes and a healthy diet is one of the main ways in which diabetes can be controlled. Type 2 diabetes is generally associated with carrying too much body weight, over 85% of people with type 2 are overweight. *Healthy eating can help control diabetes* **Guidelines for a healthy diet** o Cut down on simple, refined carbohydrates o Cut down on eating high calorie and fried foods o Choose unsaturated fats over saturated fats o Choose less or smaller portions of fatty or carbohydrate heavy foods o Include plenty of fresh vegetables and also fruit o Reduce the amount of processed foods in your diet o Watch the salt content **Cutting down on high calorie foods** Some of the highest calorie foods are those which combine relatively high amounts of carbohydrate and saturated fat. Fried foods such as the below tend to be highly calorific: o Fried rice o Samosas o Onion bhajis o Masala curries Dishes using ghee, makhan or cream will also add calories. Naan bread is quite bulky so can also push up the calories. You may ask yourself what you can eat? Look for lighter foods such as popadoms instead of naan. Curries such as bhuna or tandoori may be slightly better options for curry.

Figure 28.4 Tailored dietary advice.

Widening Success of BAME Medical and Dental Students

Reducing the attainment gap between white and BAME medical and dental students is a priority for many UK medical and dental institutions across the UK. Differential attainment is a term used to describe gaps in educational achievement between different demographic groups undertaking the same assessment. Woolf et al. [25] stated 'ethnic differences in attainment seem to be a consistent feature of medical education in the UK…and have persisted at least for the past three decades'. Wider research suggests ethnic minority students are more likely to struggle with integration into university life, report negative student experiences, less likely to access academic support avenues, and more likely to experience differential attainment in assessments [27].

Differential attainment exists across university disciplines; however, the imperative to address gaps may be more pressing in medicine and dentistry given the higher percentage of BAME students

enrolling on these courses and the growing need for a diverse workforce to address an increasingly culturally diverse patient population. At Queen Mary University of London, a large interdisciplinary project has been established to explore this further, see Figure 28.5 for an introduction into the project.

Facilitating Discussions on Discrimination Among Medical Students

The Building the Anti-Racist Classroom (BARC) student journey game was commissioned by the Re-Imagining Attainment For All projects based at Queen Mary University of London and the University of Roehampton. The game has been developed for UK university staff who are committed to or involved in developing interventions that address racial discrimination and inequalities in higher education. It can be played by both academics and members of professional services staff. The game provides learners with an interactive

Understanding and addressing differential academic outcomes and experiences among Black Asian and Minority Ethnic (BAME) undergraduate medical and dental students

Riya George, Mangala Patel, Aylin Baysan, Daniel Hartley, Diego Bunge, Daniel Uribe, Emma Kennedy, Claire Loffman and Harris Nageswaran.

Research Questions:

1. How do undergraduate medical and dental students understand the term 'BAME' and who does this include and exclude?
2. What potential differences exist between the academic outcomes of BAME and White undergraduate dental and medical students and do these potential differences persist after controlling for other social demographic factors?
3. What experiences are associated with being a BAME undergraduate medical or dental student? (Accounting for intersectional aspects of student identity i.e. gender, socioeconomic status and religion).
4. Do the findings suggest potential areas of change (i.e. institutional) that could acknowledge and support BAME undergraduate medical and dental students' experiences and outcomes?

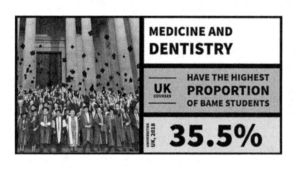 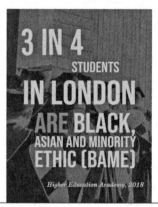

Figure 28.5 Widening success project at QMUL.

format to engage with issues around discrimination in a meaningful way and to consider potential zones of conflicts. This board game is a free resource for universities to use, further details can be found at https://barcworkshop.org/resources/student-journey-game/.

REFERENCES

1. Atkinson M, Clark M, Clay D. *Systematic Review of Ethnicity and Health Service Access for London.* Coventry: Centre for Health Services Studies, University of Warwick, 2001.
2. Bell C, Duffy M, Robinson A, Laverty C. Health inequalities Annual Report. Department of Health, 2018. Available at: https://www.health-ni.gov.uk/sites/default/files/publications/health/hscims-report-2018.pdf
3. Graham H, Kelly MP. Health inequalities: Concepts, frameworks and policy. Briefing paper. National Health Service, Health Development Agency, 2004.
4. Smith GD. Learning to live with complexity: Ethnicity, socioeconomic position and health in Britain and the United States. *American Journal of Public Health*, 2000; 90 (11): 1694–1698.
5. Nazroo JY. The structuring of ethnic inequalities in health: Economic position, racial discrimination and racism. *Public Health Matters*, 2003; 93 (2): 277–284.
6. Census General Report, Office for National Statistics, 2011. Available at: https://www.ons.gov.uk/census/2011census/howourcensusworks/howdidwedoin2011/2011censusgeneralreport

7. Kalayil S. Is it time to ditch the term BAME? *The Independent*, 2018. Available at: https://www.independent.co.uk/news/long_reads/bame-ethnic-minorities-race-identity-politics-windrush-uk-a8504961.html

8. Trevor P. Is it time to ditch the term 'Black, Asian and minority ethnic' (BAME)? *The Guardian*, 2018. Available at: https://www.theguardian.com/commentisfree/2015/may/22/black-asian-minority-ethnic-bame-bme-trevor-phillips-racial-minorities

9. Millward LM, Kelly MP, Nutbeam D. Public health interventions and research: The evidence. London: Health Development Agency, 2003. Available at: www.hda.nhs.uk/evidence

10. Bhopal R. Glossary of terms relating to ethnicity and race: For reflection and debate. *Journal of Epidemiology and Community Health*, 2004; 58: 441–445.

11. Krieger N. Embodying inequalities: A review of concepts, measures and methods for studying health consequences of discrimination. *International Journal of Health Services*, 1999; 29: 295–352.

12. Williams DR, Neighbors HW, Jackson JS. Racial and ethnic discrimination and health: Findings from community studies. *American Journal of Public Health*, 2003; 93(2): 200–208.

13. National Institute of Clinical Excellence (NICE). Health and social care directore. Quality standards and indicators – briefing paper, 2018. Available at: https://www.nice.org.uk/guidance/GID-QS10079/documents/briefing-paper

14. Robinson L. South Asians in Britain: Acculturation, identity and perceived discrimination. *Psychology and Developing Societies*, 2005; 17 (2): 181–194.

15. Hanif W, Susarla R. Diabetes and cardiovascular risk in UK South Asians; an overview. *The British Journal of Cardiology*, 2018; 25 (2): S8–S13.

16. Diabetes UK. Diabetes in the UK 2010; Key statistics on diabetes, 2010. Available at: https://www.diabetes.org.uk/resources-s3/2017-11/diabetes_in_the_uk_2010.pdf

17. Hajioff S, Mckee M. The health of Roma people: A review of the published literature. *Journal of Epidemiology and Community Health*, 2000; 54: 864–869.

18. Cook B, Wayne GF, Valentine A, Lessios A, Yeh E. Revisiting the evidence on health and healthcare disparities among the Roma: A systematic review from 2003–2012. *Journal of Public Health*, 2013; 58(6): 885–911.

19. Huang T, Shu Y, Cai YD. Genetic differences among ethnic groups. *BMC Genomics*, 2015; 16: 1093.

20. Adult Psychiatric Morbidity Survey: Survey of Mental Health and Wellbeing. England, 2014. Available at: https://digital.nhs.uk/data-and-information/publications/statistical/adult-psychiatric-morbidity-survey/adult-psychiatric-morbidity-survey-survey-of-mental-health-and-wellbeing-england-2014

21. Grey T, Sewell H, Shapiro G, Ashraf F. Harnessing diversity. Mental health inequalities facing UK minority ethnic populations: Causal factors and solutions. *Journal of Psychological Issues in Organisational Culture*, 2013; 3(S1): 146–157.

22. National Women's Council of Ireland. Out of Silence: Women's mental health in their own words. *Healthy Ireland*, 2018. Available at: https://www.nwci.ie/images/uploads/Out_of_Silence_Report_-_NWCI_-_2018.pdf

23. Szczepura A. Access to healthcare for ethnic minority populations. *Postgraduate Medicine*, 2008; 81: 141–147.

24. Kings Fund. Briefing: Access to healthcare and minority ethnic groups. 2006. Available at: https://www.kingsfund.org.uk/sites/default/files/field/field_publication_file/access-to-healthcare-minority-ethnic-groups-briefing-kings-fund-february-2006.pdf

25. Dogra N, Bhatti F, Ertubey C, Kelly M, Rowlands A, Singh D, Turner M. Teaching diversity to medical undergraduates: Curriculum development, delivery and assessment. AMEE Guide No. 103. *Medical Teacher*, 2016; 38 (4): 323–337.

26. Woolf K, Rich A, Viney R, Needleman S, Griffin A. Perceived causes of differential attainment in UK postgraduate medical training: A national qualitative study. *BMJ Open*, 2016; 6: 1–9.

27. Woolf K, McManus IC, Potts HWW, Dacre J. The mediators of minority ethnic underperformance in final medical school examinations. *British Journal of Educational Psychology*, 2013; 83: 135–159.

29

Engaging with the Health Issues of Gypsies and Travellers

ELIZABETH KEAT, MILENA MARSZALEK, HELEN JONES AND
JAMES MATHESON

More of the Travelling community is now living in housing or on settled sites and yet are still confronted with institutionalised racism.

Gypsy Travellers are among the UK's most socially excluded groups and have the worst health outcomes of any ethnic minority [1]. Governmental policy aiming to reduce health inequalities has not positively impacted the health status of the Travelling community.

Negative cultural stereotypes and harsh living conditions can further exacerbate their difficulties. Some experience a lack of essential amenities, with others not living in a fixed abode are not eligible for a variety of services. This is one of the many stereotypes that Travellers face that are not always true. More of the Travelling community is now living in housing or on settled sites and yet many are still confronted with institutional racism. Some services have not been receptive to working with Travelling communities in the past.

Literacy levels can be lower than the societal average. This leads to low health literacy as health systems frequently rely upon written letters, reports and online systems, further excluding this community and increasing their vulnerability. Contact with services can be low in this community for a variety of reasons. Services may assume the Travelling community is self-reliant and at times closed off from outside communities. Previous negative experiences associated with engaging with healthcare or general practice can lead to low expectations of healthcare and a lack of trust in services. Instances where trusted workers were withdrawn and where projects lost sustainability have contributed to these attitudes.

One of the eventual consequences of this is a lack of confidence from the Travelling community in attending services alone due to previous poor experiences or expectations of a poor service. Low literacy levels compound difficulties experienced when accessing services.

As most public health campaigns or screening invites rely upon someone having a settled address, the community may not be able to identify early symptoms or attend screenings. This may have a significant impact on prognosis. These factors contribute to the barriers obstructing adequate healthcare access in these communities.

It is for these many reasons that outreach work with the Travelling community is vital in reducing health inequalities in a long-marginalised group. Restorative work with these communities is required to build up the trust that may have been lost in the past.

CASE STUDY

Cottingley Springs

In 2013–2014, the local council performed a Joint Health Needs Assessment (JHNA) of the Travelling community-based at Cottingley Springs [2]. Cottingley Springs is a local authority Gypsy and Traveller Site in the Wortley ward, outside Leeds. The JHNA found a poor life expectancy within this group, long-term health problems, high self-reported rates of low literacy, depression and anxiety as well as barriers to healthcare access. It became the main focus area for an outreach project.

The Gypsy and Traveller Health Improvement Project aimed to establish connections between the Travelling community and health-related services in Leeds. It involved NHS services in Leeds, the city council's public health team and Leeds GATE (a local Gypsy and Traveller-led civil society organisation).

The project design enabled a two-way process that combined direct outreach work with the Travelling community and GP practices. An asset-based community development approach was used to bridge this gap and build relationships between the two, through the employment of a specialist nurse. The nurse assisted with accessing healthcare by registering community members, explaining conditions, encouraging attendance, accompanying people and helping ensure better quality appointments. A significant focus of the health advice provided by the nurse related to mental health – particularly depression and stress/anxiety. The project received funding for one year (2017–2018), but this was subsequently extended until March 2019, due to additional funding provided by the NHS Leeds Clinical Commissioning Group (CCG).

The first stage of the work involved establishing links with the community. Leeds GATE assisted with this process having provided voluntary assistance for 15 years. They accompanied outreach visits approximately two to three times a week, using their previous experiences and introductions within the community.

Rapport and Consent

Initially, rapport building involved a holistic approach to providing support. Community members received help with more general issues, such as reading letters or accompaniment to appointments. This approach allowed the nurse to be readily accepted within the community, as good relationships with one family were transferred onto another. The power balance between the health practitioner and community member lies in favour of the community. Basic social cues used in a different community may not always be appropriate in this context – extra work is required to obtain the right level of consent.

This approach is in stark contrast to the set-up of a therapeutic relationship within a conventional surgery/clinic. Usually, a healthcare professional is approached by the patient, displaying an implicit consent within the interaction. When a healthcare professional approaches a potential patient within a different community setting, the community members assume that the professional has the power and control of the consultation. The flexibility and variation from a conventional therapeutic relationship enabled the nurse to reach out to the patients in a culturally sensitive way, acknowledging the complexity of the patient's needs and the broader determinants of health. Such flexibility in comparison with the traditional structure of healthcare delivery models is key to the success of future outreach interventions in these communities.

The process of forming relationships initially can feel quite isolating. Healthcare professionals cannot enter these communities purely with the intention to provide healthcare services. There is a degree of negotiation and agenda-matching that needs to occur initially. The stores of transferrable rapport are then built for use when later providing healthcare services. This process requires a variety of skills, balancing priorities and utilising a different model of consultation.

Health Literacy

Once rapport was established, the outreach work focussed on health literacy. Within this community 78% had some or no literacy – only 3% had good literacy. This highlights some of the incredibly simple reasons for lack of access to healthcare;

for example, community members may miss appointments as they are not literate enough to use the choose and book, and then may be discharged for non-attendance. A review of the notes for these patients found that they still very much rely on a traditional medical model of healthcare. Patients are not aware of other types of therapies available to them. Medical notes were also updated to include literacy status.

Health-help cards were created to tackle the literacy issues faced in this context. These are small cards with NHS branding that patients can present which explain their literacy needs. They aim to reduce the embarrassment associated with being illiterate and also to advise the recipient of their need to adjust their service to meet the patient's need. The implementation of health-help cards will also require support from the healthcare services in which they will be used.

In the context of mental health management, patients are advised to self-refer for psychological therapy but may be unable to access this if they have literacy issues. Furthermore, cognitive behavioural therapy (CBT) is difficult for patients without literacy. The outreach workers coach people to be able to access therapeutic services and take people to their appointments. They work with services to identify barriers to access by establishing which patients have literacy problems and thus have been discharged unfairly.

Screening and Prevention

Another aspect of the work involves the promotion of preventative NHS services, such as health checks and screening. The provision of preventative services within these communities highlights their inherent gender hierarchies and the effects of these on healthcare access. On the whole, male populations were more difficult to reach as they were working during the time of outreach visits. They were less willing to discuss health which in some cases affected women's engagement. In other cases, however, female members of the community would act as the main point of contact for the dissemination of healthcare information.

Certain issues were encountered when the outreach workers were attempting to promote screening. Some women were prone to missing mammograms due to a lack of understanding

of the screening process or received the invitation in an inaccessible format. No males in the community were eligible for AAA screening as they did not reach the minimum age for eligibility, reflecting the low life expectancy within this community.

NHS health checks were performed on-site. The way in which these health checks were carried out required modification of the traditional model – the outreach nurse used a more conversational approach in light of literacy levels and their related challenges.

Preventative diabetic services offered diabetics health education in their campsites. This education was later shared amongst the community through word of mouth. Generally, health education services rely upon there being certain levels of literacy. This case study demonstrates the importance of relationship-building with a community in order to engage with people.

Vaccination

The outreach programme considered vaccination programmes, as Travellers are deemed to be a high-risk group. However logistical factors impacted their implementation.

There is a lack of clarity around which body or organisation is responsible for leading and funding vaccination. Children that are home-educated may not receive or respond to immunisation offers. Furthermore, practices will only be paid for vaccinating these groups if the patients are registered with a surgery. Unsettled communities may move from one location to another before this registration can take place. Nevertheless, the school immunisation teams have delivered community clinics twice a year on-site. These clinics focus on children who are electively home-educated as they miss the school offer for vaccination.

Leeds has also established an outreach health-visiting system. Small teams visit roadside camps to attend to communities not registered with a GP.

Complex Health Needs

A large number of the Travelling community members have complex health needs. There is often a lack of understanding of health conditions as well as the reasons for taking medicines. If management plans do not take these complex needs into account, even the simplest solutions may not work for these patients. Patients may be on medications but cannot read their tablets – in one case, thyroxine levels in a patient are chronically deranged as she cannot read the boxes with the administration instructions. This problem could have been avoided with a dosette box.

Depression and anxiety are experienced more commonly in Gypsy and Traveller communities in comparison with the rest of the population. These patients feel the stigma of the diagnosis, both within and from outside the community. Their concerns revolve around their children being taken away from them due to their mental health problems. Patients may be only willing to engage with pharmacological therapy, or sometimes have only been offered this. Due to previously mentioned literacy concerns providing psychological therapy alongside pharmacotherapy can be challenging.

Examples of good practice have emerged from a multi-disciplinary approach. Palliative care teams have worked with the outreach nurse to develop good relationships with community members and have adopted a more opportunistic approach. Research has shown a significant fear of cancer in Gypsy and Traveller communities combined with a lack of understanding of prognosis. This model of outreach work can begin to tackle these fears and preconceptions. Initiative taken by these services may encourage a similar approach to be made by other services.

Professional Attitudes

A more sensitive issue that affects healthcare work within Gypsy and Traveller communities is that of professional bias. There is a sense of fear among professionals who are reluctant to go into communities alone. Unconscious and institutional bias influences attitudes towards these communities, and this needs to be challenged. Within the context of this project, there were mixed findings regarding willingness to engage amongst those in primary care.

The project has however demonstrated positive, desirable qualities in those who engaged. Successful relationships enable the most change, and an essential foundation of trust in these relationships allows for the provision of advice in a respectful manner. The importance of soft skills in an adverse environment is highlighted, alongside awareness of our expressions, attentiveness and intuition.

Some of the practical limitations that arose from the project provide good reflective points for improvement with future outreach work. There was some difficulty with recruitment at the start, which delayed the project's delivery. Short-term funding has also limited potential progress.

Continued work with Gypsy and Traveller communities should aim for full involvement of primary care services with the provision of outreach services. Appropriate training in the complex needs of the Travelling community, tackling unconscious bias and using outreach workers are the first steps GPs can take in making their services more accessible for this marginalised group.

SUGGESTIONS FOR PRACTICE

Top Tips for Engaging with Gypsies and Travelling People [3, 4]

- *If you want to know how people prefer to be referred to – ask.*
- *Start by thinking about yourself.*

Primary care teams are not immune from conscious or unconscious bias. A recent paper published by Friends, Families and Travellers [5] found that of 50 practices, all rated good or outstanding, 24 refused to register a Traveller seeking medical help. Where it's lacking, cultural competence training can be useful and is available from a number of local and national organisations.

Think about what you hope to achieve and what limitations you have in terms of people, support, funding and time. What, realistically, can be achieved? Remember, how a project finishes can determine how future outreach projects are received.

- *Establish contact and gain community input.*

For a healthcare intervention to be relevant and well received, it is helpful to gain community input into its aims and designs as early as possible. In ideal situations an introduction can be made by people or organisations with established trust and rapport – check for relevant local organisations. If not, the local authority may be able to make introductions, especially if there is a local authority-run site for Travellers in the area. If no intermediary is available, you may have to arrive at the site and introduce yourself (as with any community intervention, considerations of lone-worker safety apply). In this instance consider the suitability of the person or people you meet; not everyone is best placed to discuss how to establish a health outreach programme in their community. In the case of some Traveller sites, they may have reached consultation fatigue, having been consulted about numerous research studies or short-term interventions without seeing much benefit.

- *Make the most of first visits.*

As with any consultation, acting with respect and starting with listening is a good way to begin. Whilst a holistic approach is appropriate, curiosity into the Travelling way of life may lead to questioning that is perceived as intrusive and inappropriate – ask about things relevant to your work. Few projects start with a blank slate, but whatever starting notions you have about your healthcare intervention, if you want it to be successful, it is important to get community advice about its relevance, acceptability and how to make it work. Better project designs come from asking, 'How do you usually?' or 'How would you like to?'. Be realistic from the start about what can be achieved and any limitations, especially duration, the project has.

Be aware that as a healthcare professional you may be regarded as a representative of the state agenda and that the state agenda has included less-welcome visits from police, bailiffs, school attendance officers and others. If a first visit meets with a guarded or hostile reception, there may be a reason for this on the day and it may be worth trying again another time. Be aware that the community can be mobile and, if your visit causes concern, they may not be there when you return. The first rule is always 'do no harm'.

Be aware that, especially in the face of behaviour change thinking, practitioners can form an inaccurate view that community members are the architects of their own poor health outcomes, via lifestyle choices etc, without taking into account wider determinants over which patients may have little control. Outsiders may not be able to form a very accurate understanding, especially quickly, about what the drivers of poor outcomes really are and that in fact community members are making the best, most logical, choices available to them [6].

- *Consider practicalities and align priorities with your community.*

Building trust and rapport takes time. It may also take time for your staff to acquaint themselves with a different culture and way of working.

Consider practicalities when working. Visiting in the morning may be inconvenient for Gypsy and Traveller women who are often at their busiest at this time. If visiting by day you may miss the men who are away at work. Be as aware of confidentiality as anywhere else. A caravan may have limited space for consultation and examination, therefore entering it may be more intrusive than consulting in other locations, but discussing medical information at the door could be inappropriate and a breach of confidentiality. Remember that where literacy levels are low, written information may be of limited value, although sometimes a reader will represent a family or group in this department (again remember confidentiality). Face-to-face communication may prove best.

Beware of creating dependency, especially if this is a time-limited intervention. Re-evaluate and reconsider if things are going wrong – adapt rather than give up if there are setbacks. If things are working, evaluate and share good practice.

- *Strategically plan how to make an exit.*

Interventions which have a long-lasting and sustainable impact are often best, especially where provision can become mainstreamed rather than time-limited additions to normal services. If your work is time or funding-limited and must come to an end, be sure to be clear from the start when and how this will happen. Early in-service development it may seem like crisis management is all-consuming but, at some point development must take priority for a service to become sustainable. Include pathways towards progress in your work, evaluate its impact and celebrate and share successes.

REFERENCES

1. Women and Equalities Committee. *Tackling Inequalities Faced by the Gypsy, Roma and Traveller Communities. Seventh Report of Session 2017–2019*. London: House of Commons; 2019.
2. Thompson N. *Leeds Gypsy and Traveller Community Health Needs Assessment*. Leeds: Leeds GATE; 2013.
3. Warwick-Booth L, Woodward J, O'Dwyer L, Di Martino S. *An Evaluation of Leeds CCG Gypsy and Traveller Health Improvement Project*. Leeds: Leeds Beckett University; 2018.
4. Jones H. *How to Engage with Gypsies and Travellers as Part of Your Work; A Guide to Best Working Practices*. Leeds: Leeds GATE; 2011.
5. Sweeney S, Worrall S. *No Room at the Inn: How Easy Is It for Nomadic Gypsies and Travellers to Access Primary Care?* Brighton: Friends, Families and Travellers; 2019.
6. Tamber PT. The Fallacy of Behaviour Change. Available from: https://www.pstamber.com/the-fallacy-of-behaviour-change/. Accessed19th May 2019.

30

The Health and Well-being of Asylum Seekers and New Refugees

REBECCA FARRINGTON AND ANNA BAILEY

Their state may have failed to protect them on a number of levels.

Forced migration is increasing across the globe and the geopolitical context of providing equitable healthcare for new arrivals is perplexing for our systems of care and our personal practice of medicine. Refugees and people seeking asylum are forced to flee their countries – places we might see in the news – due to conflict and persecution. Many arrive in the UK having been threatened, detained, beaten or tortured. Sometimes perceived as being demanding, or disengaged, many assumptions are made about asylum seekers and refugees (ASR*). They are in fact a diverse group with their own important skills, often demonstrating phenomenal resilience in the face of extreme adversity; however, they are likely to have competing priorities and health may be low on their agenda.

The much contested 'healthy migrant' effect [1], which hypothesises that those who make it to host countries are inherently the young and the healthy, fails to take into account the extremes of psychological and socioeconomic dispossession lived by ASR. The context of their migration is driven by push rather than pull factors and frequently occurs without much planning. The lack of knowledge of each other's contexts between caregivers and their recipients is another aspect of the challenge [2, 3]. The attitudes of those in positions of power can constitute further difficulty. Primary care is, however, exceptionally well placed to make a positive difference to the health of this population.

The traditional focus in learning about health in the developing world has been on communicable disease. We are now experiencing global health locally: the clinical experience of treating international residents in the UK is more around identification and management of non-communicable disease, especially long-term mental health. Depression is predicted to be the world's number one health problem by 2030 [4].

The impacts of being forced to leave your home, family, employment and culture are many. A period of adjustment is often needed; however prolonged waiting for confirmation of legal status in their host country, and the adjunctive stressors of insecurity, poverty, social isolation and separation, means for ASR this adjustment can feel difficult to attain. Asylum seekers with a current claim in-situ have no permission to work. Their financial

* This term will be used to include people seeking asylum, new refugees and those who have exhausted their asylum claim for the purposes of this chapter unless otherwise stated.

support is £5.35 per day, around half the amount given to job-seekers.

CASE STUDY

Bijan

Bijan registered with a GP surgery just after his 40th birthday. Understanding the value of knowing more about his background, the GP arranged an interpreter and a double appointment. Bijan grew up in a middle-eastern country and his early education was interrupted by war. His family are widely separated with some in Europe, some in the United States and others in various parts of the Middle East. He has little contact with them.

He has been in the UK for 11 years having fled following student protests at the university where he was studying for a PhD. Bijan has exhausted his rights to appeal his asylum claim. He sleeps in a friend's car at present, but sleep is usually interrupted by nightmares. He spends his days walking around, but he avoids the town centre as he dislikes crowds.

Until now he hasn't had any medical care in the UK. He only recently became aware of his right to register when he attended a City of Sanctuary event. His main complaint is back pain. He has lost 10kg and looks pale. He also mentions that he feels there is no point to his life because he is now 'too old to find a wife and have a family', and even if he did he 'would have nothing to offer them'.

On further questioning it becomes clear that although Bijan has daily thoughts of suicide he does not have any current plans. It is hard to identify any protective factors, but his friend, who has refugee status, seems to be supporting him with some food and shelter.

Definitions [5]

A refugee 'owing to a well-founded fear of being persecuted for reasons of race, religion, nationality, membership of a particular social group, or political opinion, is outside the country of his nationality, and is unable to or, owing to such fear, is unwilling to avail himself of the protection of that country' (Article 1, 1951 Convention Relating to the Status of Refugees).

An asylum seeker has applied to the government for refugee status and is waiting to hear the outcome. Someone who seeks asylum in the UK

is asking for protection under well-established international law (the 1951 Refugee Convention and its Protocols). Once accepted, they are granted refugee status. Sometimes this is temporary and reapplications are becoming more common.

Resettled refugees, who arrive via resettlement programmes (Gateway Programme or the Syrian Vulnerable Persons Scheme), have their status recognised by the UK government before arrival, often have a dedicated package of support to assist in orientation and integration and help to offset costs to health and social care services. Numbers in the UK are small.

Why Are These Definitions Important?

The journey to achieving legal status can take many years with multiple claims and appeals. Attempts to secure legal representation can be costly once the initial entitlement to legal aid is exhausted. During this time there may be periods of destitution, where good health is extremely difficult to maintain, and periods of detention which have been shown to be harmful [6].

Achieving refugee status moves people, sometimes only temporarily, into the position of being able to work, study, receive statutory benefits and housing rights, consider a family reunion and move forward with their lives and aspirations. All of these have a beneficial impact on health and well-being [7]. However, individuals granted refugee status face new challenges including potential homelessness, navigating the UK benefits system and difficulty securing employment [8].

At the other end of the spectrum, exhausting a claim for asylum results in destitution with no recourse to public funds (NRPF). This means reliance only on charitable sources of support for food, clothing, shelter and security. The threat of detention or deportation is a source of pervasive fear, distracting many from functioning adequately with normal daily activities. In these situations, our preventative agenda for long-term health becomes low priority for them. Short-term survival is understandably their key focus.

Entitlements to free healthcare in the NHS are complex. Currently all people ordinarily resident in the UK, including people with an active asylum claim or appeal, are entitled to free NHS care [9].

GP consultations remain free for those with NRPF, alongside a limited number of community services. All other care for those with NRPF is chargeable up front, unless it is emergency care for a life-threatening condition. This can place a moral and ethical strain on individual practitioners and can discourage all ASR from seeking care, even when they are entitled [3]. Advice on supporting patients being charged for care can be found online [10].

SUGGESTIONS FOR PRACTICE

Using a non-judgemental approach enquire regularly about the progress of an asylum claim. Be aware that both the exhaustion of a claim and the receipt of leave to remain (LTR) result in eviction from their current accommodation at short notice (21–28 days)

With LTR, the local council has an obligation to help secure accommodation, which is often initially a homeless hostel.

- *A GP letter detailing additional medical needs can be useful for prioritisation.*
- *For those with NRPF, the voluntary sector has information on where to seek shelter and food.*
- *Keep a list of local contact numbers and find out how you can issue foodbank vouchers.*
- *Consider a Section 4(2) support application on health grounds [11].*

Medicolegal Reporting (MLR)

People flee their countries for a myriad of reasons and their state may have failed to protect them on a number of levels. Persecution frequently involves torture [12] and this can be a difficult history to relate and to receive. Whilst the detail of their reasons for leaving can be helpful in gathering information to inform your care, it is important to remember that as a medical practitioner your role is not to judge them or decide the outcome of their immigration application. That said, objective reports containing medical evidence are useful for those who do make these important decisions. Individuals who have experienced torture may require more extensive medicolegal reports to support their asylum claim. These are written using the Istanbul Protocol [13] and undertaken by an independent medical practitioner who is commissioned by a legal representative.

SUGGESTIONS FOR PRACTICE

- *Document all sequelae of ill-treatment that you encounter.*
- *It is advisable to avoid giving an opinion on causation unless you have specific training on the Istanbul Protocol [13].*
- *Clearly outline your observations in letters for legal representatives in order for them to commission formal independent medicolegal reports. If this is not possible a brief printout of your consultation could be used, although be aware this may not give sufficient context.*
- *For those without legal representation your letter may help a patient or asylum adviser to access a solicitor to assist with asylum claims and appeals. Charging for these letters may take them out of reach for your patient and your discretion may be required [14–20].*

Barriers to Accessing Healthcare

The barriers mirror those from other marginalised groups.

Effective Consultations

Multiple factors contribute to building a relationship in which a patient can trust their caregiver. There are some crucial elements to the consultation that are your responsibility to influence in order to develop and maintain a trusting therapeutic relationship. These are outlined below.

Continuity of Care

Repetitive history giving is re-traumatising. Trauma-informed care [22, 23] includes longer appointments and recognition of distressed behaviour, which may indicate the need for grounding techniques [24]. If someone has disclosed to you, try to be the person who does the follow-up.

Interpretation

The responsibility for effective communication lies with you, the practitioner. There may be pressure to use inadequate interpretation on cost grounds, however, *you* must make the decision on clinical grounds. A useful toolkit has been produced by the RNZCGP [25] which includes advice on when face-to-face is preferred to telephone interpretation.

Once you have an appropriate independent interpreter in the consultation you should remain vigilant to their skill. A good interpreter does not need to make eye contact with you. They use the same rate, tone and rhythm as you, and they are comfortable with silence when you use it as a therapeutic tool. There are sometimes words and phrases that are hard to interpret directly. If they wish to clarify something with the patient, they will inform you that this is taking place.

SUGGESTIONS FOR PRACTICE

- *Observe the interaction between interpreter and patient*
  - *Do they appear uncomfortable, or overfamiliar?*
  - *Is there 'chat' taking place that is not being interpreted?*
  - *Are you receiving appropriate responses to your questions?*
- *Do not be afraid to stop and redirect the interpreter if this is happening.*
- *You may need to halt the consultation and rebook if the situation does not improve.*
- *Don't forget to feed this back to the interpreting agency.*

Cultural Sensibility [26]

Cultural competency approaches risk stereotyping and a more person-centred attitude is preferable. Given the diversity of the ASR population and the intersectionality of their issues it is very hard to generalise. This has been described as part of super-diversity [27], a concept encompassing the increased range of variables in immigrant populations in recent years. Piacentini et al call for 'a practice-evidenced research agenda promoting cultural communication across healthcare and home settings, acknowledging immigration status as a social determinant of health', making it clear that diversity 'within and between migrant populations' is often neglected [28].

Time taken to ensure excellent communication, as described above, will reap rewards beyond the basics of patient safety. Starting with a social

history can help you understand the impetus for migration and the lived experience of a person in exile. Showing genuine interest in the patient as a person helps generate trust and rapport. This will also help you gauge their level of education and literacy, alongside the social and financial resources available to them.

Stigma, discrimination and hate crimes are unfortunately common and ASR are often unaware of the pathways for reporting this or are reluctant to complain as this draws the attention of the authorities. Guidance and support through these processes is invaluable.

Communication Skills

Expectations and past experience of healthcare inevitably shapes ASRs' views of the NHS [17]. Our reliance on the patient as our partner in the consultation may be problematic for some ASR. Open questions and the Ideas, Concerns, Expectations (ICE) approach can be culturally difficult to recognise, likewise, shared management planning may cause cultural confusion. ASR patients may expect a consultation to be more prescriptive and can lose confidence in the clinician when it isn't. Framing your questions in a way that normalises them can be helpful, e.g. 'we usually ask about your preferences for treatment in this country, these are our options…'.

It is important to ask permission and use a 'warning shot' when seeking sensitive information. For example, the question, 'This may be difficult but are you able to tell me what happened?' is different to just asking "What happened?" [23] which is perceived as interrogatory. Good interpretation will take account of these nuances. Although it remains useful to give patients some autonomy, it can be difficult psychologically when someone has been ill-treated and wants to give you, the person in authority, the 'right' answer [29]. In some countries, doctors are complicit in ill-treatment and wield power as people in positions of authority. Trust is understandably a major issue for ASR [17].

Health

CHILDREN AND FAMILIES

Adverse childhood experiences (ACEs) are known to negatively impact mental health in children, on into adulthood, and have an intergenerational effect [30]. The exposure of children to frightening situations in home countries and on perilous journeys is well documented in the media. On arrival they are exposed to extremes of poverty and can become carers for parents with mental illness. The manifestation of their distress is more likely to be seen through behavioural presentations [31] such as enuresis or fear of sleeping alone.

Family separation can be very damaging and is often permanent, which may not have been anticipated before fleeing their country. The Red Cross operate an international family tracing service [32, 33]. Family reunion is a complicated process requiring refugee status, housing, and a reliable income, before even considering the cost of visa applications and legal representation. There is often a burden of expectation on the exiled family member to send money home, which is incredibly difficult to achieve.

Unaccompanied asylum-seeking children (UASC) pose specific challenges. They may have developed considerable resilience through necessity while travelling, but many have been exploited. A Dutch study showed 67% of the unaccompanied asylum-seeking girls and 14% of boys attending a clinic had experienced sexual abuse [34]. Age assessment is notoriously unreliable, and it is wise to err on the side of caution in considering safeguarding issues.

SUGGESTIONS FOR PRACTICE

- *Make sure children from new arrival families aren't being used for inappropriate duties, such as interpretation, in any setting.*
- *Check they have gained school or nursery places and as a continuation of that, check the following*
  - *Consider how they can find a low-cost uniform (sometimes through the Parent Teachers Association).*
  - *Check they are registered for free school meals and transport.*
  - *Inform the family of the role of the school nurse in psychological support.*

Mental Health

By no means do all people exposed to violence and disaster suffer consequences to their mental health, however, many do [35]. Many asylum seekers have experienced multiple traumas. They can be described in terms of pre- and post-migratory stressors [36]. Before leaving their countries, they may have been living in conditions of war, imprisonment or spent periods in hiding. Transit countries may not have had adequate healthcare and journeys can be treacherous with people witnessing multiple losses of life. Living conditions in host countries are basic and often constitute a dramatic deterioration in lifestyle. The stress of an uncertain future, the threat of hate crime and the onerous system to prove your case adds to the ongoing challenges.

Co-morbidity is common alongside post-traumatic stress disorder (PTSD), with depression and anxiety being the most prevalent conditions. PTSD can be a controversial diagnosis with some worrying about medicalising reactions to abnormal situations; however, our experience is that Complex PTSD (described below) is common with ongoing stressors, including the well-documented pressure of the asylum system [36–38].

Whilst it is important to note that not all individuals who have experienced trauma will develop PTSD, it is crucial that primary care physicians' feel equipped to diagnose the condition to facilitate referral to appropriate support services.

Definitions

POST-TRAUMATIC STRESS DISORDER (PTSD)

The new International Classification of Diseases (ICD) 11 [39] describes three key symptoms which should persist for at least several weeks following exposure to an 'extremely threatening or horrific event or series of events' and cause 'significant impairment in personal, family, social, educational, occupational or other important areas of functioning'. Symptoms include:

1) Re-experiencing the traumatic event(s) in the form of intrusive memories, flashbacks or nightmares. Often accompanied by strong physical sensations and overwhelming fear/horror.
2) Avoidance of thoughts and memories of the event(s) or activities which are reminiscent of the traumatic event(s).
3) A persistent heightened perception of threat, which may present as an enhanced startle reaction to unexpected noises and hypervigilance.

Complex PTSD (CPTSD)

ICD-11 proposals (for ratification in May 2019) include CPTSD [40]. This most commonly presents in individuals who have experienced prolonged or repetitive events from which escape is difficult or impossible (e.g., torture, slavery, genocide campaigns, prolonged domestic violence, repeated childhood sexual or physical abuse). The symptoms include the previously mentioned core PTSD symptoms and in addition

- Problems with regulation of mood.
- Beliefs about oneself as worthless, often with feelings of shame, guilt or failure related to traumatic event(s).
- Difficulties in sustaining relationships.

ASR are isolated from usual or familiar trusted sources of support. Diminished protective factors, such as social networks and employment, lead to the requirement for frequent suicide and self-harm risk assessment. Hopelessness and impulsive or risk-taking behaviour in this population may be markers of profound distress.

Diagnostic screening can be challenging as not all ASR will have a western model of psychological health, and cultural validity of your screening tool may be lacking. Boyles describes this 'therapy bureaucracy' as disruptive to the therapeutic relationship [41].

Whilst NICE describes first-line treatment for PTSD as talking therapies [42] this is often impractical. ASRs with ongoing stress may not have achieved enough stabilisation or symptom control. Medication, such as SSRIs, Mirtazapine and Trazodone, can play a part in promoting change in sleep and mood to allow participation in treatments including more purposeful or creative activity. Anxiolytics, such as β-blockers, can help where there are no contraindications. Antipsychotic and mood-stabilising medications can improve re-experiencing symptoms.

PTSD is a relapsing and remitting condition and requires a long-term approach with safety-netting. Times of additional stress are crunch points for return or worsening of symptoms. Most will recover eventually, however a significant number are left to manage a prolonged and chronic course [43]. There is also the intergenerational aspect to bear in mind when considering PTSD prognosis in the context of caring for families [44].

Physical Health

It is very unusual to see tropical illnesses. Mostly asylum seekers are physically fit, although some have neglected chronic diseases and complications from lack of access to care. Survivors of torture, combat or natural disaster may have poorlyhealed fractures, chronic infections, nerve damage and disfigurements. Female genital mutilation (FGM) is practised in a wide range of locations and has both physical and mental health ramifications. Sexual and reproductive health remains important for a group comprised mainly of young adults, sometimes in precarious relationships. Pregnancies are considered high risk [45].

Presentation of psychological distress as experience of pain is common and complex. Pain perception is formed through multiple physical and emotional influences. Links to PTSD are well-recognised and caution is required for the prescribing of analgesia [46].

SUGGESTIONS FOR PRACTICE

- *Consider a longer New Patient Check for new migrants [47] and include the following aspects*
  - *Catch up immunisation (WHO schedules).*
  - *Medication review, including use of traditional medicines or those sent from home.*
  - *Smoking, drugs and alcohol.*
  - *Tuberculosis and blood-borne virus assessment.*
  - *Sexual health and female genital mutilation.*
  - *Vitamin D screen.*
  - *Mental health assessment, including PTSD screen.*
  - *Explanation of national screening programmes.*
  - *Don't forget dental health!*

Advocacy

Tackling the underlying cause of distress can mean using your voice as a professional to facilitate change at individual and organisational levels. Creuss describes our social contract as bringing the expectation that we 'will address the problems faced by individual patients and also concern [ourselves] with issues of importance to society'. In return we 'have a legitimate right to expect to work in a system which supports, not subverts, the traditional values of the healer and the professional' [48].

On a personal level, you can show solidarity and an understanding of the patient's predicament which is therapeutic. Writing letters of support around the wider determinants of health does change the practical situation. On a population level your experiences at the grassroots are valuable to planners and policymakers. In this arena data is hard to collect. Numbers remain hidden; disenfranchised people are unheard and underrepresented. Your case studies can be key to opening up understanding in the mainstream, although maintaining confidentiality and gaining consent is imperative.

Care according to need is a fundamental tenet of the NHS. This can involve longer appointment times, providing letters without charging and prescribing rather than recommending over-the-counter (OTC) medication. Social prescribing is great as long as it doesn't incur additional or hidden costs to the ASR such as travel.

Medical organisations lobbying for policy change include Medact [49], Docs not Cops [20], Medical Justice [50] and Doctors of the World [51].

Voluntary and Community Organisations (VCO)

The expertise in the voluntary sector is considerable. Most voluntary organisations utilise people with lived experience far better than the NHS do. Practical provision can be in multiple forms from food, shelter and clothing, to purposeful activity such as music and sport, as well as advocacy, legal advice and language support. Environments are generally informal, flexible and tailored to providing a safe space. They operate a 'no door is the wrong door' policy. VCOs can, however, struggle with continuity of funding and many exist through short-term bids.

Examples of Support Organisations for Asylum Seekers

In addition, there are faith-based groups, student volunteers and political activists that help bring asylum seekers together for mutual support. There are pros and cons to encouraging people to associate with their countrymen. Some communities are highly suspicious of newcomers, particularly where there are strong political and religious divides,

others manage to be very resourceful and truly look after the concerns of their compatriots. The decision to engage will be very much on a case-by-case basis.

Vicarious Traumatisation

The risk of emotional upset from dealing with people in difficult situations is high. It is normal to have a negative reaction to a bad situation. Most of us will manage to counter this with our usual sources of support. A cup of tea with a colleague goes a long way to helping on a bad day. Sometimes a particular story will stay with us. Other times repeated exposure to inequality and injustice will frustrate us. We need to be attentive to when these feelings overload us, affecting our functioning or contributing to burnout.

Doctors often don't practice what they preach. Physical activity, eating healthily, spending time with family and friends and connecting to our communities help us relax and put our work into perspective. Recognition of when additional help is needed may come from a trusted colleague. To help facilitate this, some people prefer regular psychological supervision to touch base [52]. There are advantages to formalising this or accessing training in how to recognise it [53].

Some of the most startling inequalities in our communities are experienced by asylum seekers, particularly those with NRPF. The extremes of poverty, lack of agency, levels of discrimination and uncertain futures make their lives and health precarious. We need to remain mindful of their humanity, promoting respect and compassion, not just in our personal contact but at an organisational level.

CASE STUDY

Bijan

Bijan slowly came to trust his GP after realising they were not part of the 'authorities' and that the team, including the interpreter, would keep his case confidential. He was able to talk about his experiences of torture in prison following the protest. This included sexual assault. Although it was upsetting to hear, the GP was confident in making a PTSD diagnosis. They started treatment with Mirtazapine, which helped his nightmares, and referred him for psychological therapy. Some blood tests and imaging excluded physical reasons for his weight loss and pain, other than vitamin D deficiency. He found the food bank vouchers very helpful as he hated relying solely on his friend.

Bijan was able to take a letter from the GP to a drop-in legal advice service which resulted in a referral by a solicitor for an MLR at Freedom from Torture. He made a fresh claim for asylum and is now supported on Section 4(2) with accommodation and vouchers. Bijan has made some friends at the Art on Prescription session and hopes to be a photographer in the future if he can obtain leave to remain and permission to work.

REFERENCES

1. Lu Y. Test of the 'healthy migrant hypothesis': A longitudinal analysis of health selectivity of internal migration in Indonesia. *Soc Sci Med* [Internet]. 2008 Oct;67(8):1331–9. Available from: https://linkinghub.elsevier.com/retrieve/pii/S0277953608003225

2. Medact Manchester. Healthcare professionals' views and experiences of dealing with refugees and asylum seekers: A survey of North-West practitioners [Internet]. 2017 [cited 2019 Apr 6]. Available from: https://medactmanchester.files.wordpress.com/2017/10/medact_report_2017.pdf

3. Tomkow L, Kang C, Farrington R. Healthcare access for asylum seekers and refugees in England: A mixed methods study exploring service users' and health care professionals' awareness. 2019. *European Journal of Public Health*. doi: 10.1093/eurpub/ckz193

4. World Health Organisation. Global burden of mental disorders and the need for a comprehensive, coordinated response from health and social sectors at the country level [Internet]. 2011 [cited 2019 Apr 6]. Available from: http://apps.who.int/gb/ebwha/pdf_files/eb130/b130_9-en.pdf

5. Worthington E. *GM Asylum and Refugee Health Advocacy Group briefing*. Manchester; 2018.

6. von Werthern M, Robjant K, Chui Z, Schon R, Ottisova L, Mason C et al. The impact of immigration detention on mental health: A systematic review. *BMC Psychiatry* [Internet]. 2018 Dec;18(1):382. Available from: https://doi.org/10.1186/s12888-018-1945-y

7. Marsden R, Harris C. "We started life again": Integration experiences of refugee families reuniting in Glasgow [Internet]. British Red Cross in partnership with Scottish Refugee Council 2015 [cited 2019 Apr 6]. Available from: https://www.refworld.org/pdfid/560cde294.pdf

8. Doyle L. 28 days later: Experiences of new refugees in the UK [Internet]. 2014 [cited 2019 Apr 6]. Available from: https://www.refugeecouncil.org.uk/assets/0003/1769/28_days_later.pdf

9. NHS. Visitors who do not need to pay for NHS treatment [Internet]. https://www.nhs.uk. 2018 [cited 2019 Apr 24]. Available from: https://www.nhs.uk/using-the-nhs/nhs-services/visiting-or-moving-to-england/visitors-who-do-not-need-pay-for-nhs-treatment/

10. Docs Not Cops, Migrants Organise, Medact. Patients Not Passports - A toolkit designed to support you in advocating for people facing charges for NHS care, and in taking action to end immigration checks and upfront charging in the NHS. [Internet]. 2019 [cited 2019 Apr 24]. Available from: https://patientsnotpassports.co.uk/support/

11. www.gov.uk. Asylum support section 4(2) policy [Internet]. 2018 [cited 2019 Apr 27]. Available from: https://www.gov.uk/government/publications/asylum-support-section-42-policy

12. Freedom from torture. Where does torture happen? [Internet]. [cited 2019 Apr 30]. Available from: https://www.freedomfromtorture.org/where_does_torture_happen

13. Office of The United Nations High Commissioner for Human Rights. Istanbul Protocol Manual on the Effective Investigation and Documentation of Torture and Other Cruel, Inhuman or Degrading Treatment or Punishment [Internet]. Geneva; 2004. (Geneva PROFESSIONAL TRAINING SERIES No. 8/Rev.1 UNITED NATIONS). Available from: https://www.ohchr.org/Documents/Publications/training8Rev1en.pdf

14. NHS England. How to register with a doctor (GP) [Internet]. NHSE; 2015. Available from: https://www.nhs.uk/NHSEngland/AboutNHSservices/doctors/Documents/how-to-register-with-a-gp-leaflet.pdf

15. Language Line. Language identification card [Internet]. 2013 [cited 2019 Apr 24]. Available from: https://www.languageline.com/hubfs/LIC A4 0845.pdf

16. General Medical Council. Good medical practice [Internet]. 2013 [cited 2019 Apr 6]. Available from: www.gmc-uk.org/guidance

17. O'Donnell CA, Higgins M, Chauhan R, Mullen K. Asylum seekers; expectations of and trust in general practice: A qualitative study. Br J Gen Pract [Internet]. 2008 Dec 1;58(557):e1 LP–e11. Available from: https://bjgp.org/content/58/557/e1.abstract

18. Kang C, Tomkow L, Farrington R. Access to primary health care for asylum seekers and refugees: A qualitative study of service user experiences in the UK. Br J Gen Pract [Internet]. 2019 Feb 12;bjgp19X701309. Available from: https://bjgp.org/content/early/2019/02/11/bjgp19X701309.abstract

19. Doctors of the World. Safe Surgeries Toolkit [Internet]. 2017 [cited 2019 Apr 6]. Available from: https://www.doctorsoftheworld.org.uk/wp-content/uploads/2018/11/safe_surgeries_toolkit_A4_web_FINAL.pdf

20. Docs Not Cops. We are fighting to protect the NHS [Internet]. [cited 2019 Apr 30]. Available from: http://www.docsnotcops.co.uk/

21. NHS. HC1 form [Internet]. 2016 [cited 2019 Apr 24]. Available from: https://www.nhs.uk/NHSEngland/Healthcosts/Documents/2016/HC1-April-2016.pdf

22. Substance Abuse and Mental Health Services Administration. SAMHSA's Concept of Trauma and Guidance for a Trauma-Informed Approach [Internet]. 2014 [cited 2019 Apr 6]. Available from: https://www.nasmhpd.org/sites/default/files/SAMHSA_Concept_of_Trauma_and_Guidance.pdf

23. Tello M. Trauma-informed care: What it is, and why it's important - Harvard Health Blog [Internet]. Harvard Health Publishing. [cited 2019 Apr 6]. Available from: https://www.health.harvard.edu/blog/trauma-informed-care-what-it-is-and-why-its-important-2018101613562

24. Najavits L. Seeking Safety: A Treatment Manual for PTSD and Substance Abuse. Guilford Press; 2002.

25. Gray B, Hilder J, Stubbe M. How to use interpreters in general practice: The development of a New Zealand toolkit. J Prim Health Care [Internet]. 2012;4(1):52–61. Available from: https://www.rnzcgp.org.nz/assets/documents/Publications/JPHC/March-2012/JPHCIPGrayMarch2012.pdf

26. Betancourt J. Cross- cultural medical education: Conceptual approaches and frameworks for evaluation. Acad Med. 2003;78(6):560–9.

27. Vertovec S. Super-diversity and its implications. Ethn Racial Stud [Internet]. 2007 Nov 1;30(6):1024–54. Available from: https://doi.org/10.1080/01419870701599465

28. Piacentini T, O'Donnell C, Phipps A, Jackson I, Stack N. Moving beyond the 'language problem': Developing an understanding of the intersections of health, language and immigration status in interpreter-mediated health encounters. Lang Intercult Commun [Internet]. 2018 Jun 18;1–16. Available from: https://doi.org/10.1080/14708477.2018.1486409

29. Herman JL. Trauma and recovery [Internet]. Vol. 1992, (1992) Trauma and recovery xi, 276 pp New York, NY, US: Basic Books; US. 1992. Available from: http://ovidsp.ovid.com/ovidweb.cgi?T=JS&CSC=Y&NEWS=N&PAGE=fulltext&D=psyc3&AN=1992-97643-000%5Cnhttp://openurl.bibsys.no/openurl?url_ver=Z39.88-2004&rft_val_fmt=info:ofi/fmt:kev:mtx:journal&rfr_id=info:sid/Ovid:psyc3&rft.genre=article&rft_id=info:doi/&rft

30. Hughes K, Bellis MA, Hardcastle KA, Sethi D, Butchart A, Mikton C et al. The effect of multiple adverse childhood experiences on health: A systematic review and meta-analysis. Lancet Public Health [Internet]. 2017 Aug 1;2(8):e356–66. Available from: https://doi.org/10.1016/S2468-2667(17)30118-4

31. Cartwright K, El-Khani A, Subryan A, Calam R. Establishing the feasibility of assessing the mental health of children displaced by the Syrian conflict. Glob Ment Health [Internet]. 2015 Jun 19 [cited 2015 Oct 17];2:e8. Available from: http://journals.cambridge.org/abstract_S2054425115000035

32. British Red Cross. Find missing family [Internet]. 2019 [cited 2019 Apr 24]. Available from: https://www.redcross.org.uk/get-help/find-missing-family

33. British Red Cross. Refugee family reunion [Internet]. 2019 [cited 2019 Apr 29]. Available from: https://www.redcross.org.

uk/about-us/what-we-do/we-speak-up-for-change/improving-the-lives-of-refugees/refugee-family-reunion

34. Batista E, Wiese P, Burhorst I. The Mental Health of Asylum-seeking and Refugee Children and Adolescents Attending a Clinic in the Netherlands. [cited 2018 Apr 15]; Available from: http://journals.sagepub.com/doi/pdf/10.1177/1363461507083900

35. Kirmayer LJ, Narasiah L, Munoz M, Rashid M, Ryder A, Guzder J et al. Common mental health problems in immigrants and refugees: General approach in primary care. *CMAJ* [Internet]. 2011 [cited 2017 Nov 12];183(12):959–67. Available from: https://www.ncbi.nlm.nih.gov/pmc/articles/PMC3168672/pdf/183e959.pdf

36. Morgan G, Melluish S, Welham A. Exploring the relationship between postmigratory stressors and mental health for asylum seekers and refused asylum seekers in the UK. *Transcult Psychiatry*. 2017. 54 (5-6): 653-674

37. Refugee Action. Waiting in the Dark [Internet]. London, England; 2018. Available from: https://www.refugee-action.org.uk/wp-content/uploads/2018/05/Waiting-in-the-Dark-A4-16-May-2018.pdf

38. McColl H, McKenzie K, Bhui K. Mental healthcare of asylum-seekers and refugees. *Adv Psychiatr Treat* [Internet]. 2008 Nov 2;14(6):452–9. Available from: https://www.cambridge.org/core/product/identifier/S135551460000523X/type/journal_article

39. World Health Organisation. Post Traumatic Stress Disorder [Internet]. ICD-11 for Mortality and Morbidity Statistics (Version : 04 / 2019). 2019 [cited 2019 May 2]. Available from: https://icd.who.int/browse11/l-m/en#/http%3A%2F%2Fid.who.int%2Ficd%2Fentity%2F2070699808

40. World Health Organisation. Complex Post Traumatic Stress Disorder [Internet]. ICD-11 for Mortality and Morbidity Statistics (Version : 04 / 2019). 2019 [cited 2019 Apr 8]. Available from: https://icd.who.int/browse11/l-m/en#/http://id.who.int/icd/entity/585833559

41. Boyles J. *Psychological Therapies for Survivors of Torture*. 1st ed. Boyles J, editor. Monmouth: PCCS Books; 2017.

42. National Institute for Health Care and Excellence. Post-traumatic stress disorder NG116 [Internet]. NICE; 2018 [cited 2019 Apr 29]. Available from: https://www.nice.org.uk/guidance/ng116/chapter/Recommendations#recognition-of-post-traumatic-stress-disorder

43. Rosellini A, Stein M, Benedek D, Bliese P, Chiu W, Hwang I et al. Using self-report surveys at the beginning of service to develop multi-outcome risk models for new soldiers in the U.S. Army. *Psychol Med.* 2017;1(13): 2275-2287.

44. Menzies P. Intergenerational trauma from a mental health perspective. *Nativ Soc Work J* [Internet]. 1995;7:63–85. Available from: https://zone.biblio.laurentian.ca/handle/10219/384

45. Lewis G. The Confidential Enquiry into Maternal and Child Health (CEMACH). Why mothers die 2000–2002. The sixth report of the confidential enquiries into maternal deaths in the United Kingdom. RCOG. 2004;

46. BMA. Chronic pain : Supporting safer prescribing of analgesics [Internet]. British Medical Association. 2017. Available from: bma.org.uk

47. Shryane T. New patient checklist. Public health England [Internet]. 2019 [cited 2019 May 3]. Available from: https://migrant.health/resources/tools/new-patient-checklist-for-gps

48. Cruess SR, Cruess RL. Professionalism and Medicine's Social Contract with Society An overview of the origins of the social contract between physicians and society, with expectations and demands on both parties. *Virtual Mentor* [Internet]. 2004;6(4). Available from: https://journalofethics.ama-assn.org/article/professionalism-and-medicines-social-contract-society/2004-04

49. Skinner J. Patients Not Passports – challenging healthcare charging in the NHS [Internet]. Medact. 2019 [cited 2019 Apr 6]. Available from: https://www.medact.org/2019/resources/briefings/patients-not-passports/

50. Medical Justice. Medical justice: Charity - health rights for detainees [Internet]. [cited 2019 Apr 29]. Available from: http://www.medicaljustice.org.uk/

51. Doctors of the World. Doctors of the World [Internet]. [cited 2019 Apr 29]. Available from: https://www.doctorsoftheworld.org.uk/?utm_referrer=https%3A%2F%2Fwww.google.com%2F

52. Staten A, Lawson E. *GP Wellbeing: Combatting Burnout in General Practice.* CRC Press; 2017. 79 p.

53. Freedom from Torture. Self-care and vicarious trauma: The importance of training [Internet]. Available from: https://www.freedomfromtorture.org/news-blogs/15_10_2018/self_care_and_vicarious_trauma_the_importance_of_training

31

Homeless Healthcare

GEMMA ASHWELL

Patients find themselves in a vicious cycle.

Homelessness is an outcome at the sharp end of social and health inequalities. Housing is a key social determinant of health and a substantial body of research has shown that chronic homelessness marks a significantly increased risk of poor physical health, poor mental health and premature death. The stark reality is that in the United Kingdom the average age of death for homeless patients is just 47 for men and 43 for women [1].

Although providing housing is a vital step in addressing this appalling outcome, this alone will not resolve the underlying problems. The reasons for the premature mortality are not solely due to the conditions of homelessness itself, homeless people often die as a result of treatable medical conditions such as respiratory disease, infectious diseases, consequences of drug and alcohol dependence and cardiovascular disease [2].

Poor health in this population is also exacerbated by poor access to healthcare [3, 4]. Several studies have shown a pattern, repeated internationally, of underutilization of primary or community care services but high rates of A&E visits and acute hospital admissions [5–7]. Barriers to access and uptake of services include patient factors, such as

balancing competing priorities (food, shelter etc.) navigating healthcare systems and previous negative experiences [8].

The causes of homelessness are a combination of individual vulnerabilities and structural factors in society. Many of the risk factors that cause and sustain homelessness and lead to appalling health outcomes overlap among populations who are socially excluded [9]. Homelessness can be viewed as the most acute form of social exclusion and inequality. It can be viewed as a systems failure on a national scale [10]. In order to effectively address homelessness, as well as improving access to healthcare and the health of individuals, we could use our position to advocate for policy changes that will tackle the structural factors leading to inequalities, social exclusion and homelessness.

HOW IS HOMELESSNESS DEFINED?

Homelessness is certainly not a single entity. As well as people who are 'roofless' and sleeping outside and unsheltered, there are people who are 'houseless' and may be staying in temporary accommodation such as hostels and B&Bs or 'couch-surfing' with friends or family. From a clinical perspective it is also important to recognise people in inadequate housing, who do have a place to live but one which is unfit or unsafe for habitation. Another important situation to be aware of is those who are in insecure housing and are at imminent risk of having no place to live.

To facilitate improved research and policymaking on homelessness, the European Observatory on Homelessness have proposed the European Typology of Homelessness and Housing Exclusion (ETHOS) [11]. According to this a person is defined as homeless if they have a deficit in two out of three domains, physical, legal or social (Table 31.1).

Researchers have further defined homelessness according to duration, including chronic homelessness, intermittent homelessness and crisis or transitional homelessness [12]. Although there is overlap, risk factors for chronic homelessness such as mental health problems, substance misuse, criminal justice system history and older age are different to risks for crisis homelessness, which is usually triggered by a one-off event such as loss of a job or ill health [13].

Homelessness has negative effects on health irrespective of duration, however, people experiencing chronic homelessness have worse health outcomes than those who are intermittently or transitionally homeless. This chapter will largely be focusing on issues linked with chronic homelessness.

SUGGESTIONS FOR PRACTICE

- *Ask frequently about your patient's housing situation; be aware when patients are at risk of becoming homeless and know who to contact locally for help. Common triggers putting people at risk include*
  - *The death of a relative.*
  - *Relationship breakdown including domestic abuse.*

Table 31.1 The Theoretical Domains of Homelessness (Taken from FEANTSA)

	Physical Domain	Legal Domain	Social Domain
Homelessness			
Rooflessness	No dwelling	No legal title to a place for exclusive possession	No private and safe space for social relations
Houselessness	Has a place to live, fit for habitation	No legal title to a place for exclusive possession	No private and safe space for social relations
Housing Exclusion			
Insecure and inadequate housing	Has a place to live (not secure and unfit for habitation)	No security of title	Has space for social relations
Inadequate housing and social isolation within a legally occupied dwelling	Inadequate dwelling (unfit for habitation)	Has legal title or security of tenure, or both	No private and safe personal space for social relations
Inadequate housing (Secure tenure)	Inadequate dwelling (unfit for habitation)	Has legal title or security of tenure, or both	Has space for social relations
Insecure housing (adequate housing)	Has a place to live	No security of title	Has space for social relations
Social isolation within a secure and adequate context	Has a place to live	Has legal title or security of tenure, or both	No private and safe personal space for social relations

- *Leaving an institution such as prison or care.*
- *Rent arrears and benefit problems.*

What Are the Causes of Homelessness?

The causes of homelessness are many and complex and as discussed above, vary with the type and duration of homelessness experienced. Current thinking is that the causes are a multifaceted interplay between individual, social and structural factors [14].

Research on individual paths leading to homelessness has shown that a personal history of childhood trauma is common; including neglect, domestic abuse in the household, parental mental health issues and parental substance misuse [15]. Childhood poverty also very often predates and is a powerful predictor of adult homelessness [16]. Having been in the child welfare system is a primary risk factor for homelessness in young people (under 25 years old) and an involvement in the criminal justice system is a risk factor at any age [17, 18]. Drug and alcohol misuse have strong associations with both routes into homelessness and difficulties resolving homelessness [19].

The main protective factor preventing homelessness amongst people who may otherwise be at risk due to the above vulnerabilities is the availability of social support networks such as having a partner or being able to live as an adult in the family home.

Structural risk factors for homelessness include poverty, housing market pressures, fewer employment opportunities for low skilled workers and unfavourable welfare policies.

As Fitzpatrick et al. conclude, being able to identify these causal tendencies should focus our attention on areas where the greatest need for intervention lies [20]. At a clinical level this might mean being particularly aware of the needs of patients with the above individual vulnerabilities who also lack social support. At a societal level, being aware of the risk factors for homelessness and that they are largely outside the control of those directly affected, should inspire healthcare professionals to advocate for policy changes directed at these structural factors (Figure 31.1).

Clinical Conditions

The average age of death among homeless patients is just 47 and 43 for men and women respectively. The excessive mortality is explained not only by the conditions of homelessness itself (poor nutrition, harsh living environments, high rates of injuries); homeless people often die of treatable medical problems [21]. These include infections, ischaemic heart disease, liver disease, respiratory disease and consequences of drug and alcohol dependence. This section will look at the multiple conditions associated with excess morbidity and mortality among homeless patients and how healthcare professionals can try to reduce the burden of these.

Chronic Disease and Age-related Conditions

Chronic diseases such as asthma, COPD, diabetes and cardiovascular disease are more prevalent among homeless people compared with the general population and are typically more severe [22].

Individual Factors
Childhood trauma
Experience in care system
Experience of criminal justice system
Drug and alcohol misuse
Mental health problems

Complex interplay

Structural Factors
Poverty
Housing market pressures
Lack of employment opportunities
Welfare policies
Inequality

Figure 31.1 Risk factors for homelessness.

Reasons are thought to include lack of control over diet and living conditions, the need to prioritise basic needs over health needs, higher rates of smoking, difficulty accessing healthcare and following optimal treatment [23]. Rates of diabetes and hypertension are similar to the general population but, illustrating the above points, these are more likely to be poorly controlled in patients experiencing homelessness.

This population has also been shown to acquire age-related conditions such as falls, functional impairments and cognitive impairments 15–20 years earlier than their housed counterparts [24].

SUGGESTIONS FOR PRACTICE

- *Could you do more to diagnose and treat chronic diseases in your homeless patients?*
- *Could you do more to support smoking cessation?*

Infectious Diseases

Homeless people are particularly susceptible to infectious diseases and have an increased risk of tuberculosis, hepatitis C and HIV infection [25, 26]. The same population also experience multiple barriers to testing, treatment and adherence [27]. For example, people experiencing homelessness and symptoms of tuberculosis will present to healthcare services less and at a later stage [28]. A 2016 study of homeless people in London demonstrated a very low immunity to hepatitis B in this high-risk group and extremely poor levels of engagement in treatment for those diagnosed with hepatitis C [29]. Several studies have shown that homeless youth are more likely to engage in high-risk sexual behaviour such as unprotected intercourse and having multiple sexual partners, leading to a high prevalence of sexual transmitted infections [30, 31].

What Can Be Done in Practice?

The National Institute for Clinical Excellence (NICE) guidance recommends that homeless people should be screened for TB, hepatitis C and HIV [32]. Chest x-ray screening is a good tool for the identification of individuals with active TB in this population [33]. Use of dried blood spot testing and outreach work have been shown to improve the uptake of hepatitis C testing [34].

Hepatitis C treatment is as effective among people who inject drugs as among the general population [35]. Furthermore, newer antiviral drugs for hepatitis C with shorter courses, fewer contraindications and less side effects than traditional treatments should start to improve treatment adherence. Retention in treatment is also improved when treatment of substance misuse is provided simultaneously [36].

An accelerated hepatitis B immunization schedule has been shown to result in superior completion rates and homeless people should also be offered hepatitis A, tetanus, influenza, pneumococcus and diphtheria vaccinations [37].

Homeless drug users should be encouraged not to share injecting equipment but to use needle exchange schemes to reduce the prevalence of blood-borne viruses.

SUGGESTIONS FOR PRACTICE

- *Could you improve screening of TB and blood-borne viruses for patients experiencing homelessness?*
- *Are you offering a comprehensive immunization programme to your homeless patients?*

Unintentional Injuries

Unintentional injuries are a significant cause of morbidity and use of acute medical services in people experiencing homelessness [38]. Traumatic brain injury is an important class of unintentional injury that has been shown to be at least five times more prevalent in homeless people than the general population [39]. Studies of homelessness suggest that traumatic brain injury often occurs at a young age, before the person's first episode of homelessness [40]. Due to the risk of cognitive impairment and behavioural sequelae, traumatic brain injury is understood to be both a risk factor for becoming homeless and for remaining homeless [41]. Furthermore, studies report an apparent dose-response relation between injury severity and mental health status.

Physical and sexual assaults have also been identified as both a cause and a consequence of homelessness [42]. Research has shown that between 27% and 52% of homeless individuals were physically or sexually assaulted in the previous year [43, 44]. Homeless women and transgendered individuals are at especially high risk of severe physical and sexual assault [45].

SUGGESTIONS FOR PRACTICE

- *Consider asking patients who are experiencing homelessness about a history of traumatic brain injury.*
- *Where appropriate, assess injury severity and cognitive function.*
- *Consider referral for rehabilitation as this has been shown to improve community integration and other outcomes among people with a history of traumatic brain injury.*

Mental Health and Substance Misuse

Both mental health problems and substance misuse increase the risk of becoming homeless and are also worsened as a result of homelessness [46]. Exacerbating the issue is that these problems often occur together, termed 'dual diagnosis'.

Multiple studies have shown a high prevalence of all psychiatric conditions in homeless people compared with the general population. Homeless Link report that around 70% of people accessing homeless services in the UK have a mental health problem [47]. The homeless charity St Mungo's estimate that 64% of their clients have drug or alcohol problems [48]. A study based in three Canadian cities found that 58% of homeless women had dual diagnoses [49].

Anxiety and depression are particularly prevalent amongst people experiencing homelessness, often complicated by undiagnosed, underlying disorders including learning disabilities, traumatic brain injuries, personality disorders or compound trauma [50].

People who are homeless are also a high-risk group in relation to suicide and death from drug overdoses.

Despite this well documented morbidity, access to mental health services continues to be problematic for homeless people. A study of service provision for homeless people with mental health problems across 14 European capital cities showed low levels of input from mental health professionals, inadequate out-of-hours service provision and high levels of exclusion criteria. In spite of the high levels of dual diagnosis, almost a quarter of services reported that they would exclude a homeless person with an addiction [3].

What Can Be Done in Practice?

Be aware of patients with mental health or substance misuse problems who are at risk of becoming homeless and try to intervene to ensure they have support.

Access to appropriate mental health services is vital in reducing morbidity and premature mortality in this population. Be aware of what services are available locally and if there aren't any appropriate specialist mental health services, can you advocate on your patients' behalf for suitable services to be commissioned?

Psychologically informed environments (PIE) are intended to help staff and services understand the links between the challenging behaviour of some patients and the cumulative effects of adverse life events [51]. Psychologically informed services for homeless people (such as the Good Practice Guide) and health professionals working with people who have histories of compound trauma should be aware of the PIE guidance.

The homeless charity Pathway has also produced important guidance on mental health assessments for rough sleepers [52]. The guidance followed a serious case review into the death of a man sleeping rough with significant mental health problems who was under the care of services but had refused all help. The protocol and tools that they have produced aim to help services work more confidently with the Mental Health Act and Mental Capacity Act to assess rough sleepers who are mentally ill and at risk.

Regarding dependence on heroin and other opioids, replacement therapy has been shown to be highly effective [27]. As well as reducing illicit opioid use, it is beneficial in reducing associated risk behaviours and criminal activity. Opioid overdose prevention programmes, which train people at risk and their contacts to recognise overdose and administer naloxone to reverse the effects, have been shown to reduce heroin overdose-related deaths [53]. Educating patients who misuse opiates regarding the risk factors for drug overdoses should also be a health promotion priority (see box below).

SUGGESTIONS FOR PRACTICE

- *Could you do more to reduce the risks of opiate overdose in your patients?*

- *Advise patients not to inject alone.*
- *Advise against poly-drug use, particularly benzodiazepines, gabapentinoids or alcohol with heroin.*
- *Be aware of loss of tolerance after a period of abstinence such as discharge from prison or hospital.*
- *Provide take home naloxone and the training to recognise and treat opiate overdose.*

Accessing Healthcare

The complexity of the health needs discussed above are often seen in the context of a person lacking social support who feels ambivalent about their own self-worth and ambivalent about seeking healthcare [21]. When these factors are combined with difficulties accessing health services and previous negative experiences of healthcare and professionals, it is understandable that homeless patients present with health problems at a more advanced stage than the general population. The homeless charity, Crisis, reports that homeless people are almost 40 times more likely not to be registered with a general practitioner and are five times more likely to have had difficulty getting onto or staying on a GP's list than the housed population [54]. On the other hand, Department of Health research has shown that homeless people attend A & E five times as often as the housed population, are admitted three times as often and stay in hospital three times as long [55].

Clinicians are ideally skilled to provide holistic care and preventative care for this population, so how can barriers to accessing appropriate care be removed? (Figures 31.2–31.8)

Although people experiencing homelessness are able to access acute hospital care, problems with the care that they receive while in hospital and on discharge are widely reported. In their report, 'Safely Home' [57], Healthwatch have documented issues including homeless people feeling stigmatised and discriminated against because of their circumstances; patients being discharged before they were ready and without the right support; lack of coordination between hospitals and housing services and a lack of follow-up care. Problems cited in a report by Pathway also included delays in following protocols for methadone treatment; inadequate alcohol withdrawal treatment and inadequate analgesia [58], all of which can unfortunately lead to patients self-discharging.

These problems lead to the so called 'revolving door' of care, patients finding themselves in a vicious cycle of repeatedly going in and out of hospital without receiving the care and support needed to recover in the long term. A Department of Health report backs up this experience, showing that more

Barrier	How It Might Be Lifted
Restrictive requirement to access services	It is not a regulatory requirement to show identity documents to register with a practice; patients should not be refused registration because they don't have these.

Figures 31.2 Barriers and potential solutions.

Barrier	How It Might Be Lifted
Language or communication barriers	When giving registration or other forms in reception, always ask if patients need help filling in the forms.

Figures 31.3 Barriers and potential solutions.

Barrier	How It Might Be Lifted
Poor awareness or judgmental attitudes of staff	Provide training to ensure that all staff are aware of the specific needs of patients who are homeless and can champion their care. Involve patients who have lived experience of homelessness in your patient participation group.

Figures 31.4 Barriers and potential solutions.

Barrier	How It Might Be Lifted
Difficulty contacting the patient	Always ask about up to date address and telephone details. Avoid putting 'No fixed Abode' instead try to agree on an appropriate 'Care of Address'. Ask if they have a support worker who they see regularly and if they would be happy for the practice to contact them if needed.

Figures 31.5 Barriers and potential solutions.

Barrier	How It Might Be Lifted
Difficulty making appointments	Ask if patients have access to a phone and if not discuss how they can best make appointments.

Figures 31.6 Barriers and potential solutions.

than 70% of homeless people who were admitted to hospitals were discharged back onto the streets, sometimes prematurely and without having been treated for their underlying health problem [59].

What Can Be Done in Practice?

An admission to hospital can be a crucial opportunity to establish a homeless person's circumstances and find out the extent of their needs. It can also be a time when people are open to making positive changes in their lives if they are encouraged by compassionate, supportive care.

All hospitals should ensure they identify people who have no safe place to stay and have protocols to plan safe discharges. Many homeless people do rely on regular contact with community-based support workers, outreach programmes or primary care

Barrier	How It Might Be Lifted
Difficulty keeping appointments	Consider if some appointment flexibility or 'drop-in' appointments can be available for those whose circumstances mean getting to fixed appointments is a challenge, particularly for new patients. If they have a support worker, check if the patient would be happy with you informing the support worker about appointment and referral details.

Figures 31.7 Barriers and potential solutions.

Barrier	How It Might Be Lifted
Loss of confidence and fear of seeking healthcare	Try to make the reception and waiting areas welcoming and inclusive spaces

Figures 31.8 Barriers and potential solutions.

teams and so proactive communication between hospital staff and community staff is often vital in ensuring a safe discharge. Appropriate communication should also always involve an informative and timely discharge summary being sent to their primary care team, even when the patient may have self-discharged. To avoid unnecessary self-discharges before the patient is fit, it is important for patients who are addicted to opioids to be safely prescribed sufficient substitute medication. If they have been treated with methadone or subutex while in hospital, it is obviously imperative that arrangements are made with the community drug services prior to discharge.

The charity Pathway tries to assist with all the issues mentioned in this section. Pathway started in London in 2009 and at the time of writing includes teams in 11 hospitals across the UK. The aims are to identify homeless people at an early stage of their admission, establish their needs and collaborate with hospital staff and community services to support them while in hospital and facilitate a safe, comprehensive plan for their discharge. Hopefully this excellent service will continue to expand.

The Homelessness Reduction Act came into effect in April 2018 and imposes a 'duty to refer' to public authorities including hospitals and GP surgeries, to notify the Local Housing Authority of any person who they consider may be homeless or at risk of homelessness. This should provide an opportunity to improve collaboration between health services and the housing authorities in their areas (Figures 31.9–31.11).

SUGGESTIONS FOR PRACTICE

Effective Consultations

Pendleton described the consultation as the central act of medicine [60]. For homeless populations the consequences of healthcare consultations can be particularly profound; people who are homeless feel they are treated as though they are worthless, compounding loss of confidence and social isolation [61]. Conversely, when someone is ready to seek healthcare they are very responsive when a doctor does listen, show concern and the professionalism to give non-judgemental and personalised healthcare [62].

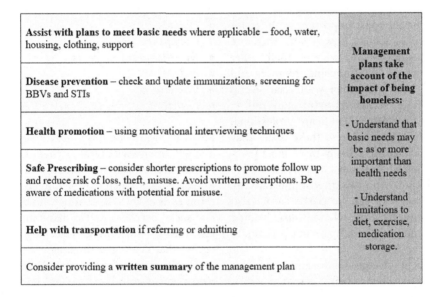

Agenda setting – what do they wish to address first?	**Maintaining a positive therapeutic relationship:**
Living conditions- housing, food, water, clothing, safe storage for medication	
Support – family, friends, support workers check consent to contact and record contact details	- Establish mutual trust
Substance use – smoking, alcohol, drugs, amount and frequency	- Nonjudgmental - Respect for the
Safety assessment – risks of abuse	individual - Trauma
Update contact details- at every visit, may need to agree on a care of address	informed
Examination – understand that they may be reluctant or embarrassed to be examined	

Figures 31.9 Considerations for practice.

Assist with plans to meet basic needs where applicable – food, water, housing, clothing, support	**Management plans take account of the impact of being homeless:**
Disease prevention – check and update immunizations, screening for BBVs and STIs	- Understand that basic needs may be as or more
Health promotion – using motivational interviewing techniques	important than health needs
Safe Prescribing – consider shorter prescriptions to promote follow up and reduce risk of loss, theft, misuse. Avoid written prescriptions. Be aware of medications with potential for misuse.	- Understand limitations to diet, exercise,
Help with transportation if referring or admitting	medication storage.
Consider providing a **written summary** of the management plan	

Figures 31.10 Considerations for practice.

Continuity of care: Building a trusted relationship can be as important as clinical care	**Comprehensive safety-netting:** Building in flexibility, anticipating that rigid plans may not be feasible
Look after yourself and ensure you have sufficient support	

Figures 31.11 Considerations for practice.

Earlier in the chapter the accumulation of disadvantage that can lead to homelessness was discussed. It is vital to recognise the effects of this personal history, for example someone who has experienced compound trauma from an early age may understandably have difficulty developing trusting relationships and managing emotions.

Caring for homeless patients can be as much about establishing and maintaining a positive relationship as about clinical expertise. The key ingredients for such a relationship include a trauma-informed approach, building mutual trust, showing respect for the individual and taking a non-judgmental approach.

At the start of a consultation, one way of showing respect and empowering a patient who may be used to feeling disempowered is to make an extra effort to set the agenda together, ensuring that they are given a choice about which issues they want to prioritise.

Many consultation models advocate understanding the personal and psychosocial context of the illness. It is hard to think of a patient group for whom this advice is more relevant. Homeless individuals will often be balancing competing priorities such as shelter, food and money. Rae and Rees describe how the daily priorities of a person experiencing homelessness will alter the importance they attach to their health, with a trend towards neglecting their health until crisis point when they have fewest resources. Understanding that healthcare may not be the most important problem for individuals unless acutely unwell, and therefore incorporating strategies to address their other basic needs such as food, housing, finances and clothing, will help strengthen your relationship and promote more successful treatment overall.

The extent to which a healthcare professional will be able to directly address these issues may obviously be limited. It is likely to be most practical to find out what, if any, support they have in place and know who to signpost and refer to. Peer support workers can be particularly valuable in building trusting relationships, helping with social issues and accompanying patients to appointments.

With frequent changes of location and loss or theft of mobile phones being common issues, ensure that at each appointment you check details to contact the patient and if applicable, their support worker. If the patient doesn't have a fixed address, ask for a 'care of' address and number. Discuss with them if they are happy to consent for you to contact their support workers directly if needed.

For safety reasons it is worth carefully considering the amount of medications that you prescribe at a time. Take account of the patient's wishes and transportation to the surgery or pharmacy as well as the risks of loss, theft, overdose and misuse. For the most vulnerable patients reducing to even daily prescribing can be appropriate. Prescribing short durations can also sometimes be helpful in promoting follow-up. Consider the safe storage of medications for patients who are sleeping rough or staying in hostels or shelters. Handwritten prescriptions are rarely used these days, printed or ideally electronic scripts have less potential for forging and are certainly safer options. Do try to keep up to date with medications with the potential for misuse, this includes medications that can be used as adjuncts to street drugs as well as those that can be diverted to raise money for other purposes. Having a practice prescribing policy that covers the above points can help to promote consistency and avoid conflict.

SUGGESTIONS FOR PRACTICE

- *The following is a list of medications which have potential for diversion or misuse.*
- *Benzodiazepines,*
- *Opioids,*
- *Gabapentin and pregabalin,*
- *Nutritional supplements,*
- *Z-drugs,*
- *Clonidine,*
- *Cyclizine.*

Please be aware that this is not a comprehensive list and will change with location, trends and time.

This section has shown there is a lot to cover in a consultation which may be limited to around ten minutes, is likely to be dealing with complex health and social needs, as well as maintaining a trusting relationship. The term housekeeping is used to recognise that dealing with patients can be stressful and healthcare professionals need to look after their own states of mind and feelings no less diligently than those of their patients. In their study of resilience among doctors, Stevenson et al found that those who thrive while working in areas of social disadvantage were 'sustained by a deep appreciation and respect' for the population they work with, they celebrated small gains and were not overwhelmed by the larger context of social disadvantage.

REFERENCES

1. Thomas B. Homelessness kills: An analysis of the mortality of homeless people in early twenty-first century England. Crisis head office [Internet]. 2012 [cited 2019 Jun 8]. Available from: https://www.crisis.org.uk/media/236798/crisis_homelessness_kills2012.pdf

2. O'Connell JJ. Premature mortality in home-less populations: A review of the literature premature mortality in homeless popula-tions: A review of the Literature. National Health Care for the Homeless Council [Internet]. 2005 [cited 2019 Jun 8]. Available from: https://www.nhchc.org/wp-content/uploads/2011/10/Premature-Mortality.pdf

3. Canavan R, Barry MM, Matanov A, Barros H, Gabor E, Greacen T et al. Service provision and barriers to care for homeless people with mental health problems across 14 European capital cities. *BMC Health Serv Res* [Internet]. 2012 Dec 27 [cited 2019 Jun 8];12(1):222. Available from: https://bmchealthservres.biomedcentral.com/articles/10.1186/1472-6963-12-222

4. Baggett TP, O'Connell JJ, Singer DE, Rigotti NA. The unmet health care needs of home-less adults: A national study. *Am J Public Health [Internet]*. 2010 Jul [cited 2019 Jun 8];100(7):1326–33. Available from: http://www.ncbi.nlm.nih.gov/pubmed/20466953

5. Verlinde E, Verdée T, Van de Walle M, Art B, De Maeseneer J, Willems S. Unique health care utilization patterns in a home-less population in Ghent. *BMC Health Serv Res [Internet]*. 2010 Dec 19 [cited 2019 Jun 8];10(1):242. Available from: http://www.ncbi.nlm.nih.gov/pubmed/20723222

6. Bharel M, Lin W-C, Zhang J, O'Connell E, Taube R, Clark RE. Health care utiliza-tion patterns of homeless individuals in Boston: Preparing for Medicaid expan-sion under the Affordable Care Act. *Am J Public Health [Internet]*. 2013 Dec [cited 2019 Jun 8];103(S2):S311–7. Available from: http://www.ncbi.nlm.nih.gov/pubmed/24148046

7. O'Carroll A, O'Reilly F. Health of the home-less in Dublin: Has anything changed in the context of Ireland's economic boom? *Eur J Public Health [Internet]*. 2008 Oct 1 [cited 2019 Jun 8];18(5):448–53. Available from: http://www.ncbi.nlm.nih.gov/pubmed/18579577

8. Håkanson C, Öhlén J. Illness narratives of people who are homeless. *Int J Qual Stud Health Well-being* [Internet]. 2016 [cited 2019 Jun 8];11:32924. Available from: http://www.ncbi.nlm.nih.gov/pubmed/27914194

9. Fitzpatrick S, Bramley G, Johnsen S. Pathways into multiple exclusion homeless-ness in seven UK cities. *Urban Stud [Internet]*. 2013 Jan 27 [cited 2019 Jun 8];50(1):148–68. Available from: http://journals.sagepub.com/doi/10.1177/0042098012452329

10. Blackburn P. Streets of shame: Homelessness and the NHS – tomes of tragedies. *Doctor* [Internet]. 2019;7–13. Available from: https://www.bma.org.uk/features/streetsofshame/

11. On the way home? FEANTSA monitor-ing report on homelessness and home-less policies in Europe 3 [Internet]. [cited 2019 Jun 8]. Available from: https://www.feantsa.org/download/on_the_way_home-16908290734892551038.pdf

12. Kuhn R, Culhane DP. Applying cluster analysis to test a typology of homelessness by pattern of shelter utilization: Results from the analysis of administrative data. *Am J Community Psychol [Internet]*. 1998 [cited 2019 Jun 8];26(2):207–32. Available from: http://repository.upenn.edu/spp_papersURL:http:http://dx.http://repository.upenn.edu/spp_papers/96

13. Fazel S, Geddes JR, Kushel M. The health of homeless people in high-income coun-tries: Descriptive epidemiology, health consequences, and clinical and policy rec-ommendations. *Lancet [Internet]*. 2014 [cited 2018 Feb 6];384:1529–40. Available from: https://0-ac-els--cdn-com.wam.leeds.ac.uk/S0140673614611326/1-s2.0-S0140673614611326-main.pdf?_tid=01837fc6-0b63-11e8-ac6c-00000aab0f02&acdnat=15179 38229_6ae3752d1b92af7b0ed3b6101cc2be1c

14. Fitzpatrick S. Explaining homeless-ness: A critical realist perspective. *Housing, Theory Soc [Internet]*. 2005 Apr [cited 2019 Jun 8];22(1):1–17. Available from: http://www.tandfonline.com/doi/abs/10.1080/14036090510034563

15. England PH. *Evidence Review: Adults with Complex Needs (With a Particular Focus on Street Begging and Street Sleeping)*. About Public Health England.

16. Bramley G, Fitzpatrick S. Homelessness in the UK : Who is most at risk ? *Hous Stud [Internet]*. 2018;3037:1–21. Available from: http://doi.org/10.1080/02673037.2017.1344957

17. Dworsky A, Napolitano L, Courtney M. Homelessness during the transition from foster care to adulthood. *Am J Public Health [Internet]*. 2013 Dec [cited 2019 Jun 8];103(S2):S318–23. Available from: http://www.ncbi.nlm.nih.gov/pubmed/24148065

18. Greenberg GA, Rosenheck RA. Jail incarceration, homelessness, and mental health: A national study. *Psychiatr Serv [Internet]*. 2008 Feb [cited 2019 Jun 8];59(2):170–7. Available from: http://www.ncbi.nlm.nih.gov/pubmed/18245159

19. Patterson ML, Somers JM, Moniruzzaman A. Prolonged and persistent homelessness: Multivariable analyses in a cohort experiencing current homelessness and mental illness in Vancouver, British Columbia. *Ment Heal Subst Use [Internet]*. 2012 May [cited 2019 Jun 8];5(2):85–101. Available from: http://www.tandfonline.com/doi/abs/10.1080/17523281.2011.618143

20. Fitzpatrick S, Pawson H, Bramley G, Wilcox S, Watts B. The homelessness monitor: England 2015 [Internet]. 2015 [cited 2019 Jun 8]. Available from: https://www.crisis.org.uk/media/237031/the_homelessness_monitor_england_2015.pdf

21. Standards for commissioners and service providers: Self assessment tool for primary care providers. The Faculty for Homeless and Inclusion Health of the College of Medicine. 2013 [cited 2018 Mar 6]; Available from: http://www.pathway.org.uk/wp-content/uploads/2014/01/Standards-for-commissioners-providers-v2.0-INTERACTIVE.pdf

22. Lee TC, Hanlon JG, Ben-David J, Booth GL, Cantor WJ, Connelly PW et al. Risk factors for cardiovascular disease in homeless adults. *Circulation [Internet]*. 2005 May 24 [cited 2019 Jun 14];111(20):2629–35. Available from: http://www.ncbi.nlm.nih.gov/pubmed/15897342

23. Zerger S. A preliminary review of literature chronic medical illness and homeless individuals. Prepared for interfaith house mini-continuum of care for chronically medically ill homeless adults: Phase one planning grant [Internet]. 2002 [cited 2019 Jun 14]. Available from: www.nccconline.org

24. Brown RT, Kiely DK, Bharel M, Mitchell SL. Geriatric syndromes in older homeless adults. *J Gen Intern Med [Internet]*. 2012 Jan 31 [cited 2019 Jun 14];27(1):16–22. Available from: http://www.ncbi.nlm.nih.gov/pubmed/21879368

25. Raoult D, Foucault C, Brouqui P. *Reviews: Infections in the homeless*. 2001;1(September).

26. Aldridge RW, Story A, Hwang SW, Nordentoft M, Luchenski SA, Hartwell G et al. Morbidity and mortality in homeless individuals, prisoners, sex workers, and individuals with substance use disorders in high-income countries: A systematic review and meta-analysis. *Lancet (London, England) [Internet]*. 2017 Nov 10 [cited 2018 Feb 6];391(10117):241–50. Available from: http://www.ncbi.nlm.nih.gov/pubmed/29137869

27. Luchenski S, Maguire N, Aldridge RW, Hayward A, Story A, Perri P et al. What works in inclusion health: Overview of effective interventions for marginalised and excluded populations. *Lancet (London, England) [Internet]*. 2017 Nov 10 [cited 2018 Feb 6];391(10117):266–80. Available from: http://www.ncbi.nlm.nih.gov/pubmed/29137868

28. Story A, Murad S, Roberts W, Verheyen M, Hayward AC, London Tuberculosis Nurses Network. Tuberculosis in London: The importance of homelessness, problem drug use and prison. *Thorax [Internet]*. 2007 Aug 1 [cited 2019 Jun 15];62(8):667–71. Available from: http://www.ncbi.nlm.nih.gov/pubmed/17289861

29. Story A, Hayward A, Aldridge R. Co-infection with hepatitis C, hepatitis B, HIV and latent TB infection among homeless people in London. *Journal of Hepatology*, 2016;64(2):S455–6.

30. Rew L, Fouladi RT, Land L, Wong YJ. Outcomes of a brief sexual health intervention for homeless youth. *J Health Psychol [Internet]*. 2007 Sep [cited 2019 Jun 15];12(5):818–32. Available from: http://www.ncbi.nlm.nih.gov/pubmed/17855465

31. Greene JM, Ennett ST, Ringwalt CL. Prevalence and correlates of survival sex among runaway and homeless youth. *Am J Public Health* [Internet]. 1999 Sep

[cited 2019 Jun 15];89(9):1406–9. Available from: http://www.ncbi.nlm.nih.gov/pubmed/10474560

32. Identifying and managing tuberculosis among hard-to-reach groups [Internet]. 2012 [cited 2019 Jun 15]. Available from: www.nice.org.uk/

33. Paquette K, Cheng MP, Kadatz MJ, Cook VJ, Chen W, Johnston JC. Chest radiography for active tuberculosis case finding in the homeless: A systematic review and meta-analysis. *Int J Tuberc Lung Dis [Internet]*. 2014 Oct 1 [cited 2019 Jun 15];18(10):1231–6. Available from: http://www.ncbi.nlm.nih.gov/pubmed/25216838

34. Jones L, Bates G, McCoy E, Beynon C, McVeigh J, Bellis MA. Effectiveness of interventions to increase hepatitis C testing uptake among high-risk groups: A systematic review. *Eur J Public Health [Internet]*. 2014 Oct 1 [cited 2019 Jun 15];24(5):781–8. Available from: http://www.ncbi.nlm.nih.gov/pubmed/24158318

35. Ryder SD. Chronic hepatitis C - what do the new drugs offer and who should get them first? *Clin Med [Internet]*. 2015 Apr 1 [cited 2019 Jun 15];15(2):197–200. Available from: http://www.ncbi.nlm.nih.gov/pubmed/25824075

36. Dimova RB, Zeremski M, Jacobson IM, Hagan H, Des Jarlais DC, Talal AH. Determinants of hepatitis C virus treatment completion and efficacy in drug users assessed by meta-analysis. *Clin Infect Dis [Internet]*. 2013 Mar 15 [cited 2019 Jun 15];56(6):806–16. Available from: http://www.ncbi.nlm.nih.gov/pubmed/23223596

37. Wright NMJ, Tompkins CNE. How can health services effectively meet the health needs of homeless people? *Br J Gen Pract*. 2006;56(April):286–93.

38. Mackelprang JL, Graves JM, Rivara FP. Homeless in America: Injuries treated in US emergency departments, 2007–2011. *Int J Inj Contr Saf Promot [Internet]*. 2014 Jul 3 [cited 2019 Jun 15];21(3):289–97. Available from: http://www.ncbi.nlm.nih.gov/pubmed/24011180

39. Silver JM, Kramer R, Greenwald S, Weissman M. The association between head injuries and psychiatric disorders: Findings from the New Haven NIMH Epidemiologic Catchment Area Study. *Brain Inj [Internet]*. 2001 Jan 3 [cited 2019 Jun 15];15(11):935–45. Available from: http://www.ncbi.nlm.nih.gov/pubmed/11689092

40. Hwang SW, Colantonio A, Chiu S, Tolomiczenko G, Kiss A, Cowan L et al. The effect of traumatic brain injury on the health of homeless people. *CMAJ [Internet]*. 2008 Oct 7 [cited 2018 Feb 6];179(8):779–84. Available from: http://www.ncbi.nlm.nih.gov/pubmed/18838453

41. Topolovec-Vranic J, Ennis N, Colantonio A, Cusimano MD, Hwang SW, Kontos P et al. Traumatic brain injury among people who are homeless: A systematic review. *BMC Public Health [Internet]*. 2012 Dec 8 [cited 2019 Jun 15];12(1):1059. Available from: https://bmcpublichealth.biomedcentral.com/articles/10.1186/1471-2458-12-1059

42. Stein JA, Leslie MB, Nyamathi A. Relative contributions of parent substance use and childhood maltreatment to chronic homelessness, depression, and substance abuse problems among homeless women: Mediating roles of self-esteem and abuse in adulthood. *Child Abuse Negl [Internet]*. 2002 Oct [cited 2019 Jun 15];26(10):1011–27. Available from: http://www.ncbi.nlm.nih.gov/pubmed/12398858

43. Larney S, Conroy E, Mills KL, Burns L, Teesson M. Factors associated with violent victimisation among homeless adults in Sydney, Australia. *Aust N Z J Public Health [Internet]*. 2009 Aug [cited 2019 Jun 15];33(4):347–51. Available from: http://www.ncbi.nlm.nih.gov/pubmed/19689595

44. Newburn T, Rock P. Living in fear: Violence and victimisation in the lives of single homeless people. 2004 [cited 2019 Jun 15]; Available from: https://scholar.google.com/scholar_lookup?hl=en&publication_year=2005&author=R+Newburn&author=P+Rock&title=Living+in+fear%3A+Violence+and+victimisation+in+the+lives+of+single+homeless+people

45. Kushel MB, Evans JL, Perry S, Robertson MJ, Moss AR. No door to lock. *Arch Intern Med [Internet]*. 2003 Nov 10 [cited 2019 Jun 15];163(20):2492. Available from: http://www.ncbi.nlm.nih.gov/pubmed/14609786

46. Adapting your Practice: General recommendations for the care of homeless patients [Internet]. [cited 2019 Jun 15]. Available from: http://www.nhchc.org/wp-content/uploads/2011/09/GenRecsHomeless2010.pdf

47. Support for single homeless people in England [Internet]. [cited 2019 Jun 15]. Available from: https://www.crisis.org.uk/media/237833/moving_on_2017.pdf

48. A future. Now homeless health matters: The case for change [Internet]. 2014 [cited 2019 Jun 15]. Available from: https://www.mungos.org/app/uploads/2017/12/A_Future_Now.pdf

49. Torchalla I, Strehlau V, Li K, Krausz M. Substance use and predictors of substance dependence in homeless women. *Drug Alcohol Depend [Internet]*. 2011 Nov 1 [cited 2019 Jun 15];118(2–3):173–9. Available from: http://www.ncbi.nlm.nih.gov/pubmed/21498010

50. Homelessness Guidance for Mental Health Professionals. Making the most of your support. Let's end homelessness together. 2017. https://www.homeless.org.uk/

51. Psychologically informed services for homeless people Good Practice Guide. 2012 [cited 2018 Feb 6]. Available from: http://www.pathway.org.uk/wp-content/uploads/2013/05/Psychologically-informed-services-for-Homeless-People.pdf

52. Mental Health Service Assessments for Rough Sleepers: Tools and Guidance [Internet]. 2017 [cited 2019 Jun 16]. Available from: https://www.pathway.org.uk/wp-content/uploads/RSTG-2017-FINAL.pdf

53. McDonald R, Strang J. Are take-home naloxone programmes effective? Systematic review utilizing application of the Bradford Hill criteria. *Addiction [Internet]*. 2016 Jul 1 [cited 2019 Jun 16];111(7):1177–87. Available from: http://doi.wiley.com/10.1111/add.13326

54. Crisis. *Critical Condition Homeless People's Access to GPs* [Internet]. London; 2002 [cited 2016 Dec 3]. Available from: http://www.crisis.org.uk/data/files/document_library/policy_reports/gp_mediabrief.pdf

55. Office of the Chief Analyst D. Healthcare for Single Homeless People Office of the Chief Analyst [Internet]. 2010 [cited 2019 Jun 16]. Available from: https://www.housinglin.org.uk/_assets/Resources/Housing/Support_materials/Other_reports_and_guidance/Healthcare_for_single_homeless_people.pdf

56. How to register with a doctor (GP) [Internet]. [cited 2019 Jun 16]. Available from: www.england.nhs.uk

57. England H. Safely home: What happens when people leave hospital and care settings? [Internet]. 2015 [cited 2019 Jun 16]. Available from: www.healthwatch.co.uk

58. Hewett N, Halligan A, Boyce T. A general practitioner and nurse led approach to improving hospital care for homeless people. *BMJ [Internet]*. 2012 Sep 28 [cited 2019 Jun 16];345(sep28 2):e5999–e5999. Available from: http://www.ncbi.nlm.nih.gov/pubmed/23045316

59. Improving hospital admission and discharge for people who are homeless. Analysis of the current picture and recommendations for change [Internet]. 2012 [cited 2019 Jun 16]. Available from: https://www.homeless.org.uk/sites/default/files/site-attachments/HOSPITAL_ADMISSION_AND_DISCHARGE._REPORTdoc.pdf

60. Pendleton D, Schofield T, Tate P, Havelock P. *The New Consultation: Developing Doctor-Patient Communication*. Oxford: Oxford University Press; 2003.

61. Rae BE, Rees S. The perceptions of homeless people regarding their healthcare needs and experiences of receiving health care. *J Adv Nurs [Internet]*. 2015 Sep 1 [cited 2018 Mar 11];71(9):2096–107. Available from: http://doi.wiley.com/10.1111/jan.12675

62. Bunkers SS. The lived experience of feeling cared for: A human becoming perspective. *Nurs Sci Q [Internet]*. 2004 Jan 18 [cited 2019 Jun 16];17(1):63–71. Available from: http://journals.sagepub.com/doi/10.1177/0894318403260472

63. Jones A. Caring for people experiencing homelessness in primary care. In: Gill P, Wright N, Brew I, editors. *Working with Vulnerable Groups*. London: Royal College of General Practitioners; 2014. p. 39–54.

64. Neighbour R. *The Inner Consultation*. Second edition. London: CRC Press; 2005.

65. Stevenson AD, Phillips CB, Anderson KJ. Resilience among doctors who work in challenging areas: A qualitative study. *Br J Gen Pract [Internet]*. 2011 Jul [cited 2018 Apr 7];61(588):e404–10. Available from: http://www.ncbi.nlm.nih.gov/pubmed/21722448

32

Veterans' Health

MICHAEL BROOKES

A sense of self-reliance and resilience which coupled with the high value placed on personal physical fitness may make veterans reluctant to accept health problems.

Veterans are defined as anyone who has served at least for one day in Her Majesty's Armed Forces (Regular or Reserve) or Merchant Mariners who have seen duty on legally defined military operations [1].

However, former service personnel do not always identify themselves as veterans. In a survey of 202 people who left the military, only half considered themselves to be veterans [2]. Definitions used by ex-service personnel do not always align with the official UK government definition or public perceptions of veterans, which tend to focus on older veterans. The term 'service leaver' is often better understood by the public and preferred by former service personnel.

There were approximately 2.56 million veterans living in the UK in 2016. Approximately 60% of veterans were over the age of 65 and 90% were male [3]. A practice with an average list size of 7,292 [4] patients, will look after approximately 350 veterans. About 18,000 people leave the services each year to return to civilian life. Of those, approximately 2,000 have been discharged on medical grounds.

WHAT MAKES VETERANS DIFFERENT?

Risk of Ongoing Health Problems

Many people associate service-related health problems with severe injuries sustained during combat operations or post-traumatic stress disorder (PTSD). Veterans may also experience less visible occupational health problems such as hearing loss, which is over three times more likely to occur in veterans under 75 than in the general population, depression and anxiety [5].

Cultural Differences

Military training instils a sense of self-reliance and resilience into service personnel which, coupled with the high value placed on personal physical fitness may make veterans reluctant to accept health problems or seek help.

Traditionally in the services, alcohol has been used to cope with the intense psychological stress of battle and also to mediate the transition from the heightened experience of combat to routine safety [6]. Fear et al [7] found excessive alcohol consumption was more common in the UK armed forces than in the general population even after taking age and gender differences into account.

Transition from Military to Civilian Life

Early service leavers tend to be entitled to less support than other service leavers in the transition to civilian life. Early service leavers are at particular risk from mental health and social problems such as unemployment and homelessness. It is known that ex-service personnel are at a greater risk of experiencing homelessness than the civilian population. The Combined Homelessness and Information Network (CHAIN) contains information about rough sleepers in London. The CHAIN annual report 2017–2018 found that 7% of rough sleepers were former service personnel [8].

The Military Covenant

The Military Covenant is an understanding between the nation and those who serve in the military. In return for the commitment of those who serve in the armed forces, their willingness to forgo certain civil liberties and put themselves in harm's way (personnel in Iraq and Afghanistan are 150 times more likely to be killed at work than their civilian counterparts in the UK), the nation promises to help and support them when they are in need. The impact of the covenant and the role it plays in healthcare is discussed later in this chapter.

COMMON HEALTH PROBLEMS EXPERIENCED BY VETERANS

Mental Health

The commonest types of mental health problems associated with service life include PTSD, depression, anxiety and substance misuse.

Whilst 'Gulf War Syndrome' is not recognised as a specific disease it has been officially accepted as an umbrella term to cover accepted conditions linked to the 1990–91 Gulf War conflict [9]. Conditions include psychiatric illnesses and multi-system diseases. Research has not identified a discrete disease specific to Gulf War veterans.

A 2010 study of 10,000 serving personnel found lower than expected levels of PTSD. About 4% of respondents reported PTSD; 19.7% reported common mental health disorders such as depression and anxiety were reported by 19.7%; this is comparable to the general population rate of about 20% [10]. In addition, 13% reported alcohol misuse. Male service personnel are about twice as likely as their civilian counterparts to be dependent on alcohol; female service personnel are five times as likely. Recent service leavers appear to be continuing their drinking pattern into civilian life [11]. PTSD was more likely to be reported by reservists and regulars in a combat role. Interestingly the experience of mental health problems did not seem related to the number of deployments [12]; those who left the services early seemed to be at a higher risk of mental health problems compared to those who serve for longer periods. There may be a higher suicide rate in veterans under the age of 25, particularly in the first two years after discharge [13].

With overall low levels of PTSD, a service leaver is much more likely to present with more common mental health disorders such as anxiety, depression or alcohol misuse.

Around 7,000 service personnel who served in the 1990–1991 Gulf War conflict are in receipt of war pensions or other assistance due to a variety of injuries or illnesses causally linked to the conflict. These conditions have been grouped under the term 'Gulf War Syndrome'. This represents about 13% of the personnel deployed during the conflict. Interestingly, there is no current evidence in the UK of a new Gulf War Syndrome arising from more recent conflict in Iraq and Afghanistan, although there is a rise in post-conflict psychiatric disorders being reported in the USA [14].

LONG TERM INJURIES

Chronic Pain

Between 2001 and 2018, there were 329 personnel who experienced traumatic or surgical amputation as a result of injuries sustained in either Iraq or Afghanistan [15].

Approximately 15% of amputees experience phantom limb pain. Phantom limb pain is more common after a traumatic amputation of an arm, particularly if the amputation was delayed.

Sexual Problems and Fertility Issues

Some servicemen experience injuries which affect their fertility. The government has committed to providing up to three cycles of IVF treatment for veterans with injury-related infertility problems.

Some servicemen choose to bank sperm prior to deployments. The cost of doing this should be met by the individual. The NHS will meet the cost of ongoing storage if the serviceman develops an injury-related infertility problem.

Psychological Adjustment

There can be difficulties for veterans adjusting to physical injuries. These may include anxieties about their appearance and how others might perceive them personally and professionally. There may be relationship difficulties caused by functional difficulties as well as worry about bodily appearance.

Injured veterans may develop unhelpful behaviours such as avoiding social contact, intimate relationships and being self-conscious and defensive.

Factors which are predictive of a good adjustment include having a good social network, good social and communication skills, having a positive outlook and being involved in treatment decisions. An individual's outcome will be associated with their *perception* of the severity of the injury and the importance of their appearance in relation to their standing in society. Educational attainment, visibility of the injury and clinical severity do not seem to correlate with the ability to adjust psychologically.

Veterans Exposed to Nuclear Testing

Between 1952 and 1967, the UK tested nuclear weapons at several sites including Australia, Christmas Island in the Pacific and Nevada in the USA. The tests involved over 22,000 service personnel and there are believed to be about 1,500 service personnel alive today who witnessed the tests. Veterans or families may raise health issues associated with the testing.

TRANSFER ARRANGEMENTS ON DISCHARGE FROM THE SERVICE

When a service leaver with serious injuries is due to be discharged from rehabilitation and into the care of the NHS, the CCG responsible for the area where the service leaver is due to reside should commission a multi-disciplinary team (MDT) meeting about three months before the discharge date. Ideally, the MDT should have contributions from both health and social care to ascertain and make plans for a personalised care package. The injured veteran may be eligible for NHS continuing care. NHS continuing care is a package of ongoing healthcare provided outside hospital and organised and funded by the NHS. This is in contrast to social care which is the responsibility of the local authority.

PROSTHETIC CENTRES

A review of the care of veterans who had lost a limb or limbs found a significant discrepancy between the services provided by the NHS and the MOD. A veterans' prosthetics programme was developed to implement the findings of the report, which included national commissioning of prosthetics services and the rationalisation of services into nine specialised multi-disciplinary centres in the UK.

It is known that patients with a good quality prosthesis which minimises the difference to pre-amputation functioning adjust better. The NHS prosthetic service is obliged to offer veterans with amputations replacement prostheses which are of the same or better technological standard than their original prosthesis.

Veterans wishing to access the programme should do so via their local Disablement Service Centre.

IMPROVING CARE OF VETERANS

SUGGESTIONS FOR PRACTICE

- *Learn more about the particular needs of those serving, their families and veterans by completing a free online learning module at www.e-lfh. org.uk/programmes/armedforces.*
- *Identify veterans.*
- *Learn more about the Practice Military Veteran Accreditation Scheme.*

In the UK, primary care information technology systems use Read codes to detail various conditions and information in a patient's records. There are specific codes pertaining to previous military service. A study of over 40,000 patients at several primary care centres noted the prevalence of military veterans with a Read code in their records was 8.7%. After a period of brief training for staff at the practices using an online training module, and an advertising campaign to encourage veterans to make their status known, the number of veterans identified and coded increased nearly 200% [16]. The identification of veterans and knowledge of their specific health issues from increased awareness through staff training seeks to improve the overall health of service leavers. This principal has been crystallised in collaboration between the Royal College of General Practitioners and NHS England [17]. The scheme is called the Military Veteran Aware Accreditation and encourages primary care providers to identify a lead for veterans' health. The lead will have received extra training in the health needs of veterans or may be a veteran themselves. The lead will encourage the identification and recording of veterans as well as acting as a link for patients and colleagues to access the various support services available.

Veterans' Mental Health Programmes

The NHS Veterans' Mental Health Transition, Intervention and Liaison Service (TILS) is a dedicated, locally-based service for veterans and those leaving the services. It provides a range of treatments including help to recognise the early signs of mental health problems and access to early support. TILS can also provide treatment for more complex mental health problems and psychological trauma.

The NHS Veterans' Complex Mental Health Treatment Service (CTS) is an enhanced service for service leavers experiencing complex mental health problems related to their time in the military, which have not improved with earlier treatment. CTS provides intensive care and treatments such as occupational and trauma-focused therapies and support for drug and alcohol dependency.

To access the NHS veterans' mental health programmes, a veteran may contact the TILS directly or be referred by their GP or a service charity.

The NHS Military Covenant

The Armed Forces Covenant is a statement of the moral obligation which exists between the nation, the government and the armed forces in return for the sacrifices they make. It is enshrined in law in the Armed Forces Act 2011. There are two main strands to the covenant:

- No current or former member of the armed forces or their families should be at a disadvantage compared to other citizens in the provision of public or commercial services.
- Special consideration is appropriate in some cases, particularly for those who have been injured or bereaved.

The NHS Constitution was updated in 2015 to strengthen this accountability by stating that 'the NHS will ensure that in line with the Armed Forces Covenant, those in the armed forces, reservists, their families and veterans are not disadvantaged in accessing health services in the area they reside' [18].

SUGGESTIONS FOR PRACTICE

- *When referring a veteran to secondary care, ensure that their veteran status is in the referral letter, as they may be entitled to priority care under the NHS Military Covenant.*
- *Encourage veterans take out an armed forces network membership.*

There are nine regional networks closely aligned to military regional structures. The networks meet regularly to ensure collaborative work between local and regional people, the NHS, the Ministry of Defence, local authorities and service charities.

The networks aim to shape how each region develops and delivers care to veterans, serving soldiers and their families as well as providing feedback to the NHS, Ministry of Defence and Department of Health on their current delivery strategies.

- The War Pension Scheme is available to those with an injury or illness sustained on or before 5 April 2005.
- The Armed Forces Compensation Scheme is available to those with an injury or illness

sustained on or after 6 April 2005. Applications can be made while serving for injuries or illness after 6 April 2010.

- Useful resources:
- The NHS has some comprehensive information for current and ex-service personnel.
  - www.nhs.uk/using-the-nhs/military-healthcare/
- SSAFA (The Armed Forces Charity)
  - www.ssafa.org.uk
- The Royal British Legion.
  - www.britishlegion.org.uk
- Army Welfare Service.
  - www.army.mod.uk/personnel-and-welfare
- Combat Stress.
  - www.combatstress.org.uk
- MOD Legacy Health.
  - www.gov.uk/guidance/support-for-war-veterans
- British Limbless Ex-Servicemen's Association.
  - www. blesma.org
- British Nuclear Test Veterans' Association.
  - www.bntva.com

REFERENCES

1. Veterans UK. A guide to Veterans Services. London: Ministry of Defence; 2017. Available from: https://www.gov.uk/government/organisations/veterans-uk
2. Burdett H, Woodhead C, Iversen A et al. "Are you a veteran?" Understanding of the term "Veteran" among UK ex-service personnel: A research note. *Armed Forces and Society*. 2013; 39(4): 751–759.
3. Ministry of Defence. Annual population survey UK armed forces veterans residing in Great Britain 2016. London: Ministry of Defence; 2017.
4. Kaffash J. Why GP practice list sizes are on the rise. *Pulse Magazine*; 2015. Available from: http://www.pulsetoday.co.uk/political/practice-boundaries/why-gp-practice-list-sizes-are-on-the-rise/20010188.article
5. The Royal British Legion. A UK household survey of the ex-service community. The Royal British Legion; 2014. Available from: https://www.vfrhub.com/article/a-uk-household-survey-of-the-ex-service-community/
6. Jones E, Fear N. Alcohol use and misuse within the military: A review. *International Review of Psychiatry*. 2011; (23): 166–172.
7. Fear N, Iversen A, Meltzer H. Patterns of drinking in the UK armed forces. *Addiction*. 2007; (102): 1749–1759.
8. CHAIN. CHAIN Annual Report Greater London, April 2017–March 2018. London: Greater London Authority; 2018. Available from: https://s3-eu-west-1.amazonaws.com/files.datapress.com/london/dataset/chain-reports/2018-06-28T08%3A37%3A29.68/Greater%20London%20bulletin%202017-18.pdf
9. Hansard. Defence written statement C128WS. 24 Nov 2005. Available at: https://publications.parliament.uk/pa/cm200506/cmhansrd/vo051124/wmstext/51124m01.htm#51124m01.html_spmin1
10. Office of National Statistics. Measuring National Wellbeing. London: Office of National Statistics; 2016. Available at: https://www.ons.gov.uk/peoplepopulationandcommunity/wellbeing/articles/measuringnationalwellbeing/2016#how-good-is-our-health
11. Hoptoft M, Hull L, Fear N et al. The health of UK military personnel who deployed to the 2003 Iraq war: A cohort study. *The Lancet*. 2006; (367): 1731–1741.
12. Fear N, Jones M, Murphy D et al. What are the consequences of deployment to Iraq and Afghanistan on the mental health of the UK armed forces? A cohort study. *The Lancet*. 2010; (375): 1783–1797.
13. Kapur N, While D, Blatchley N et al. Suicide after leaving the UK armed forces: A cohort study. *PLoS Med*. 2009; e1000026.
14. Greenberg N, Wessely S. Gulf War Syndrome: An emerging threat or a piece of history. *Emerging Health Threats Journal*. 2008; (1): e10.
15. Ministry of Defence. Amputation statistics 1 April 2013–31 March 2018. London: Ministry of Defence; 2018. Available from: https://assets.publishing.service.gov.uk/government/uploads/system/uploads/attachment_data/file/728224/20180612_Amputation_Statistic_O_v2.pdf

16. Finnegan A, Jackson R, Simpson R. Finding the forgotten: Motivating military veterans to register with a primary healthcare practice. *Military Medicine*. 2018; 183 (11–12): e509–e517.

17. NHS England. GP Practices across the country to become veteran friendly. London: NHS England; 2018. Available from: https://www.england.nhs.uk/2018/07/gp-practices-across-the-country-to-become-veteran-friendly/

18. Department of Health and Social Care. The NHS constitution for England. London: Department of Health and Social Care; 2015. Available from: https://www.gov.uk/government/publications/the-nhs-constitution-for-england/the-nhs-constitution-for-england

33

Working with People in Contact with the Criminal Justice System and in Secure Environments

CAROLINE WATSON

Half of prisons are rated as inadequate or needing improvement in their provision.

Many people in contact with the criminal justice system, including those in prison, are affected by socioeconomic, psychological and biological factors that lead to health inequalities, and they represent the spectrum of population types covered in other chapters. The majority of health needs and inequalities affecting people in prison will have originated prior to being taken into the custodial setting [1] however there are adverse environmental and social factors associated with prisons that may have a detrimental impact on health, some of which may persist or be exacerbated beyond release causing a deterioration of health when they are back in the community setting.

Health inequalities may start in-utero or early childhood and accumulate over the years. Adverse childhood experiences (ACEs) may include direct harm through neglect, physical, emotional or sexual abuse, or effects of exposure to poor living conditions and domestic violence [2]. Poverty and unemployment, both linked with poor mental and physical health, may be transferred across generations [3].

The Ministry of Justice reported in 2012 that 29% of adults (53% of women and 27% of men) in prison experienced childhood abuse, 24% were looked-after children (compared to 2% of the general population) and 41% (compared to 14% of the general population) observed violence in the home [4]. A survey published by Public Health Wales NHS Trust and Bangor University in 2019 found that more than 8 in 10 adult males in prison had experienced at least 1 ACE and nearly half had experienced 4 or more [2].

Further figures from the Ministry of Justice in 2012 showed that social characteristics associated with poor educational achievement (regular truancy, permanent school exclusion, lack of qualifications), unemployment and poverty were all of greater prevalence in the prison population compared to the general population [5, 6].

Isolation and poor relationships may be present prior to prison but may occur or deteriorate as a result of being taken into custody and persist following release. The impact of separating parents from their children during periods in custody can be significant, particularly if the main caregiver is separated. This can result in changes in health to both parent and child. Often separation will have negative influences on the health of both parent and child, persisting beyond the period of separation, however, if the relationship has been an abusive one, there may be an opportunity for an improvement in the child's health if they are placed in a more secure and stable home environment. It is possible that the period in custody may result in positive changes in parental health too, particularly if there is an opportunity to start a journey of recovery from substance misuse or to receive education in healthy living, parenting skills and other qualifications leading to improved employment prospects.

Biological factors leading to health inequalities include gender and ethnicity as well as biological changes resulting from negative emotional responses to stressful circumstances and lack of control.

There is an over-representation of ethnic minority groups in the prison population (26%) compared to the general population (14%) which has an impact on the prevalence of some chronic diseases, e.g. heart disease, seen more commonly in South Asian men. Foreign nationals (non-UK passport holders) form 12% of the prison population and may have a higher prevalence of some conditions e.g. post-traumatic stress disorder (PTSD) and HIV and lower rates of immunisation. Armed forces veterans are less likely to go to prison than the general population for all types of crimes except sexual offences [7]. Negative socioeconomic factors (instability of relationships, housing, finance and unemployment) and mental health problems (anxiety disorders, including PTSD and problem drinking) are risk factors for offending behaviour in veterans [8]. Those veterans in prison are more likely to have committed violent or sexual offences and to report issues with alcohol or drug abuse, anger management, anxiety, depression and PTSD [8, 9].

Women make up 5% of the prison population but around 10% of those sent to prison each year.

Around 60% are sentenced to less than 6 months and over 70% of those serving sentences of less than 12 months are reconvicted within a year [1, 10]. Over half of women in prison report having experienced abuse as a child and many have high levels of mental health needs, with the numbers of incidences and individual women involved in self-harm and self-inflicted death increasing. Under 1% of children in England are in care, but they make up 38% of those in secure training centres and 42% of those in young offender institutions [1, 11].

Of those in contact with the criminal justice system, 7% have a learning disability (LD) compared to 2% of the general population and in 2016–2017, a third of those entering prison were found to have a learning disability or difficulty on assessment [1, 12]. Of those in prison with learning difficulties or disabilities, 80% have difficulty accessing written prison information and difficulties expressing themselves. They are more likely to have broken prison rules, to have been restrained and to have spent time in segregation than other residents. In 2009, at the request of the government, Lord Bradley published a report recommending the development of a liaison and diversion programme, in order to better identify those individuals with vulnerabilities who would be suitable for diversion away from the criminal justice system. In 2010, the programme was set up in police custody and courts, employing practitioners to screen, assess and refer to health and social care, where appropriate, those with vulnerabilities facing criminal charges. Given the difficulties faced in prison by those with mental health and LD, there is also a need for community primary care teams to identify early the needs of vulnerable patients in order to reduce the risk of a crisis point being reached. Those individuals who are not suitable to remain in the community due to the severity of their crime but whose suitability for prison is in question may be transferred to secure units under the Mental Health Act for further assessment or treatment. The current Department of Health guidelines (2011) state that the maximum transfer time from doctors approving transfer is 14 days [13]. At present, due to a number of factors, including pressure on suitable beds, it takes on average 100 days for transfer, during which time mental and physical health are likely to further deteriorate [14].

The number of people in prison aged 60 and over has tripled in the last 15 years and this age group is the fastest growing in the prison estate [15]. There are 4 main profiles of people in this age group: those repeatedly imprisoned, those with a long sentence who have grown old in prison, those with first-time convictions and short sentences and those with first-time long sentences, possibly for historic sex or violent offences. Each group will have different needs. Some evidence suggests that people age up to 10 years quicker while in prison [16] and a study in Ontario showed reduced life expectancy and increased mortality in prison residents compared to the general population, but with a greater relative mortality in younger and in female residents [17]. The Prison Reform Trust suggests that this accelerated ageing may be due to poverty, poor diet, inadequate access to healthcare, smoking, alcohol and other substance misuse causing chronic health problems either prior to or during time in prison, as well as the psychological stresses associated with life in prison [18].

Although there are similarities in health needs seen across the prison estate, the prison population is not uniform and therefore there will be expected variations in health needs according to the type and category of prison. Category A, B, C, D (ranked from high to low security), remand, local, resettlement, and training prisons will have differing turnover rates and may hold people reflective of the local demographics or house those drawn from across the country. One example of this variation in health needs according to category and type can be seen in 2 prisons in the east of England, which are 12 miles apart. One, a category B prison with local and resettlement functions, houses young adult and adult male residents. It has a high turnover of people, a significant number of whom require support with substance misuse. Gang culture in the local communities from which the population is drawn is reflected in the prison and this can lead to issues with debt, bullying and violence with consequent trauma, mental health needs (e.g. anxiety, depression, PTSD) and self-harm. Another example is a category C training prison that houses people who have committed sexual offences. Many of the residents have long sentences and the population is more settled with a high burden of chronic disease. The number of residents with substance misuse issues is much

lower than at the category B local prison and those engaged with the substance misuse team tend to be further down the path to recovery. Violence levels and trauma are much lower too, but there is a high daily requirement for escorts to hospital for chronic and complex morbidities together with suspected cancer. Bed-watch hours for patients requiring inpatient hospital treatment are higher at the category C prison which houses an older population than the Category B local prison. It also has greater need for palliative care, a higher proportion of patients with dementia and greater need for social care provision.

The category C prison provides level 2 healthcare, which means that there is onsite healthcare provision during the day but access to healthcare at night is from offsite out-of-hours urgent care providers. The Category B prison has level 3 healthcare, with 24-hour nursing cover, a doctor on site until late evening during the week and weekend mental health and medical cover, to meet the needs of the incoming reception patients. This Level 3 healthcare provision attracts referrals from Level 2 prisons across the region who have residents in need of greater nursing input and monitoring during the night.

As illustrated above, healthcare provision is driven not only by specific patient population needs but by duration of stay and commissioned level of healthcare. At the time of writing, the prison estate is undergoing a reconfiguration process, which is likely to further differentiate healthcare priorities and provision. Reception prisons, which will house residents for up to 10 days, are likely to have a major function in screening for immediate risk and identification of initial urgent health priorities. This is likely to be in contrast with training prisons with long-stay populations, who will be commissioned to identify and manage existing and emerging chronic and complex health issues. As well as different needs found in any snapshot across the prison estate, there are population trends that emerge over the course of time. There is legislation that requires regular health needs assessments in all prisons in the UK to ensure that services provided within each establishment meet the needs of the specific population and reflect any changes in the demographics. The expectation is that this will be achieved through integrated working between the prison and healthcare providers. There is also an obligation to promote continuity of health and social care on release from prison.

MEDICAL, SOCIAL AND PSYCHOLOGICAL ISSUES OF PEOPLE IN CONTACT WITH THE CRIMINAL JUSTICE SYSTEM

Clinical Conditions

There is very little published data on chronic disease prevalence amongst people in prison, but it is known that socioeconomic disadvantage is associated with chronic diseases which share key behavioural risk factors (smoking, problem drinking, unhealthy diet, physical inactivity) [19]. Co-morbidities increase in prevalence with age and a coordinated approach is required to effectively screen for, identify and manage the increasing burden of chronic disease in the ageing UK prison population. Currently, NHS health-screening criteria in prisons exclude a large proportion of people on remand or with short sentences, and therefore there is a risk that disease in these populations will remain unidentified or undertreated.

LONG-TERM AND CHRONIC CONDITIONS

Asthma and COPD are common in people coming into prison and may be poorly controlled or more severe than in the general population due to smoking, poor living conditions, neglect of health needs or difficulty accessing healthcare prior to prison. Coronary heart disease is more common in smokers, lower socioeconomic groups and some ethnic minority groups (e.g. South Asian) and therefore the estimated prevalence is higher in prisons than in the general population.

The prevalence of diabetes in prison is similar to that in the wider community however, control may be worse due to poor dietary choices and difficulties adhering to treatment plans prior to and after entering prison. Some health needs assessment data suggests that epilepsy in prison is more common than expected [34]. This is possibly due to an over-representation of people who have sustained head injuries or who have learning disabilities with associated epilepsy, or it may be due to an over-reporting or misclassification of withdrawal seizures or symptoms reported by residents in an attempt to obtain antiepileptic medication with desirable and potentially addictive effects.

In addition to chronic diseases, older prison residents are at greater risk of falls, physical frailty requiring assistance to complete activities of daily living and of cognitive impairment. It is therefore important to screen for these age-related conditions in order to identify and provide appropriate care. At present, even once needs are identified, there may be barriers to accessing appropriate investigations and care, particularly if escorts to hospital are required. This is a growing problem in some prisons where inadequate allocation of officers for escorts prevents all except urgent referrals (i.e. 2-week wait referrals) being taken out to attend their secondary care appointments.

SUGGESTIONS FOR PRACTICE

- *Address under-identification of chronic conditions (non-communicable diseases)*
  - *Use screening templates in first night reception and secondary screening in line with NICE guidance on physical and mental health of prisoners.*
  - *Provide NHS health screening for those eligible.*
  - *Consider NHS health screening for people on remand or serving short sentences (who currently fall outside eligibility criteria).*
- *Establish a coordinated approach to managing long-term conditions*
  - *Train nurses to specialise in long-term conditions.*
  - *Establish nurse-led chronic disease clinics.*
  - *Train staff in the use of Read coding for chronic diseases to ensure figures reported for HJIPs accurately reflect the delivery of services for long-term conditions.*
  - *Monitor hospital outpatient escorts to ensure access to routine appointments is not unacceptably compromised by demand for emergency escorts (for 2-week referrals and A & E) or other staffing constraints.*
  - *Consider the use of telemedicine to reduce number of escorts sent to hospital for appointments.*
- *Develop a coordinated approach to smoking cessation support*
  - *Train healthcare assistants to deliver smoking cessation support.*

- *Create a patient group directive (PGD) for nicotine replacement therapy (NRT).*
- *Train 'health champions' to deliver peer-led smoking cessation support.*
- *Develop a coordinated approach to identifying physical frailty, falls risk and cognitive impairment*
  - *Train nurses to use validated tools to screen for falls risk, physical impairments and cognitive impairment.*
  - *Identify a team member to coordinate referrals to social care, occupational therapist or physiotherapist where physical needs have been identified.*
  - *Agree a clear pathway for further investigation and management of people in prison with identified cognitive impairment.*

Infectious Diseases

There are higher rates of infectious diseases (including HIV, hepatitis and tuberculosis) among people in prison compared to the general population. This is partly due to high-risk lifestyle choices including sexual behaviour and substance misuse behaviour with the associated risk of hepatitis C and hepatitis B but also due to lower rates of immunisation, poor living conditions and the number of foreign nationals in prisons who originate from countries where hepatitis B and C are endemic.

NICE guidance for physical health in prisons [20] sets out the requirements for screening for infectious diseases. Comprehensive coverage is most likely to be achieved through the primary and secondary screening process and through offering opt-out blood-borne virus (BBV) screening and chlamydia testing to those eligible.

SUGGESTIONS FOR PRACTICE

- *Address under-identification of infectious diseases*
  - *Use screening templates at first night reception and secondary screening that identify risk behaviour and symptoms suggestive of infectious diseases, in line with NICE guidance on physical health of prisoners.*
  - *Offer opt-out BBV screening at secondary screenings.*
  - *Develop a pathway to follow up and further investigate those who have screen-positive results.*

- *Consider dried blood spot (DBS) testing for BBVs to overcome venous access difficulties in people with a history of IV drug misuse.*
- *Consider offering screening for BBVs and TB in the community to those known to participate in high-risk behaviour and those recently released from prison.*
- *Establish a coordinated approach to immunisation*
  - *Offer an opt-out hepatitis B vaccination programme to be initiated at secondary screenings.*
  - *Identify, at secondary screenings, people who have not received a full course of vaccinations in the community (including DTP, MMR and menC) and those who are eligible for specific vaccines either because of age or risk due to chronic disease (influenza, pneumococcal vaccination).*
  - *Develop PGDs for vaccine administration.*
  - *Consider training a nurse to oversee the vaccination programme and healthcare assistants or pharmacy technicians to deliver vaccines.*
  - *Consider identifying those in the community practice population who have not completed primary vaccination schedules and those with high-risk behaviour including substance misuse and recent release from prison.*
  - *Consider offering hepatitis A and B vaccinations in the community to all patients with a history of drug misuse.*
  - *Consider training prison residents to be health champions to raise awareness of the importance of completing vaccination courses and to deliver harm reduction advice with regards to high-risk behaviour (drug taking, multiple sexual partners) that leads to infectious diseases.*
- *Develop a coordinated approach to delivering harm-minimisation advice and follow up for people who have screened positive for infectious diseases*
  - *Consider training a nurse to specialise in infectious diseases to coordinate the follow up of those patients who have screened positive for present or past infection with hepatitis B and C, Chlamydia, HIV or TB.*
  - *Consider using this specialist nurse to deliver harm reduction advice or to train HCAs and those taking blood from prison residents to deliver harm reduction advice.*

Cancer, Palliative and End-of-Life Care

People in prison are at greater risk of cancers associated with smoking (1 in 3 cancers), alcohol and deprivation. Although the prison estate is now smoke-free, it is not yet clear what impact this will have on the incidence of smoking-related cancers as the rates of smoking of people entering prison are likely to be more than double the general population. The prevalence of all cancers is increasing among the prison population due to increasing numbers of older people in prison.

Referral of patients with suspected cancer on the 2-week pathway (following NICE cancer referral guidelines) should be well coordinated, with escorts prioritised to avoid a delay in diagnosis and to ensure equivalence of care. Referral targets should be audited to identify whether any delays are attributable to prison, healthcare or hospital factors.

Since cancer treatment is usually delivered in secondary care, for each newly diagnosed case there will be a significant impact on prison escorts, bed watches and potentially the prison regime due to deployment of staff away from their scheduled duties. This can be particularly difficult for high-security prisons (for whom any escort to hospital is very high risk and requires high numbers of escorting officers), and for those prisons with a large number of older residents.

The number of deaths from natural causes in prison has significantly increased in the past few years, largely due to the rising number of older people serving sentences, some of whom may be eligible for compassionate release but many of whom will not. Where compassionate release is not granted, equivalence of care must be provided, with comparable social care and end-of-life nursing together with a choice regarding surroundings. This is challenging in terms of security and cost if input is required from community services, and therefore there is an argument to ensure prison nursing staff are adequately trained in delivering high-quality palliative care, with support from palliative care specialists.

SUGGESTIONS FOR PRACTICE

- *Identification of cancer*
  - *Ensure a coordinated approach to screening for cancers, equivalent to that offered in the community (bowel, breast, cervical programmes).*
  - *Refer all patients with suspected cancer onto a 2-week pathway, following NICE guidance.*
  - *Audit 2-week referrals to identify whether targets are met or whether there are commissioning needs to be addressed.*
- *Management of diagnosed cancer*
  - *Prioritise escorts for patients requiring access to hospital for regular cancer treatment.*
  - *Negotiate with the prison to increase the number of escorts for the period of cancer treatment in order to continue to allow access to secondary care for non-urgent cases.*
- *Palliative care*
  - *Consider training a nurse to specialise in delivering end-of-life nursing care, to facilitate social care referrals to the local council for people who are dying in custody, and to facilitate support for families.*
  - *Build good links with local specialist palliative care services in order to ensure equivalence of holistic physical, mental, emotional and spiritual care of the dying patient and to support families, prison healthcare staff and other prison residents affected by the death.*

Physical Injuries

Violence in prisons has escalated significantly in the past 5 years, affecting both prison residents and staff. Both physical and sexual assaults on people in prison have increased, together with self-inflicted harm incidents, which are disproportionately high among the female population but increasing among men. Physical assaults may be related to bullying and debt, gang-related issues and drugs. Injuries may require X-rays, scans, suturing or even surgery. Unscheduled additional escorts to hospital due to injuries place a significant burden on prison staffing and non-urgent escorts for planned outpatient appointments may have to be cancelled as a result. In some prisons, X-ray facilities are available on site, reducing the need for hospital escorts. Appropriately trained healthcare staff, competent in assessing injuries and suturing, can also decrease the burden of unscheduled escorts and a bespoke accredited emergency care training course for use in prisons is currently being developed.

Mental Health and Substance Misuse

MENTAL HEALTH

Statistics show that 9 out of 10 people in prison in the UK have evidence of mental health problems (including substance misuse) although only around half have a diagnosis. This is significantly higher than in the general population. Problems with sleep, anxiety and depression are particularly common, and greater in those on remand and approaching release. Personality disorders are present in around 70% of men and 50% of women, which is 12 times higher than in the general population. Psychotic disorders are 16 times higher in prison that in the general population, 7% of people in prison have a severe enduring mental illness and 12–15% have 4–5 co-existing mental health disorders [21].

Given the high prevalence of mental health disorders and the stresses associated with imprisonment, there is a need for all staff to be psychologically informed and equipped to deliver a coordinated approach with high-level communication skills, conveying empathy and a non-judgemental attitude. This is particularly important when engaging with residents who struggle to form trusting relationships with others as a result of adverse childhood experiences. Between 2010 and 2017, the capacity of prison officers to effectively manage the emotional well-being of those in custody was challenged by a reduction of 23% of front-line operational staff as part of a benchmarking process, which occurred in the face of growing numbers of people in prison. A significant number of experienced staff left the prison service at this time. Since then, the number of officers has increased, however, staff retention remains problematic and this has resulted in a largely younger and inexperienced workforce, managing complex issues in an increasingly dangerous environment.

Pressure on mental health services has also had an impact on the well-being and safety of those in prison. Prisons and Probation Ombudsman (PPO) investigations and House of Commons discussions in 2016 highlighted shortfalls in mental healthcare delivered to those in the criminal justice system. Particularly bleak statistics were reported: nearly 1 in 5 of those diagnosed with a mental health problem received no care from a mental health professional while in prison; no mental health referral was made in 29% of deaths by suicide where it was indicated that mental health needs had been identified; only 32% of transfers from prison to secure hospitals under the Mental Health Act in 2016–2017 were within the recommended 14-day timeframe [18].

Despite this negative picture, there are many people who are picked up on screening and engage successfully with mental health and substance misuse teams during their time in custody, make improvements in their mental health and take steps in their recovery journey when previously their lives had been in chaos.

Self-harm and Suicide

Self-harming behaviour may or may not be associated with mental illness and/or suicidal intent. It is more common in women and multiple incidents may be carried out by the same individual. Common forms of self-harm seen in prisons include cutting, punching, head-banging, attempted hanging, mutilation of body parts, burning, overdosing, substance misuse, withholding food or medicine and ingestion of non-edible substances. Problems and motivations underlying self-harm range widely, from an inability to moderate emotions or a maladaptive response to a perceived unmet need (e.g. not getting tobacco) to the anniversary of a significant event or a psychosis associated with underlying mental illness or illicit substance use.

Self-inflicted deaths are around 10 times more likely in prison than in the general population, with around a quarter of these occurring in the first 30 days and over half of these within the first week. Of people who die in prison by their own hand, 70% have had mental health needs identified prior to their death and new psychoactive substance (NPS) intoxication has been implicated in 56 of 79 self-inflicted deaths in prison between 2013 and 2016, largely due to acts of impulsivity [29].

People identified to be at risk of suicide or self-harm in prison are managed through assessment care in custody and teamwork (ACCT). The approach involves multi-disciplinary teamwork to assess static and dynamic risk factors in order to plan and deliver tailored support.

Learning Disabilities and Difficulties

SUBSTANCE MISUSE

Substance misuse is a major cause of poor health and can lead to both acquisitive and violent crime. Of people entering prison, 70% report using drugs in the community; 51% of these admit dependence and 35% intravenous use. Problem drinking is reported by 36% of people coming into prison and alcohol dependence by 16% [30]. Tackling substance misuse within the criminal justice system is therefore a significant public health issue and affords the opportunity to benefit both individuals in prison, through addressing health and lifestyle problems that accompany their substance misuse, and the community in which they come from and to which they will return.

Heroin and cocaine use account for the majority of drug-related deaths. The risk of opioid-related death is especially high within 4 weeks of initiating or stopping opiate substitute treatment (OST) and within the first 4 weeks of leaving prison due to increased access to illicit drugs, chaotic use, use of concurrent sedating substances including alcohol and benzodiazepines together with a loss of tolerance to opioids.

Harm reduction can reduce morbidity and mortality associated with drug use. For those coming into prison with opioid dependence, OST is initiated in reception in order to minimise withdrawals and stabilise opioid use. Methadone is usually the drug of choice for OST in prison, since buprenorphine is at greater risk of diversion and there are operational implications, due to the time required for officers to supervise sublingual buprenorphine administration. Although both medications are equally efficacious, and therefore equivalent care is being delivered, buprenorphine is more widely used in the community, is titrated more safely and is often preferred over methadone by those being treated. Addiction support is delivered through the psychosocial substance misuse team, working in close partnership with the clinical substance misuse team.

For some people serving longer sentences, it can be appropriate to agree a plan to withdraw OST following a period of stabilisation. For others, stopping OST increases the risk of relapse into harmful illicit drug use while in prison and after release, with its associated health risks. It should not therefore be mandatory to reduce and stop OST in prison, but it is good practice to review OST on a regular basis. Some people who have stopped OST while in prison may request 'retoxification' back onto OST prior to release to reduce their risk of relapsing into illicit drug use. Others may express a wish to come off OST prior to release to avoid attending community drug clinics and mixing with previous drug-using acquaintances, or prior to a parole board hearing in order to increase the likelihood of release or transfer to a lower category prison.

Needle exchange programmes available in the community for those continuing to inject after leaving prison reduce transmission of BBVs and training in the administration of naloxone for those at highest risk of overdose (those with a history of injecting drugs) can reduce the risk of death due to opioid overdose. There are no current specific recommendations in the orange guidelines 2017 as to whether prisons or community drug services should offer naloxone training and kits, however, if group training were to be offered in prison, the number of those trained in harm reduction and the use of naloxone would increase the proportion of the injecting community being trained and able to deliver life-saving treatment.

Cocaine can cause death through direct cardiovascular and cerebrovascular problems including intracranial bleeding or thrombosis and cardiac arrest. It can also increase the risk of self-harm and suicide due to psychological effects including psychosis and severe depression, particularly during times of increased vulnerability associated with entering and leaving prison.

Integrated teamwork is important in the assessment and delivery of care to people coming into prison with substance misuse problems. Immediate risk and needs are identified in reception by the substance misuse nurse. If medication is required to assist withdrawal, it will be initiated in reception, in collaboration with the prison GP. Regular monitoring for withdrawal will then be undertaken during the first few days in prison for those stabilising on medication, or if there is some uncertainty about whether or not a prescription will be required to alleviate symptoms of withdrawal. In addition to clinical input, psychosocial support is an important aspect of the pathway to recovery from substance misuse. Management of opioid dependence has been referred to above. Further details of treatment for all types of substance misuse, including alcohol misuse can be found in the *Drug Misuse and Dependence: UK Guidelines on Clinical Management 2017* [22]. For some substances, including cocaine, NPS and cannabis there are no specific medications recommended to alleviate withdrawal symptoms.

While time in prison offers opportunities to tackle substance misuse, it can also be a place where illicit use and dependence starts. NPS – of which there are 4 main categories: synthetic cannabinoid receptor agonists (SCRAs), stimulants, depressants and hallucinogens – have become an increasing problem in the community and in prisons. There is a global market for NPS (SCRAs – mostly 'spice') targeted at UK prisons, available in herbal, powder and liquid forms. Liquid form may enter prisons sprayed onto letters or children's pictures and herbal NPS has started to be secreted in vapes rather than mixed with tobacco following the introduction of smoke-free prisons across the country. SCRAs are usually taken for the effects of euphoria, disinhibition or relaxation but they may cause side effects including convulsions, paralysis, tachycardia, hypotension or hypertension, psychosis, extreme bizarre behaviour, agitation and aggression. The unpredictability of their effects and relatively low cost has made NPS popular in prisons and they have been suspected or known to have been linked to a number of deaths, the majority of which have been due to impulsive acts of self-inflicted harm while intoxicated. An NPS toolkit for use in prisons has been developed and symptomatic treatment remains the mainstay of management of intoxication with NPS [23].

If there is a report of suspected intoxication, the affected person should be assessed urgently by the emergency nurse (and, if necessary by the duty doctor) and their medication should be reviewed. If someone is suspected of being intoxicated when they present for medication administration, it is recommended that prescribed medication should be withheld until their presentation improves and a medication review undertaken as a matter of clinical urgency. It is not recommended practice to stop or withhold medication as a punitive action, however, if someone is suspected of misusing or diverting prescribed medication, this may be changed to a liquid formulation and administered under supervision with a plan to review ongoing clinical need.

Certain prescribed medicines are at risk of misuse, diversion and dependence in prison, particularly those with psychoactive effects. They include sedating antidepressants, antipsychotics, strong analgesics including opioids and gabapentinoids, hypnotics, anxiolytics and certain antiepileptics. Illicitly circulating prescribed medicines have the potential to cause significant harm since they may be taken in uncontrolled doses by treatment-naïve people for whom they are not clinically indicated. They may interact with other medicines that are being appropriately prescribed to a person or react with illicit substances that are also being used. When taken in this way, there is a risk of dangerous side effects, drug interactions, dependence and death. There is also the potential for bullying, debt and violence due to the high prices commanded by such medicines. In order to reduce these risks, medicines with psychoactive effects should be prescribed judiciously and taken under supervision (see to take – STT) or in association with compliance checks. It is also recommended that initial confirmation of prescribing in the community through the medication reconciliation process is followed up with planned medication reviews to assess ongoing clinical need. Guidance on safer prescribing in prisons has been produced by the RCGP and a prison pain formulary has been written along with other guidance to inform the management of pain, which is a particular problem in prisons, requiring a multidisciplinary approach [24–26].

SUGGESTIONS FOR PRACTICE

- *Physical injuries and violence*
  - *Arrange communication skills training, including de-escalation techniques.*
  - *Arrange breakaway training for all staff.*
  - *Train and update medical staff (nurses and doctors) in suturing and dealing with minor injuries.*
  - *Consider commissioning on site X-ray facilities (particularly for high-security estates).*
- *Mental health and learning disabilities*
  - *Arrange training for all clinical staff in self-harm and suicide and ACCT.*
  - *Arrange training for all staff in communication and support to equip them to adopt a*

psychologically informed approach to care for people who have experienced complex trauma in their lives.

- *Restructure mental health team service delivery to meet 5-day assessment targets for all referrals.*
- *Substance misuse*
  - *Encourage integrated multi-disciplinary teamwork (MDT) between prison and healthcare teams to ensure patient safety and continuity of care, particularly at the interfaces between community, police custody, courts and prisons.*
  - *Arrange NPS training for all clinical staff.*
  - *Ensure work between the substance misuse and prison drug strategy teams is integrated to reduce the risks from illicit drug use in prison.*
  - *Raise awareness of dependence on prescribed medicines and the need for safe judicious prescribing of medicines with psychoactive effects, encouraging the use of RCGP's* Safer Prescribing in Prisons, *prison pain formulary,* Opioids Aware *and other local and national guidance.*

Health Promotion

Health promotion is both an individual and a public health issue. Taking personal responsibility for their own health while in the community is often low on the agenda of those who come into prison. Smoking rates are higher, and the prevalence of alcohol and drug misuse issues and lifestyle-related illnesses is greater than in the general population. Prison Service Order 3200 (PSO 3200) requires a whole prison approach to build the physical, mental and social health of those in prison, to prevent deterioration of health while in custody and to help those in prison develop healthy behaviours to continue on release. Every contact between staff and those serving time in prison can provide an opportunity to promote healthy change and there is a variety of support available, not only from officers and healthcare staff but also the chaplaincy team, counsellors, mental health and substance misuse teams, and peers. The PSO identifies 6 major areas for the promotion of health: mental health and well-being; smoking; healthy eating and nutrition; healthy lifestyle choices including relationships, sex and activity; substance misuse.

Barriers to health promotion in prison include regime constraints and staffing levels which can limit time out of cell and opportunities for exercise. Canteen choices are often unhealthy and budget constraints on food (£2.02 per person per day in 2015–2016) limit what can be provided. The prison environment itself can be detrimental to mental health. This is compounded by overcrowding, violence, bullying and an intolerance to people with vulnerable attributes, among both prison residents and staff.

SUGGESTIONS FOR PRACTICE

- *Communicating health promotion*
  - *Use every contact with people in prison, starting with first night reception and secondary screening to offer tailored information about healthy lifestyle choices including diet, exercise, smoking, substance misuse, safe sexual practice, healthy relationships and behaviour choices to promote mental health and well-being.*
  - *Consider delivering health messages and health education campaigns through prison TV and poster campaigns.*
  - *Make connections with the prison and St Giles Trust to develop a coordinated approach to peer adviser training so that prison residents can be trained to provide health promotion (health champions), coaching and mentoring, practical and emotional support to peers, and undertake intermediary 'prisoner voice' roles to shape service provision.*
  - *Healthy eating and nutrition.*
  - *Offer a coordinated approach between prison and healthcare to ensure a range of healthy balanced meals and those suitable for different specific medical problems.*
  - *Offer advice about the dangers of obesity and the benefits of choosing healthier meal options and snacks from the canteen (prison list of items available for ordering).*
- *Smoking*
  - *Train members of the healthcare team (e.g. HCAs) and health champions to deliver smoking cessation advice and promote the benefits of a smoke-free lifestyle.*

- *Draw up a PGD for the provision of a choice of NRT.*
- *Offer harm reduction advice for those who to continue to smoke vapes and e-cigarettes.*
- **Mental health and well-being**
  - *Train all staff to equip them to understand complex trauma and adverse childhood experiences and the difficulties with engagement and maladaptive behaviour that it can generate.*
  - *Train staff to support positive behavioural change and reduce the need for crisis management.*
  - *Consider offering mood management groups, relaxation, mindfulness, yoga and promote the benefit of exercise.*
- **Healthy lifestyle choices and screening**
  - *Offer DBS screening for BBV and testing for chlamydia (in under 24s) at secondary screening, on an opt-out basis.*
  - *Offer hepatitis B vaccination on an opt-out basis and initiate the vaccination schedule at secondary screening.*
  - *Train staff to deliver NHS health checks to those who are eligible and arrange a coordinated approach to physical health-screening programmes recommended in NICE guidance.*
  - *Offer sexual health promotion within a safe welcoming environment, including access to advice for those wishing to consider transition of gender.*
  - *Offer harm reduction advice and barriers e.g. condoms and dental dams to reduce transmission of STIs between people who engage in sexual activity while in prison.*
- **Substance misuse**
  - *Offer harm reduction advice and information about the health implications of substance misuse, including the dangers of NPS.*

Social Care

The Social Care Act (2014) sets out the responsibilities for provision of social care in prisons and since 1 April 2015, social care needs have been the responsibility of the local authority in which the prison is situated. Prison service instruction (PSI) 15/2015 (adult social care), PSI 16/2015 (adult safeguarding in prison) and PSI 17/2015 (prisoners assisting other prisoners) clarify processes and roles, including the distinction between personal care, with which other prison residents may assist, and intimate care which should be provided by a professional caregiver.

Social care needs are not limited to the older person in prison or to physical health however, the ageing prison population has led to a significant increase in demand for social care and highlighted the fact that many older buildings in the prison estate are not suitable for accommodating people with disabilities due to structural constraints e.g. narrow cell doorways, residences accessible only by stairs. Referrals to the local authority for assessment of entitlement to social care should be made by members of the healthcare team as soon as needs are identified.

All those in prison are entitled to housing and benefits advice and, if sentenced, to structured support with release planning. There is no compensation or financial help at the point of release, however, for those held on remand who are acquitted or for those who are refugees and do not have UK status. This places those who have lost housing or jobs while in prison at particular risk of spiralling debt and further inequalities in health. Those with parenting responsibilities and their families can be supported through the third sector e.g. the Ormiston Trust; however, statutory agency involvement will be required if there are issues of safeguarding.

SUGGESTIONS FOR PRACTICE

- *Refer to the local authority as soon as potential care needs are identified.*
- *Ensure good communication with prison staff if vulnerabilities in a resident are identified.*
- *Refer any safeguarding concerns according to the Trust Safeguarding Policy.*

Justice System Specific Ethical and Practical Issues

PRISON ESTATE BUILDINGS AND OVERCROWDING

Overcrowding has been a problem in prisons since 1994, despite building projects to increase capacity due to the expanding prison population. Many prison cells designed for single occupancy are now shared, and have been adapted only by adding in a bunk bed. This requires residents to share toilet facilities and to eat in proximity to these. Cells, particularly in older prisons, may be affected by damp or pest infestation (e.g. cockroaches or rats) and may be located below ground level with poor natural light. These conditions may all contribute to a deterioration in both physical and mental health of those in prison, particularly when people are required to spend up to 22 hours each day locked up.

Safety in Prisons

Safety has deteriorated in prisons over the past 7 years. Self-harm and the number of prisoner-on-prisoner and prisoner-on-staff assaults are at highest-ever levels. The number of deaths in custody rose again in 2018, with an increase in self-inflicted deaths and in homicides [31]. More than a quarter of self-inflicted deaths occur within 30 days of arrival in prison, half of these occurring within the first week and it is therefore important to assess for static and dynamic risk factors from when a person first arrives in prison, to communicate effectively any concerns over someone's presentation and to use the ACCT where this is needed to keep someone safe.

Issues at the Interface between Community and Prison and on Transfer between Prisons

Good communication is necessary for delivering safe effective integrated care throughout a person's journey from the community, during their time in prison and on to transfer or release back into the community. It is particularly important at the interfaces between community, police custody, courts and prisons in order to transfer relevant information relating to health and risk between and within teams.

Of immediate importance in reception into prison are details of past and current risk of deliberate self-harm and suicide, medical conditions including mental illness and substance misuse and any prescribed medicines, particularly those that would put the person at risk if omitted e.g. insulin. Information relating to risk of deliberate self-harm, suicide and any medications administered

in police custody is contained in the person escort record (PER). Confirmation of OST script details (if not administered in police custody) can be obtained from community pharmacies, if they are open during reception hours, and details of other prescribed medicines can be accessed on the summary care record, if the NHS number is known and the record is up to date. It is important to obtain further information from community services within the next few days, with the consent of the person coming into prison. It is now recommended by NHSE that the community general practice with whom a patient is registered should stop their repeat prescriptions while a patient is in prison, in order to reduce the risk posed by ongoing collection of medicines by patient representatives while they are in prison.

Transfer to court, to another prison or back to the community are times where patient safety and delivery of effective continuing care rely on good communication about a person's risk, health and medication, outstanding hospital appointments and planned care. Without this information, omission of medication, delays in diagnosis and delays in treatment can result in potentially poorer health outcomes. Planning for release and resettlement should involve supporting those in prison to register with a GP in the community and setting up appointments with community substance misuse and mental health services where required. It is very important to ensure the timely transfer of a comprehensive discharge summary, with information provided by prison primary care, and mental health and substance misuse teams (where involved). This should include any new diagnoses, investigations and treatment undertaken while someone was in prison and any changes made to their medication. Without this discharge information, there is a risk that medicines will be inappropriately re-prescribed that have been stopped while in prison will be inappropriately re-prescribed, including dependence forming medicines, and that continuity of care and patient safety will be compromised.

Rehabilitation, Resettlement and Community Response

Reoffending by people recently released from prison cost the economy between £9.5 and £13 billion in 2007–2008 [32]. 49% of adults released from prison are reconvicted within one year (66% of those with sentences less than 12 months) and it has been shown that community sentences are more effective at reducing reconviction than short prison sentences [18]. Factors protective against reoffending include employment, housing, family support while in prison and on release, access to children, receiving treatment for drug and alcohol misuse and qualifications. Prisons are required to provide purposeful activity during the working day, including education, vocational training or jobs to assist in the rehabilitation of those in custody. Inspections have however rated almost half of prisons as inadequate or needing improvement in their provision of effective learning, skills and work and found that 31% of local prisons and 37% of young adult prisons provide less than 2 hours out of cell time a day [33].

There is a need for the general population to accept that the majority of those in prison, rather than being removed from community responsibility, are on a journey through a system and will need multifaceted support, starting prior to release, in order to successfully reintegrate back into the community and play a part with social responsibility. It is important to inform the general population that improving the health of those in prison (e.g. by screening for infectious diseases and treating hepatitis C) will impact positively on the general population and is a public health responsibility.

Only 27% of people leaving prison have a job to go to on release [27] and those seeking work can face discrimination by potential employers. This has led to some employers, including the civil service, removing the need to disclose convictions at the initial application stage. Other employers e.g. Halfords and Timpsons, provide training for people in prisons and extend this beyond release while others, including National Grid and Balfour Beatty, link in through the system of release on temporary licence (ROTL), providing connections with community employers. The Clink Charity offers opportunities for gaining experience and qualifications in the food and hospitality industry and offers mentoring schemes and support after release which has been shown to reduce reoffending by 41% [28]. As well as providing employment opportunities, ROTL offers the opportunity for those reaching the end

of long sentences to reconnect with their families, to find accommodation and to volunteer in their local community. Effective relational connections are important in successful resettlement and in addition to those provided by employment or family, faith communities can be another source of support.

Equivalence

It is agreed that healthcare delivered in the secure setting should be 'equivalent' to that provided in the community but, until now, there has been no definition of equivalence. In July 2018, the Royal College of General Practitioners published a position statement defining 'equivalence of care in secure environments in the UK', endorsing the right of those living in secure environments to healthcare provision and access that provides equitable health outcomes. It highlighted the fact that 'equivalence' does not mean 'the same' provision and that different approaches may be required across the prison estate in order to meet differing needs. It underlined the complexity in managing the primary duty of care to an individual patient while working within the constraints of security and regime requirements. For example, requesting an escort for emergency access to hospital for one person may necessitate rescheduling the routine hospital appointment of another if numbers of officers are insufficient to facilitate both escorts and continue the regime in the prison.

While the ethical principle of independence and duty of the healthcare professional to their patient must be upheld, it is also recognised that an integrated multi-disciplinary partnership between healthcare providers, security teams and community services will be most likely to achieve an equivalent outcome for the patient.

REFERENCES

1. Prison Reform Trust. Bromley Briefings - Prison Factfile Autumn 2018.
2. Public Health Wales NHS Trust, Bangor University. Ford K, Barton ER et al. *Understanding the prevalence of adverse childhood experiences (ACEs) in a male offender population in Wales: The Prisoner ACE Survey.* 2019. ISBN 978-1-78986-053-5.

3. British Medical Association. *Health at a price. Reducing the impact of poverty. A briefing from the board of science*, June 2017.

4. Ministry of Justice (2012) *Prisoners' Childhood and Family Backgrounds*, London: Ministry of Justice.

5. Ministry of Justice (2012) *The Pre-custody Employment, Training and Education Status of Newly Sentenced Prisoners*, London: Ministry of Justice.

6. Ministry of Justice (2012) *Accommodation, Homelessness and Reoffending of Prisoners*, London: Ministry of Justice.

7. Royal British Legion. Literature review: UK veterans and the criminal justice system. https://www.rblcdn.co.uk/media/2280/lit-rev_ukvetscrimjustice.pdf

8. Short RML, Dickson H, Greenberg N, MacManus D (2018) Offending behaviour, health and wellbeing of military veterans in the criminal justice system. *PLOS One*, 13(11). https://doi.org/10.1371/journal.pone.0207282

9. The Howard League for Penal Reform (2011) *Report of the Inquiry into Former Armed Service Personnel in Prison*. ISBN 978-1-905994-36-6

10. Ministry of Justice (2019) *Offender Management Statistics Bulletin, England and Wales; Quarterly July to Sept 2018*.

11. HM Inspectorate of Prisons (2017) *Children in Custody 2016–17*, London: HM Stationery Office.

12. NHS England (2016) *Strategic Direction for Health Services in the Justice System*: 2016–2020, London: NHS England.

13. Department of Health. Secure Services Policy Team (April 2011) *Good Practice Procedure Guide*. The transfer and remission of adult prisoners under s47 and s48 of the Mental Health Act.

14. Watkins S. NHS Benchmarking Network (January 2019) *Waiting times for Prison mental health hospital transfer and remission. Analysis of NHS England Specialised Commissioning and Health & Justice, and Her Majesty's Prison and Probation Services audits*.

15. Ministry of Justice (2018) *Offender Management Statistics Prison Population 2018*, London: Ministry of Justice

16. HM Inspectorate of Prisons (2004) '*No Nroblems – Old and Quiet': Older Prisoners in England and Wales*. A thematic review by HM Chief Inspector of Prisons.

17. Kouyoumdjian FG, Andreev EM, Borschmann R et al. (2017) Do people who experience incarceration age more quickly? Exploratory analyses using retrospective cohort data on mortality from Ontario, Canada. *PLoS One*, 12(4):e0175837.

18. Prison Reform Trust. Bromley Briefings - Prison Factfile Autumn 2017.

19. Plugge E, Martin R, Hayton P. Prisons and Health 10. Non-communicable diseases and Prisoners. WHO/Europe.

20. National Institute for Health and Care Excellence (2016) Physical health of people in prison. NICE guideline (NG57). nice.org.uk/guidance/ng57

21. Singleton N, Meltzer H, Gatward, R, Coid J, Deasy D (1998) *Psychiatric Morbidity Among Prisoners in England and Wales*, London, The Stationery Office.

22. Drug misuse and dependence: UK guidelines on clinical management. Clinical Guidelines on Drug Misuse and Dependence Update 2017 Independent Expert Working Group (2017)

23. Public Health England (2015) New psychoactive substances (NPS) in prisons. A toolkit for prison staff.

24. RCGP Safer Prescribing in Prisons Guidance for clinicians - second edition - January 2019

25. NHS England (2015/17) Prison Pain Management Formulary and Implementation Guide

26. Faculty of Pain Medicine (2015) Opioids Aware. rcoa.co.uk/faculty-of- pain-medicine/opioids-aware

27. National Offender Management Service Annual Report 2014/15: Management Information Addendum Ministry of Justice Information Release

28. Thompson H. The Clink Restaurants Reduce Re-offending by 41% (14/11/16) https://www.bighospitality.co.uk/article/2016/11/14/the-clink-restaurants-reduce-prisoner-re-offending-by-41-per-cent

29. Prison Reform Trust. Bromley Briefings - Prison Factfile Summer 2018.

30. 6 Drugs in prisons - www.publications.parliament. https://publications.parliament.uk/pa/cm201213/cmselect/cmhaff/184/18409.htm

31. Ministry of Justice (2019) Safety in Custody Statistics, England and Wales: Deaths in Prison Custody to December 2018 Assaults and Self-harm to September 2018.

32. Prison Reform Trust. Bromley Briefings - Prison The Facts Summer 2014.

33. HM Inspectorate of Prisons (2017) Life in prison: Living Conditions. A findings paper.

34. Health and Social Care Needs Assessment HMP BEDFORD AND HMP & YOI CHELMSFORD (September 2015) Tamlyn R. Claire Cairns Associates Ltd with Revolving Doors Agency.

34

Mental Health and Primary Care Management of Complex Psychiatric Conditions

JENNY DRIFE

Practitioners have a unique opportunity to provide longitudinal and holistic care to those experiencing mental distress.

In the UK, one in four adults and one in ten children experience some degree of mental health problem in any year, and mental disorders account for the largest single burden of disease (22.8%) as measured by disability adjusted life years [1]. But these disorders are not spread equally through society: the degree of socioeconomic deprivation a person experiences is proportionally linked to the likelihood of their developing a mental disorder [2]. The reasons for this are complex:

- People from lower socioeconomic groups are more likely to be exposed to risk factors for mental disorder, including stressful life events, food insecurity, lack of adequate housing, and unemployment [3].
- There is a strong association between experiencing four or more adverse childhood experiences (ACE) and developing mental illness as an adult [4].
- Wilkinson and Pickett have shown that rates of mental illness are higher in countries, like the

UK, where income is unequally distributed [5] and argue that mental distress can be related to low social status, stigma and shame [6].

Meanwhile, the British Medical Association reported in 2017 that three out of four people with a mental health problem receive little or no treatment [7].

People from disadvantaged communities may face specific barriers to engaging with a community mental health team, including:

COMMUNICATION

Mental health teams may send out opt-in letters, which are easily missed if the patient is couch-surfing or sleeping rough, or if they have poor literacy. Increasingly, appointments are made or confirmed by text message, which will not work if the person frequently changes their phone number or rarely has credit or charge on their phone.

COMPLEXITY

Mental health services can seem bewilderingly complex even to other professionals, let alone patients. Patients may face assessments with several different professionals and have to repeat their history multiple times. This, along with a low threshold for discharge back to the GP, can engender a sense of distrust in psychiatric services, which may add to a longer standing distrust of professionals stemming from childhood experiences.

LONG WAITING TIMES

This is particularly for psychological therapy. This can mean that those with itinerant lifestyles, or ambivalent engagement, never get seen.

Comorbidities

The life expectancy of people with severe mental illness is up to 20 years less than that of the general population [8]. Cardiovascular disease, type 2 diabetes, some communicable diseases including HIV/AIDS and tuberculosis, injuries, and gynaecological morbidity have all been shown to be more common in people with mental health conditions [9]. Possible reasons for this association are that:

- Mental disorders (or their treatment) affect the rate of health conditions.
- Other health conditions affect the rate of mental disorders.
- Mental disorders affect the treatment and outcome of other health conditions.

People with mental health conditions are many times more likely to engage in behaviours that present a risk to their physical health; for example, 42% of tobacco consumption in England is by people with a mental disorder – but only a minority receive a smoking cessation intervention [6].

There are also strong links between substance misuse and mental health problems: an estimated 70% of people in community drug treatment, and 86% of people in community alcohol treatment, experience mental health problems [10]. However, the current separation of secondary psychiatric care from substance misuse services does not allow the two to be easily assessed or treated in parallel. There is currently a drive from Public Health England and NHS England to address this, but the reality is that at present these most vulnerable patients often find themselves bouncing between services and potentially excluded from both [11].

SUGGESTIONS FOR PRACTICE

- *Remember that primary care services are uniquely placed to offer holistic and continuous mental health support.*
- *When referring on give as much information as possible about why you are making the referral at this point. If you are concerned about risk – to the patient or to others – make it explicit. Include detail about how best the team can contact the client.*
- *Forewarned is forearmed – try to understand as much as possible about the model of secondary mental health care in your area, what the threshold is for accepted referrals, what the intersection is with substance misuse services, and so on. Referrals that are knocked back result in frustration for patient and practitioner alike.*

Depression

There is a well-established association between depression and disadvantage [12]. Poverty, debt, unemployment, and social isolation are all associated with depression [13] and this effect is long standing: children exposed to socioeconomic disadvantage are more likely to develop depression as adults [14].

ASSESSMENT

It has been suggested that depressive illness is not detected by GPs in up to half of cases, and that those patients in whom it is missed are likely to be diagnosed with, and treated for, a physical illness [15]. It is wise to keep the possibility of depression in mind in all consultations, regardless of the overt focus of the meeting.

Despite considerable campaigns to breakdown stigma about mental health, ingrained attitudes can remain, and this may be particularly true in some ethnic groups [16]. Men in particular may find it hard to talk to a GP about their mood [17] and it should also be borne in mind that depression in men can present differently, with irritability, aggression, and increased alcohol consumption often characteristic [18].

SUGGESTIONS FOR PRACTICE

- *Consider screening for depression in all consultations. The Patient Health Questionnaire 9 (PHQ-9), a nine-item self-administered instrument, was not developed as a screening tool but can be useful. An even shorter version, the PHQ-2, has only twp questions:*
  1. *Over the past two weeks, have you felt down, depressed, hopeless?*
  2. *Over the past two weeks, have you felt little interest or pleasure in doing things?*

Treatment

The NICE guidelines for depression in adults [19] gives clear advice on treatment

Mild depression:
Watching and waiting', then antidepressants or cognitive behavioural therapy (CBT). Both are equally effective.

Moderate depression:
Antidepressants and CBT as adjunctive treatment.

Severe depression:
Refer psychiatrist, consider hospitalisation and/or antidepressants

However, situations can be more complex.

SOCIAL FACTORS

Low mood can seem a natural reaction to an intolerable situation: extreme poverty, for example, or lengthy waits for asylum status to be resolved. It is all too easy for the professional to feel overwhelmed by the details: be alert, here, to the possibility of high levels of empathy leading to burnout [20]. Rating scales can be helpful in retaining objectivity and focusing on biological symptoms of depression and can also be used to monitor the effects of treatment.

SUBSTANCE MISUSE

Assessing depression in the context of substance misuse can be difficult, and treatment more so. Alcohol, for example, is associated with low mood, but it can be very difficult to tease out whether the depression is secondary to the drinking, or vice versa. In the former case the mood disorder should resolve within two to four weeks of stopping drinking, without the need for antidepressants [21]. There is some evidence that motivational interviewing can be particularly helpful in reducing drinking in patients who are depressed or anxious [22]. Change is more likely to happen if you have fostered a supportive style in which the patient can be open about their drinking [23].

LACK OF AVAILABILITY OF THERAPY

In England, since 2008, the focus for psychological therapy from the NHS has been the Improving Access to Psychological Therapies programme, or IAPT. This provides rapid access to time-limited treatment, particularly CBT, for depression and anxiety. However, IAPT services often have exclusion criteria including suicide risk, history of self-harm, or psychosis, and so it can be difficult for clients with complex needs to access therapy. Other forms of therapy can have long waits: in 2018 the BMA reported that 3,700 patients in England waited more than six months for talking therapies, 1,500 of them for over a year [24].

SUGGESTIONS FOR PRACTICE

If you have prescribed antidepressants and they do not seem to be working, ask yourself:

- *Has it been long enough?*
  Ensure you measure from the time when the patient actually started taking the medication. Antidepressants can take a month to work, which is a long time to keep taking medication without seeing an effect: it can help to warn the patient of this.
- *Is it the correct diagnosis?*
  Is there a resolvable social stressor that has prompted this? Is there alcohol or drug use that's affecting mood? Are there symptoms of psychosis?
- *Is the patient taking the medication?*
  Non-adherence with antidepressants has been shown to be up to 50% [25]. Unless you have created an atmosphere in the consulting room where the patient feels able to disclose non-adherence, appointments can quickly become frustrating for all involved
- *Is this the right medication?*
  Consider switching antidepressant, initially to another SSRI or well tolerated newer-generation antidepressant. Carefully consider side effects and overdose risks before prescribing second-line treatments such as venlafaxine or tricyclic antidepressants, particularly if there are comorbidities. Combinations of antidepressants,

or augmentation with lithium or antipsychotics, are the next step but should generally be undertaken with input from a psychiatrist.

Post-traumatic Stress Disorder

Post-traumatic stress disorder (PTSD) may occur not just in those who have experienced war or torture, but following other forms of torture including abuse or assault; the state of homelessness can itself also lead to PTSD [26].

Symptoms of PTSD include:

- Re-experiencing (flashbacks, nightmares, or intrusive images or sensations).
- Avoidance and/or emotional numbing.
- Hyper-arousal (including hyper-vigilance, anger and irritability).

The PTSD Checklist – Civilian Version (PCL-C) can be a useful screening tool: it has good diagnostic utility [27], is freely available and is self-administered (but be aware of difficulties caused by poor literacy or language barriers).

SUGGESTIONS FOR PRACTICE

- *Make your consulting room sensitive to the patient's needs: seeing a doctor may itself provoke traumatic memories and these may be heightened if the setting is noisy or busy.*
- *Avoid trying to fit too many questions, particularly about the nature of the traumatic event, into one appointment. Consider a follow-up, especially after a disclosure.*

Treatment for PTSD, as recommended by NICE, should include psychological therapy in the form of trauma-focused CBT [28]. It is worth being aware of how readily available this is in the area you work in. Specialist services, such as Freedom from Torture, are available in some areas but may have specific inclusion criteria for referrals and long waits. Discussing this openly with the patient will avoid raising unrealistic expectations. There may also be peer support groups available, particularly in areas with large populations of ethnic groups who have been affected by large-scale events but bear in mind that there may be individual reasons why your patient does not want to access these.

Drug treatment of PTSD – in the form of an SSRI – is recommended by NICE if the patient prefers it; practically it may seem the only option available, particularly initially. However, progress may be slow; beware the urge to 'fix' things with changes to medication at each visit.

Complex PTSD

Complex PTSD is expected to be included in the 11th revision of the WHO's *International Classification of Diseases* (ICD-11), due to come into effect in 2022. It is a form of PTSD from exposure to cumulative traumas, particularly in childhood, and is described as an 'enhanced form of PTSD' [30]. Clinical features are those seen in PTSD plus three additional symptom clusters: emotional dysregulation, negative self-cognitions and interpersonal difficulties. There is considerable overlap with between complex PTSD and borderline personality disorder (and the former may be a diagnosis that is more acceptable to the patient). However, the two are thought to be distinguishable conditions [31].

Personality Disorder

Personality disorder is controversial. The diagnosis is often disliked by patients, who can feel it implies criticism or judgement [32], and has long been linked to stigma from medical personnel [33]. A recent study of GPs found they felt patients with a diagnosis of personality disorder were poorly served by the NHS [33].

However, personality disorder – which has a 4% prevalence in the general population – is commonly seen in those in touch with health services: about 25% of those in primary care and 50% of those in psychiatric outpatients [34]. It is also linked with death, on average, 18–19 years earlier than should be. This is thought to be not just because of suicide and homicide but also because of comorbidities including cardiovascular and respiratory disease. Tyrer suggests that this may partly be due to difficulties in relationships with health care professionals, as well as lifestyle factors such as increased rates of smoking, drinking and drug abuse [31].

There is reason to be optimistic: personality disorder is no longer thought to be static across the lifespan [36], and recent literature shows that the serious behaviours associated with personality disorder, such as suicide attempts and aggression, can improve markedly with treatment [37]. However, interpersonal problems and a disordered sense of self often continue.

SUGGESTIONS FOR PRACTICE

- *Promote consistency and boundaries. Can you arrange for the patient to see the same practitioner at set appointments, e.g. once a fortnight, or once a month?*
- *Regular discussion at practice meetings or supervision groups can help to keep the practitioner alert to changes which may signify increase in risk, such as a change to more dangerous methods of self-harm. When these happen, reconsider the need to refer to secondary care and make any changes clear in the referral.*
- *Work collaboratively with the patient: in crisis planning, goal setting and shaping decisions about treatment.*
- *Beware the temptation to try to fix things with medication. NICE guidelines for treatment of borderline personality disorder are to only use psychotropics for comorbid conditions, such as depression, rather than the BPD itself.*

Pregnancy and Post-natal Period

Pregnancy can bring considerable extra worries, particularly if there are concerns about finances, living space, and pressures on relationships, which can lead to the development or exacerbation of mental health problems. This can affect men as well as women. Be aware also that there is an increased incidence of intimate partner violence in pregnancy in disadvantaged groups: in some studies of low income, predominately single women, this has been estimated at up to 50%, compared with rates of 3–9% in more general studies [38].

The Marmot review showed a clear social class gradient for post-natal depression, with an incidence of 20% in the lowest socioeconomic quintile compared with 7% in the highest [39]. In society as a whole, one in five mothers suffers from depression, anxiety or psychosis during pregnancy or in the first year after childbirth. It is crucial that this is addressed: suicide is the second-leading cause of maternal death, and mental health problems in the

mother can have significant effects on the social, emotional, and cognitive development of the child [40]. However, women may be reluctant to disclose any difficulty in coping with their baby, particularly if they or people they know have previously had babies taken into care. Sensitive and sympathetic inquiry is key.

Lack of social support is a strong predictor of post-natal depression. Sadly the number of children's entres – introduced in the 2000s with the aim of improving outcomes for children and their families in disadvantaged communities – has fallen by as much as a third since 2010 and those that remain often have a reduced range of services [42].

SUGGESTIONS FOR PRACTICE

- *Some GP surgeries have set up baby and toddler groups within the practice, which provides both an outlet for mothers and an easy way for the practice to keep in touch with new families.*

Care Proceedings

Losing children to care proceedings can be psychologically devastating for the mother. Sadly, this process is often repeated: a recent study estimated that 24% of women involved in family court proceedings will return with subsequent pregnancies or children, usually within a short space of time (the average in the study was 17 months) [42]. Historically these women have been given little formal support but in recent years there have been new initiatives: Pause is an organisation that works with women who have experienced, or are at risk of, repeat removals of children from their care; the Family Drug and Alcohol Court National Unit is a court model which takes a problem-solving approach that aims to help parents avoid repeated patterns. These are not currently available in all areas.

SUICIDALITY

There are strong links between suicide and disadvantage, a tragic fact which is perhaps not unexpected: many factors which follow a socioeconomic gradient, such as alcohol and substance use, poorer social networks, unemployment, and mental disorders, can also be contributors to death by suicide. Sadly, there is evidence that socioeconomic inequality is increasingly resulting in suicide across Europe [45].

It is imperative that the risk of suicide is held in mind. *The Five Year Forward View for Mental Health* reported in 2016 that a quarter of people who took their life had been in contact with a health professional, usually their GP, in the week before they died, while most had been in contact in the previous month [46]. The same report found that more than a quarter of people who died by suicide had been under the care of a mental health team in the preceding 12 months – which means that the majority did not have such support.

If someone discloses suicidal thoughts in a consultation, consider:

- Are they already under the care of a mental health team? Do they have a crisis plan outlining what should happen if the risk of suicide increases? If they have a named care coordinator, contact them for immediate advice.
- If they do not have a named care coordinator, ask are the risks high enough that they need urgent psychiatric attention?

There may be a high immediate risk if the patient:

1. States an intent to end their life,
2. Has thought of a plan, and has a timeframe,
3. Has access to the means,
4. Has made preparatory acts such as saying goodbyes or giving away possessions or pets.

In these cases you will need to understand the local mental health team's crisis arrangements. Many areas now have a centralised phone number which patients or professionals can call for urgent advice. In other areas the best advice may be to attend A&E to seek psychiatric care.

Once again in reality, the situation can be less straightforward: the patient may not wish to seek further help, and the degree of risk can be less clear-cut. They may have been in a similar situation before and sought help, only to feel unsatisfied with the response.

Try to work out a plan that you and the patient both feel happy with: will they agree to a phone call the following day, an appointment next week? Can they undertake to go to A&E if they feel more at risk later?

SUGGESTIONS FOR PRACTICE

- *Be aware that such consultations may bring about complex emotions for the professional, including feelings of frustration and impotence as well as empathy. Can your practice build space in to the working day or week to discuss these feelings as a group?*
- *In the event that a patient dies by suicide, practitioners can experience strong feelings of guilt or shame which may be complicated by concerns that their involvement with the patient will be scrutinised or criticised. It can be useful to talk to someone who can help to look at the situation objectively, either within the practice or elsewhere. If these feelings continue, seek help. The GP Health Service provides confidential support for GPs in England with any level of mental health concern.*

Psychosis

Psychosis is associated with significant social exclusion, and while some of this may be a consequence of the illness (the so-called 'downward drift' of schizophrenia) it appears likely that causal mechanisms are also at play [47]. There is evidence of an association between socioeconomic disadvantage and first-episode psychosis; it has been suggested that this partially explains the increased incidence of schizophrenia in the black Caribbean population in the UK [48].

ASSESSMENT

Psychosis, unless very florid, may be difficult to pick up in a short appointment. Both lack of insight and paranoia may prevent a person from disclosing symptoms; even if this is not the case, people with schizophrenia are more likely to encounter stigma than those with most other mental illnesses [49], which can make open discussion very difficult. If in doubt it is wise to invite the person back for a second appointment.

Additionally, schizophrenia does not always present with the classic symptoms of delusions and hallucinations. Negative symptoms such as social withdrawal, apathy, and blunted emotion can be mistaken for depression or signs of substance misuse. The description of 'simple schizophrenia' in the ICD-10 includes 'considerable social impoverishment' and states that 'vagrancy may ensue' [50]; in fact, with rates of psychosis 4–15 times higher among the homeless population and 50–100 times higher among the street homeless, the possibility of psychotic illness should always be considered in this group.

MANAGEMENT

If you suspect first-episode psychosis, referral to the local early intervention team is always appropriate: NICE guidelines state that antipsychotics should not be started in a first presentation unless it is done in consultation with a psychiatrist [51]. In reality this may present difficulties, particularly if the patient does not have an address: in some areas this is a stipulation for early intervention teams. Referral may not be straightforward if it is unclear whether or not this is indeed a first episode, as is often the case with homeless people with itinerant lifestyles.

Pragmatically, in some cases it may be felt that the benefits of initiating antipsychotic treatment in primary care, and the risks of not doing so, outweigh the risks of prescribing. It is important to consider some of the points below.

SUBSTANCE MISUSE

Always enquire about the use of substances if a patient is presenting as psychotic, but don't assume that use implies causation: opiates, for example, can have an antipsychotic effect and may be used to reduce symptoms.

In other cases you may be unfamiliar with the psychotropic effect of the drug in question, particularly in the case of novel psychiatric substances. It is sensible to be open about this fact and always to explore with the patient what happens when they use: this non-judgemental approach can be refreshing and illuminating for both parties.

DIVERSION OF MEDICATION

Antipsychotics can have a street value, particularly those with sedation as a side effect. If you suspect this, perhaps reconsider the wisdom of prescribing, but also consider a less sedating drug.

MONITORING

Antipsychotics can have significant health effects and NICE guidance should be followed in terms of monitoring. If the patient declines to engage with

such monitoring, there should again be consideration of the risks and benefits of continuing to prescribe, and the result documented. One important consideration is the potential for QTc prolongation with many antipsychotics, which is increased with the concurrent use of crack cocaine or methadone. In these circumstances every attempt should be made to obtain an ECG.

CASE STUDY

Owen

Owen's mother was a drinker and his father suffered from mental health problems. He was raised mainly by grandparents, and spent some time in local authority care. He was bullied at school and truanted from an early age. Owen started drinking and smoking cannabis at the age of 11, and later progressed to using crack and heroin. During his first custodial sentence in a young offenders' institution he started hearing voices, and self-harmed in response to this.

Since then Owen has had several more prison spells. He has also had two admissions to psychiatric hospital, where he has received a diagnosis of drug-induced psychosis. He has not attended follow-up appointments with his local mental health team and has not engaged with the drug and alcohol team. Recent benefit problems led to losing his accommodation, so he is now couch-surfing or occasionally sleeping rough.

LEARNING EXERCISE

- Owen's trajectory to psychosis and homelessness started long before he reached adulthood. Think about how your practice could have intervened, from the time of his mother's pregnancy onwards.
- Owen is likely now to be distrustful of authority. The services he is involved with change frequently – can you provide consistency? Can you have a system where he sees the same professionals at every appointment?
- He may not receive appointment letters. He may not be able to read them if he does. Can you develop a system where you are informed of appointments, and alert him to them?
- If he does get to appointments he may find that he falls through the net between drugs and

mental health. If you have many patients in this situation, think about how far you can go to plug the gap. Can you offer opiate substitute prescribing? Can you initiate antipsychotics?

REFERENCES

1. McManus S, Meltzer H, Brugha T, Bebbington P, Jenkins R. *Adult Psychiatric Morbidity in England, 2007. Results of a Household Survey*. Health and Social Information Centre, Leeds; 2009.
2. Campion J, Bhugra D, Bailey S, Marmot M. Inequality and mental disorders: Opportunities for action. *The Lancet*. 2013;382(9888):183–4.
3. Patel V, Lund C, Hatheril S, Plagerson S, Corrigall J, Funk M et al. Mental disorders: Equity and social determinants. In: Blas E, Kurup AS, editors. *Equity, Social Determinants and Public Health Programmes*. Geneva: World Health Organization; 2010. p. 115–34.
4. Hughes K, Bellis MA, Hardcastle KA, Sethi D, Butchart A, Mikton C, Jones L, Dunne MP. The effect of multiple adverse childhood experiences on health: A systematic review and meta-analysis. *The Lancet Public Health*. 2017;2(8):e356–66.
5. Wilkinson R, Pickett K. *The Spirit Level: Why Equality is Better for Everyone*. Penguin; 2010.
6. Pickett K, Wilkinson R. Inequality: An underacknowledged source of mental illness and distress. *British Journal of Psychiatry*. 2010;197:426–8.
7. British Medical Association 2017: Breaking down barriers – the challenge of improving mental health outcomes. Royal College of Psychiatrists: Whole-person care: From rhetoric to reality—achieving parity between mental and physical health. Royal College of Psychiatrists, London; 2013.
8. Prince M, Patel V, Saxena S, Maj M, Maselko J, Phillips MR, Rahman A. No health without mental health. *The Lancet*. 2007;370:859–77.
9. Public Health England 2017: Better care for people with co-occurring mental health and alcohol/drug use conditions - A guide for commissioners and service providers.
10. Care Quality Commission (2015) Right here, right now – http://www.cqc.org.uk/sites/default/files/20150611_righthere_mhcrisis-care_summary_3.pdf
11. World Health Organization and CalousteGulbenkian Foundation. *Social Determinants of Mental Health*. World Health Organization, Geneva; 2014.
12. Marmot M. *Fair Society, Healthy Lives (The Marmot Review)*. [online] UCL Institute of Health Equity; 2010. https://www.local.gov.uk/marmot-review-report-fair-society-healthy-lives
13. Gilman SE. Review: There is marked socioeconomic inequality in persistent depression. *Evidence-Based Mental Health*. 2003;6:75.
14. Stirling AM, Wilson P, McConnachie A. Deprivation, psychological distress, and consultation length in general practice. *British Journal of General Practice*. 2001;51(467):456–60.
15. Marwaha S, Livingston G. Stigma, racism or choice. Why do depressed ethnic elders avoid psychiatrists? *Journal of Affective Disorders*. 2002;72(3):257–65.
16. Moller-Leimkuhler AM. Barriers to help-seeking by men: A review of sociocultural and clinical literature with particular reference to depression. *Journal of Affective Disorders*. 2002;71(1–3):1–9.
17. Branney P, White A. Big boys don't cry: Depression and men. *Advances in Psychiatric Treatment*. 2008;14:256–62.
18. National Institute for Health and Care Excellence (2009, updated 2016) (Depression in adults: Recognition and management NICE Guideline 90).
19. Zenasni F, Boujut E, Woerner A, Sultan S. Burnout and empathy in primary care: Three hypotheses. *Br J Gen Pract*. 2012; 62(600):346–7.
20. McIntosh C, Ritson B. Treating depression complicated by substance misuse. *Advances in Psychiatric Treatment*. 2001;7(5):357–64.
21. Satre DD, Delucchi K, Lichtmacher J, Sterling SA, Weisner C. Motivational interviewing to reduce hazardous drinking and drug use among depression patients. *Journal of Substance Abuse Treatment*. 2013;44(3):323–9.

22. Miller WR, Rollnick S. *Motivational Interviewing: Helping People Change.* Guilford Press; 2012.

23. BMA: The Devastating cost of Treatment Delays 2018.

24. Sansone RA, Sansone LA. Antidepressant adherence: Are patients taking their medications? *Innovations in Clinical Neuroscience.* 2012;9(5–6):41–6.

25. Hopper EK, Bassuk EL, Olivet J. Shelter from the storm: Trauma-informed care in homelessness services settings. *The Open Health Services and Policy Journal.* 2010;3(1).

26. Weathers FW, Litz BT, Herman DS, Huska JA, Keane TM. The PTSD Checklist (PCL): Reliability, validity, and diagnostic utility. In Annual *Convention of the International Society for Traumatic Stress Studies,* San Antonio, TX 1993 Oct 24 (Vol. 462).

27. National Institute for Health and Care Excellence (2018) *Post Traumatic Stress Disorder* (NICE Guideline 116).

28. Cloitre M, Stolbach BC, Herman JL, Kolk BV, Pynoos R, Wang J, Petkova E. A developmental approach to complex PTSD: Childhood and adult cumulative trauma as predictors of symptom complexity. *Journal of Traumatic Stress.* 2009;22(5):399–408.

29. Giourou E, Skokou M, Andrew SP, Alexopoulou K, Gourzis P, Jelastopulu E. Complex posttraumatic stress disorder: The need to consolidate a distinct clinical syndrome or to reevaluate features of psychiatric disorders following interpersonal trauma? *World J Psychiatry.* 2018;8(1):12–9.

30. Cloitre M, Garvert DW, Weiss B, Carlson EB, Bryant RA. Distinguishing PTSD, complex PTSD, and borderline personality disorder: A latent class analysis. *European Journal of Psychotraumatology.* 2014;5(1):25097.

31. Wood H, Bolton W, Lovell K, Morgan L. Meeting the challenge, making a difference: Working effectively to support people with personality disorder in the community. 2014.

32. Lewis G, Appleby L. Personality disorder: The patients psychiatrists dislike. *The British Journal of Psychiatry.* 1988;153(1):44–9.

33. French L, Moran P, Wiles N, Kessler D, Turner KM. GPs' views and experiences of managing patients with personality disorder: A qualitative interview study. *BMJ Open.* 2019;9(2):e026616.

34. Tyrer P, Reed GM, Crawford MJ. Classification, assessment, prevalence, and effect of personality disorder. *The Lancet.* 2015;385(9969):717–26.

35. Newton-Howes G, Clark LA, Chanen A. Personality disorder across the life course. *The Lancet.* 2015;385(9969):727–34.

36. Bateman AW, Gunderson J, Mulder R. Treatment of personality disorder. *The Lancet.* 2015;385(9969):735–43.

37. Alhusen JL, Ray E, Sharps P, Bullock L. Intimate partner violence during pregnancy: Maternal and neonatal outcomes. *J Womens Health (Larchmt).* 2015;24(1):100–6. doi:10.1089/jwh.2014.4872.

38. Marmot M. *Fair Society Healthy Lives (The Marmot Review).* [online] UCL Institute of Health Equity; 2010.

39. Mental Health Taskforce. The Five Year Forward for Mental Health. 2016. Available at: https://www.england.nhs.uk/wp-content/uploads/2016/02/Mental-Health-Taskforce-FYFV-final.pdf

40. O'Hara MW, Swain AM. Rates and risk of postpartum depression—a meta-analysis. *International Review of Psychiatry.* 1996;8(1):37–54.

41. Broadhurst K, Alrouh B, Yeend E, Harwin J, Shaw M, Pilling M, Mason C, Kershaw S. Connecting events in time to identify a hidden population: Birth mothers and their children in recurrent care proceedings in England. *The British Journal of Social Work.* 2015;45(8):2241–60.

42. *Samaritans, Dying from inequality* 2017.

43. Das-Munshi J, Thornicroft G. Failure to tackle suicide inequalities across Europe. *British Journal of Psychiatry.* 2018;212(6):331–2. doi:10.1192/bjp.2018.80.

44. Lorant V, de Gelder R, Kapadia D, Borrell C, Kalediene R, Kovács K et al. Socioeconomic inequalities in suicide in Europe: The widening gap. *The British Journal of Psychiatry.* Cambridge University Press; 2018;212(6):356–61.

45. Mental Health Taskforce. The Five Year Forward for Mental Health. 2016. Available at: https://www.england.nhs.uk/wp-content/uploads/2016/02/Mental-Health-Taskforce-FYFV-final.pdf

46. Selten JP, Booij J, Buwalda B, Meyer-Lindenberg A. Biological mechanisms whereby social exclusion may contribute to the etiology of psychosis: A narrative review. *Schizophrenia Bulletin*. 2017;43(2):287–92.

47. Morgan C, Kirkbride J, Hutchinson G, Craig T, Morgan K, Dazzan P et al. Cumulative social disadvantage, ethnicity and first-episode psychosis: A case-control study. *Psychological Medicine*. 2008;38(12):1701–15.

48. Crisp A, Gelder M, Goddard E, Meltzer H. Stigmatization of people with mental illnesses: A follow-up study within the Changing Minds campaign of the Royal College of Psychiatrists. *World Psychiatry*. 2005;4(2):106–13.

49. Timms P, Perry J. Sectioning on the street – futility or utility? *BJPsych Bulletin*. 2016;40(6):302–5. doi:10.1192/pb.bp.115.052449.

50. National Institute for Health and Care Stirling AM, Wilson P, McConnachie A. Deprivation, Excellence. *Psychosis and Schizophrenia in Adults: Prevention and Management*. [London]: NICE; 2014 (Clinical guideline [CG178])

51. Stirling AM, Wilson P, McConnachie A. Deprivation, psychological distress, and consultation length in general practice. *British Journal of General Practice*. 2001.

PART 4

Successful Models of Learning and Practice

35

A GP Curriculum for Health Equity

TOM RATCLIFFE AND DOMINIC PATTERSON

Rise up against the organisation of misery.

GP educators are almost universally drawn from front-line practice. As such, they will have directly observed social determinants of health and how the effects of these lead to unequal health outcomes. Higher rates of mental health problems, early onset of chronic disease and multi-morbidity, the long-term effects of early life trauma, the impact of poor housing, homelessness, poverty, violence, and a myriad other issues are translated from cold statistics to the often bleak and painful reality of peoples' lives.

Michael Marmot's call to arms, 'rise up against the organisation of misery' [1], has real resonance. Whilst the human experiences GPs witness are not without colour, hope and happiness, it is impossible not to imagine an alternative reality where more individuals, families and communities are enabled to reach their full potential. International comparisons of child well-being, health outcomes in more equal societies and evidence that tackling health inequity delivers real benefits indicate that many patients' life chances and experiences could be significantly improved.

Allied to the moral imperative to address health inequity is the recognition that we need to do more to ensure that medical education is accountable to the societies who fund, support and ultimately employ the professionals that emerge from clinical training. Whilst up until now social accountability in medical education has mostly been considered in the context of undergraduate programmes, it is hard to argue that the concepts are not also relevant to postgraduate education.

In 1995, the World Health Organisation defined social accountability in medical education as follows: 'The obligation for medical schools to direct their education, research and service activities towards addressing the priority health concerns of the community, region and/or nation they have a mandate to serve' [2].

Published in 2010, the global consensus statement on social accountability developed the concept further, summarising the challenge:

The 21st Century presents medical schools with a different set of challenges: improving quality, equity, relevance and effectiveness in healthcare delivery; reducing the mismatch with societal priorities; redefining roles of health professionals; and providing evidence of impact on people's health status. [3]

A curriculum for health equity will underpin postgraduate GP medical education's response to this challenge.

CAN PRIMARY CARE MAKE A DIFFERENCE TO HEALTH INEQUITY?

In 2013, the World Organisation of Family Doctors' health equity workshop explored how primary care can address health inequity. The key role played by strong, sustainable primary care was highlighted, as well as the need for the development of a curriculum for health professionals [4]. It is estimated that access to good quality medical care, most of which is being or could be delivered by primary care, can reduce inequalities in health outcomes between the poorest and most affluent by as much as 15% [5]. Primary care is therefore a key determinant of health in our communities [6].

HOW CAN A POSTGRADUATE GP MEDICAL EDUCATION HELP?

Medical education can both influence workforce distribution and instil the knowledge, skills and attitudes clinicians require to address health inequity. Therefore, it should impact on both equity of access and quality of care. It is extremely difficult to establish a causal link between educational interventions and health outcomes, particularly when these are likely to be separated in time and subject to multiple confounding factors. There is a strong *prima facie* case, a consensus across academics, royal colleges, educators and trainees and nothing in the way of published counterargument that medical education can and should do more to address health inequity.

The Institute of Health Equity [13] describe in detail the role that doctors can play in addressing the social determinants of health and working towards health equity, making a specific call for better education and training for health professionals, which should include:

- Improved access to training and education;
- The teaching of practical skills and competencies to address health equity;
- Knowledge of social determinants of health; and
- The use of e-learning and community involvement in education.

The conclusion of the *Lancet*'s commission on medical education for the 21st century, which describes how medical education can, amongst other things,

address inequity was similar: 'Students should be trained on competencies that tackle the social determinants of health such as communication, partnership and advocacy skills' [14]

The Royal College of Physicians has produced a report on how the social determinants of health can be tackled through culture change, advocacy and education, stating:

> Learning on health promotion, health inequalities, disease prevention and the social determinants of health should be made more engaging, be embedded as a vertical strand throughout medical education and be considered a key outcome of the process. The structure of postgraduate medical training of all doctors must be examined, to see how opportunities to engage with the social determinants of health can be better incorporated through practice, research and secondments.[15]

Much like the primary care workforce in general, training capacity – the potential and mechanism to produce a future workforce – tends to be unevenly and unfairly distributed [16]. There is evidence to show that students who train in underserved areas or with populations in need are more likely to work there in the future [17–18], and it follows that programmes which promote learning in such environments may in turn address the inverse care law to which general practice is currently subject.

Assuming the workforce can be maintained and equitably distributed, it must also be ensured clinicians are capable and resilient enough to work in the areas of highest need. Qualitative research has shown that GP trainees have an appetite for working in more socioeconomically deprived areas but feel they need help in acquiring the necessary knowledge and skills to survive these challenging posts [19].

DOES THE CURRENT WORKFORCE HAVE THE KNOWLEDGE, SKILLS AND ATTITUDES NEEDED TO TACKLE HEALTH INEQUITY?

In 2016, Health Education England surveyed 103 GP specialist trainees at all stages of training in Yorkshire and Humber. The vast majority thought knowing about health inequity, multi-morbidity and care of vulnerable groups is important for GPs. They identified the following specific learning needs:

- Understand the health problems affecting vulnerable groups;
- Improve competence around communicating effectively with marginalised / vulnerable groups;
- Understand the inverse care law and its impact on healthcare delivery;
- Increase awareness of local community groups working to tackle health inequalities;
- Understand the role of GPs in policy-formation / commissioning / public health relating to health inequity; and
- Understand the UK social security and benefits system.

Exploration of GP and student attitudes towards poverty indicates recognition that a lack of financial and other resources impacts on health and there is a role for health professionals in identifying gaps in access and care. In what appears to be the only published research on GP attitudes to poverty, semi-structured interviews were conducted with 21 GPs in Belgium, revealing some practitioners' quite negative and paternalistic attitudes, particularly regarding patients' approaches to their own health. However, the GPs did feel that responding to the health needs of their patients, specifically around poverty, was certainly part of their role [20].

Participatory research has been used to explore the attitudes of patients living in poverty towards access to and provision of healthcare, as well as the views of healthcare professionals [21]. Together, patients and healthcare professionals concluded the education and training of medical staff should include a focus on improving practitioners' awareness of the effects of living in poverty and barriers to accessing healthcare.

David Blane at the University of Glasgow has explored the attitudes of GP trainers, those who supervise and educate trainee GPs in practices, in an area of high health inequality in Scotland. This revealed many trainers, though they identify this as a key issue, don't discuss health inequalities with their trainees. They were also conscious that knowledge of such issues isn't well tested in

assessments to become a GP. Blane concludes there is a need for more learning in environments of deprivation and inequality [22]. This call for more experiential learning with socioeconomically deprived communities has been consistent, with others concluding there is a need for training capacity to be increased in such areas, partly to address historical workforce inequalities [23].

Others have argued that the traditional GP role needs to be extended both to improve population health and to make practitioners more resilient by tapping into existing non-medical resources in the community; a workforce for the most deprived communities needs to include not just competent and committed clinicians, but also individuals who are strong community advocates [24].

As to the effectiveness of learning interventions on modifying clinician behaviour around addressing health inequity, there is no published evidence other than a small study of paediatric trainees in the USA. However, this did demonstrate that education on social determinants of health can change learner-practitioner behaviours and lead to a greater awareness and exploration of the social determinants of health [25–26].

IS A POSTGRADUATE GP CURRICULUM FOR HEALTH EQUITY NEEDED?

On the basis of evidence, primary care can make a difference to health inequity and the consensus is that postgraduate GP training needs to do more to address this topic. There is a strong argument that a GP curriculum for health equity to underpin learning and the delivery of medical education is needed. But isn't this just replicating what is already in place?

The Royal College of General Practitioners (RCGP) produces the curriculum for postgraduate GP training in the UK, which sets out what is required to practise as a GP: the required 'knowledge, skills and qualities' [27]. It acts as the foundation for the training and assessment of new GPs and so, understandably, it is extremely long and broad in its scope. Anecdotally, whilst the curriculum determines the assessments of knowledge and competence for GP training, trainees and educators rarely access it when planning or undertaking learning activities. Furthermore, there are important gaps (for example there is nothing specifically in the current RCGP curriculum about the health-care of homeless people) and nowhere are the various strands of suggested learning around health inequalities pulled together into a coherent and readily usable curriculum for health equity.

WHAT SHOULD BE IN A POSTGRADUATE GP CURRICULUM FOR HEALTH EQUITY?

To answer this question, a Delphi study was undertaken in which the thoughts of 28 participants drawn from a range of backgrounds [primarily general practice, inclusion healthcare, academia, medical education and public health] were distilled down into a final curriculum covering knowledge, skills and attitudes. Each of these areas was then subdivided into core and extended capabilities [Figure 35.1 through 35.3].

HOW SHOULD THE CURRICULUM BE DELIVERED?

Having accepted the moral argument for addressing health inequalities and that primary care and medical education can both contribute to this process, the GP curriculum for health equity becomes a blueprint for ensuring social accountability. Much can be achieved through the existing training structures. What is needed, and what the curriculum set out above provides, is a little more focus.

The majority of learning, teaching and supervision of GP trainees in the UK is conducted at practice level and within GPs' and trainees' locality. Day-to-day learning revolves around seeing patients, debriefing these encounters with a trainer or experienced GP, reflecting on practice and undertaking workplace-based assessments. All of these provide rich opportunities for learning about health inequity. For example, one might take a situation where a trainee expresses frustration with a patient who is not adhering to their medical treatment and explore why this might be by reflecting on the patient's social circumstances, any psychological distress, the impact of past trauma and then broaden this out to make the link between the social conditions the patient and their family have experienced and the long-term health outcomes for the individual and the local population. Such reframing exercises could build empathy, permit deeper understanding of peoples' lives and enable

the trainees to acquire skills and attitudes to make them a GP capable of tackling health inequity.

At the practice level, trainees might be engaged in looking at equity of outcomes for patients using existing sources of data (easily accessible in the NHS) or undertaking their own 'health equity audit'. They could also be asked to reflect on how easy or difficult it is for disadvantaged or socially excluded groups to access primary care and suggest approaches to improving access and quality. Within the community, there will almost certainly be statutory and non-statutory providers offering patients help with social care needs, homelessness, mental health problems, domestic violence, drug and alcohol problems and numerous other issues. Trainees could learn a great deal and enhance their own practice by learning about these community resources, referring to them and spending time out of general practice and embedded in non-NHS settings.

The organisation of training at locality level can include workshops to help educators improve their focus on health equity and social accountability, could provide supplementary training around health inequalities or, as is the case in some areas, provide training placements in specialist inclusion health settings or entire schemes that are focussed on the needs of marginalised groups. This could enable trainees to acquire the extended capabilities set out in the curriculum.

At regional and national level, resources can be pooled to provide more intensive supplementary resources such as e-learning modules, repositories for patient narratives to be used in training and courses or workshops that bring larger numbers of educators, statutory and non-statutory health and social care providers, patients and trainees together to learn about health equity. There should also be an assurance process that enables regional training bodies, local training schemes, practices and individual GP trainers to demonstrate that the education they are providing is accountable to the needs of their population.

Finally, high stakes assessment at the point of entry and exit from GP training should include material relevant to health equity to ensure that trainees have the potential to and/or have developed the capabilities set out in the curriculum. This should encompass selection for GP training, workplace-based assessment and the nationally mandated and delivered assessments for progression to certificate of completion of training (Advanced Knowledge Test and Clinical Skills Assessment).

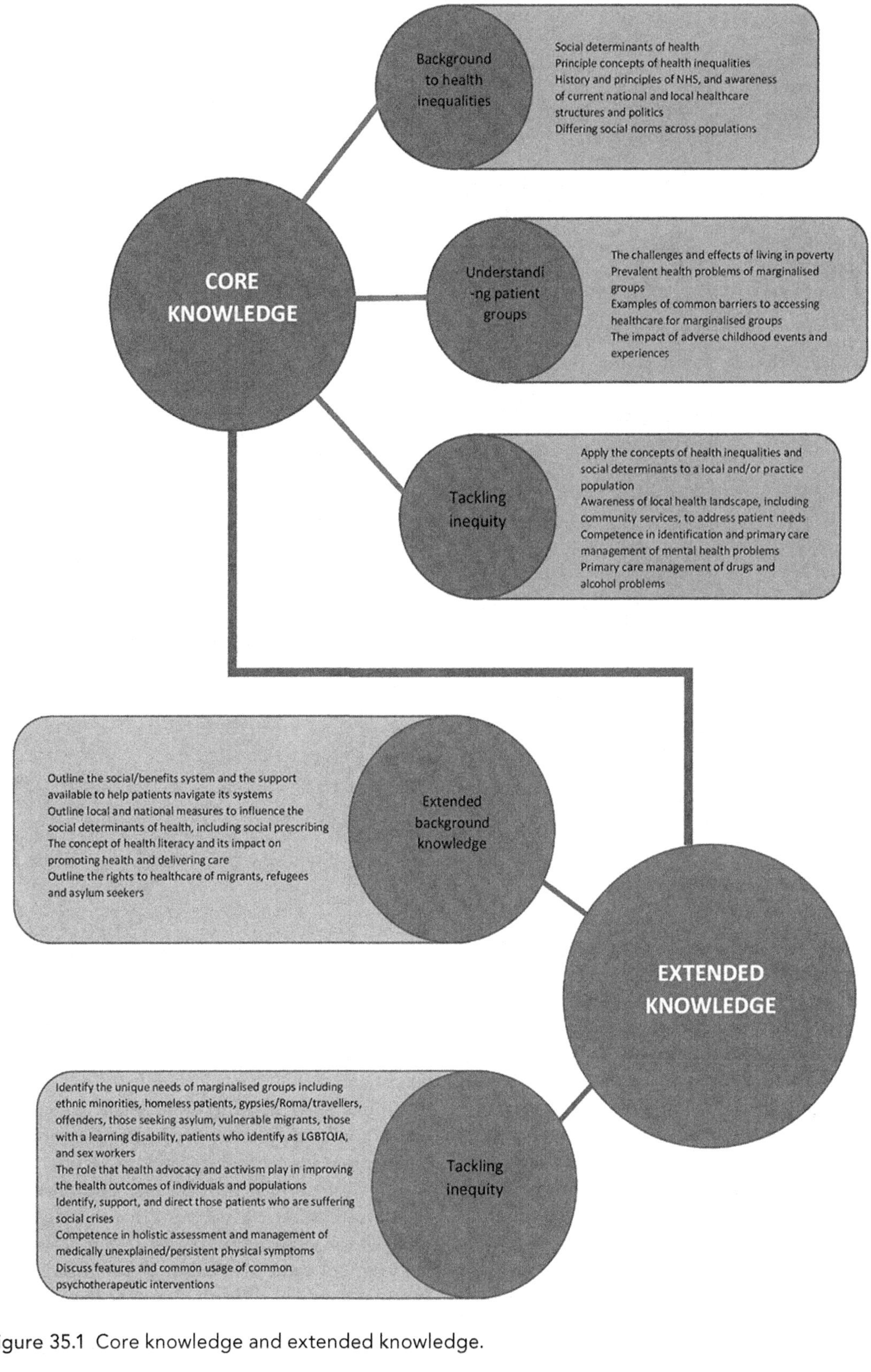

CORE KNOWLEDGE

Background to health inequalities

Social determinants of health
Principle concepts of health inequalities
History and principles of NHS, and awareness of current national and local healthcare structures and politics
Differing social norms across populations

Understanding patient groups

The challenges and effects of living in poverty
Prevalent health problems of marginalised groups
Examples of common barriers to accessing healthcare for marginalised groups
The impact of adverse childhood events and experiences

Tackling inequity

Apply the concepts of health inequalities and social determinants to a local and/or practice population
Awareness of local health landscape, including community services, to address patient needs
Competence in identification and primary care management of mental health problems
Primary care management of drugs and alcohol problems

Extended background knowledge

Outline the social/benefits system and the support available to help patients navigate its systems
Outline local and national measures to influence the social determinants of health, including social prescribing
The concept of health literacy and its impact on promoting health and delivering care
Outline the rights to healthcare of migrants, refugees and asylum seekers

EXTENDED KNOWLEDGE

Tackling inequity

Identify the unique needs of marginalised groups including ethnic minorities, homeless patients, gypsies/Roma/travellers, offenders, those seeking asylum, vulnerable migrants, those with a learning disability, patients who identify as LGBTQIA, and sex workers
The role that health advocacy and activism play in improving the health outcomes of individuals and populations
Identify, support, and direct those patients who are suffering social crises
Competence in holistic assessment and management of medically unexplained/persistent physical symptoms
Discuss features and common usage of common psychotherapeutic interventions

Figure 35.1 Core knowledge and extended knowledge.

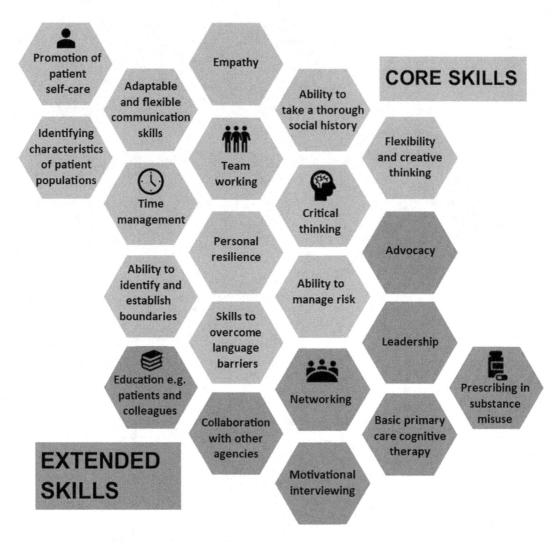

Figure 35.2 Core skills and extended skills.

HOW CAN WE MEASURE SUCCESS?

Kirkpatrick provides a well-known and widely used hierarchy for evaluating medical education [28]. At the base of the pyramid, it starts by simply checking learners have participated in the activity. At the levels above this, it looks at the measurement of satisfaction with the educational activity, followed by confirmation learning has taken place (i.e. the results of formal assessment) and then confirmation of a change in professional behaviour. At the apex, it concludes with a demonstration that patient care has been improved.

Evaluation at the lower levels of the hierarchy is relatively straightforward. It is well within current capabilities of educators at all levels to require that all GP trainees progressing through postgraduate education for general practice receive a series of educational interventions focussed on health inequity and then evaluate satisfaction. This in itself, implemented widely, would represent an achievement for local or regional providers of postgraduate GP education.

Things then become more challenging. One could conceivably analyse whether learning has taken place via workplace-based assessment and scrutiny of performance against questions and cases in summative assessment that relate specific areas of the curriculum described here. However, working out the contribution of particular interventions would be difficult. It may be that multiple datasets collected over time can provide supporting evidence of educational effectiveness and the benefit of the curriculum.

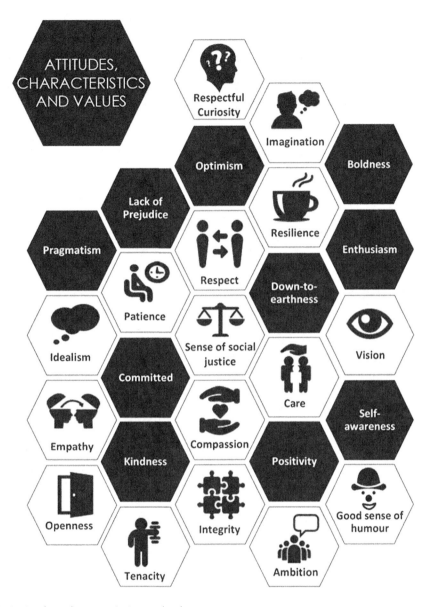

Figure 35.3 Attitudes, characteristics and values.

We then move up to the apex. As set out above, there is scant published evidence indicating that professional behaviour changes following educational interventions relating to health equity. One might measure the locations that trainees choose to practice in with the aim that primary care capacity is more equitably distributed but making a link between this and delivery of the curriculum would be difficult because of multiple biases and confounding factors. If trainees could link specific quality improvement exercises back to activities relating to or inspired by the curriculum, this might provide some evidence at the top of the hierarchy (improved patient care). Linking measures of patient care to changes in GP behaviour back to medical education around health equity is nigh on impossible. One might attempt this by comparing cohorts who have and have not received education governed by the curriculum according to time or location of training to outcome measures such as patient enablement and quality of life. Such measures were used in evaluating the GP delivered CARE Plus programme in Glasgow for complex patients living in socioeconomically deprived neighbourhoods [29]. The ultimate aim of tackling health inequity is arguably outside even Kirkpatrick's ambitious hierarchy as it would require evidence of medical education interventions leading to a shift in population health many years after the initial intervention!

The GP curriculum for health equity described here and published on the Fair Health website will provide a concise and renewed focus on health equity in postgraduate GP education. There is a strong consensus around the need for improved education in this area and this project dovetails with the need to show that medical education is accountable to the society it serves. In this case, the curriculum described above has the bold aim of ensuring better medical care for the poorest in society whose health outcomes are unfair and morally unacceptable.

Putting the curriculum into action will require a concerted effort at all levels: effective feedback and learning at the GP coalface, high quality educational resources within local training schemes, support for educators and learners within regional bodies delivering postgraduate medical education and renewed focus on health equity in standard-setting, curriculum development and assessment nationally. It may also require us to fundamentally re-evaluate the role of the GP as both a clinician and community advocate.

REFERENCES

1. Marmot, M. (2015). *The Health Gap: The Challenge of an Unequal World*. London: Bloomsbury.
2. Boelen, C., and Heck, J. (1995). *Defining and Measuring the Social Accountability of Medical Schools*. Geneva: World Health Organization. (Unpublished document WHO/HRH/95.7, available on request from Division of Organization and Management of Health Systems, World Health Organization, 1211 Geneva 27, Switzerland.)
3. Global Consensus for Social Accountability of Medical Schools (2010) [online]. Available at: http://healthsocialaccountability.org/. [Accessed: 1 April 2018].
4. Shadmi, E., Wong, W., Kinder, K., Heath, I., and Kidd, M. (2014). Primary care priorities in addressing health equity: Summary of the WONCA 2013 health equity workshop. *International Journal for Equity in Health*, 13(1).
5. Schroeder, S. (2007). We Can Do Better – Improving the Health of the American People. *New England Journal of Medicine*, 357(12), 1221–1228.
6. Dussault, G., and Franceschini, M. (2006). Not enough there, too many here: Understanding geographical imbalances in the distribution of the health workforce. *Human Resources for Health*, 4(1).
7. Mclean, G., Guthrie, B., Mercer, S.W., and Watt, G.C.M. (2015). General practice funding underpins the persistence of the inverse care law. *British Journal of General Practice*. 799–805.
8. Centre for Workforce Intelligence. (2014). *In-depth review of the General Practitioner workforce*. [Online]. Available at: https://www.gov.uk/government/uploads/system/uploads/attachment_data/file/507493/CfWI_GP_in-depth_review.pdf. [Accessed: 6 July 2017].
9. Hobbs, F.D.R. et al. (2016). Clinical workload in UK primary care: A retrospective analysis of 100 million consultations in England, 2007–14. *The Lancet*, 387, 2323–2330.
10. Pedersen, A.F., and Vedsted, P. (2014). Understanding the inverse care law: A register and survey-based study of patient deprivation and burnout in general practice. *International Journal for Equity in Health*, 13, 121. Asaria, M. (2015). Unequal socioeconomic distribution of the primary care workforce: Whole-population small area longitudinal study. *BMJ Open*, 6, e008783. doi:10.1136/bmjopen-2015-008783. NAO. (2015). *Stocktake on access to GP*.
11. Hogg, C., and Sharpe, N. Inverse Care Law of Yorkshire and Humber General Practice? [online]. Available at: https://yorkshiredeependgp.org/2017/12/27/inverse-care-law-for-yorkshire-and-humber-general-practice/. [Accessed: 17 May 2018].
12. Tudor-Hart, J. (1971). The inverse care law. *The Lancet*, 297, 405–412.
13. Thomas, S. (2016). *Doctors for Health Equity. The Role of the World Medical Association, National Medical Associations and Doctors in Addressing the Social Determinants of Health and Health Equity Reference*. London: UCL Institute of Health Equity.

14. Frenk, J. et al. (2010). Health professionals for a new century: Transforming education to strengthen health systems in an interdependent world. *The Lancet*, 376, 1923–1958.

15. Royal College of Physicians. (2010). *How Doctors Can Close the Gap. Tackling the social determinants of health through culture change, advocacy and education.* [Online]. London. Available at: https://www.rcplondon.ac.uk/news/doctors-can-promote-fairness-and-equality-health. [Accessed: 6 July 2017].

16. Health Education England, internal analysis of GP training capacity for Yorkshire and Humber, 2016.

17. Tavernier, L., Connor, P., Gates, D., and Wan, J. (2003). Does exposure to medically underserved areas during training influence eventual choice of practice location? *Medical Education*, 37(4), 299–304.

18. VanderWielen, L., Vanderbilt, A., Crossman, S., Mayer, S., Enurah, A., Gordon, S., and Bradner, M. (2015). Health disparities and underserved populations: A potential solution, medical school partnerships with free clinics to improve curriculum. *Medical Education Online*, 20(1), 27535.

19. Nadeem, T., and Ramsay, A. Yorkshire and Humber GP Trainees want to work in areas of socio-economic deprivation. [online]. Available at: https://yorkshiredeependgp.org/2017/12/27/yorkshire-and-humber-gp-trainees-want-to-work-in-areas-of-greater-socioeconomic-deprivation/. [Accessed 17 May 2018].

20. Willems, S. (2005). The GP's perception of poverty: A qualitative study. *Family Practice*, 22(2), 177–183.

21. Hudon, C., Loignon, C., Grabovschi, C., Bush, P., Lambert, M., Goulet, É., Boyer, S., De Laat, M., and Fournier, N. (2016). Medical education for equity in health: A participatory action research involving persons living in poverty and healthcare professionals. *BMC Medical Education*, 16(1).

22. Blane, D., Hannah, H., McLean, G., Lough, M., and Watt, G. (2013). Attitudes towards health inequalities amongst GP trainers in Glasgow, and their ideas for changes in training. *Education for Primary Care*, 24(2), 97–104.

23. Russell, M., and Lough, M. (2010). Deprived areas: Deprived of training? *British Journal of General Practice*, 60(580), 846–848.

24. Zakaria, S., Johnson, E., Hayashi, J., and Christmas, C. (2015). Graduate Medical Education in the Freddie Gray Era. *New England Journal of Medicine*, 373(21), 1998–2000.

25. Klein, M., Alcamo, A., Beck, A., O'Toole, J., McLinden, D., Henize, A., and Kahn, R. (2014). Can a video curriculum on the social determinants of health affect residents' practice and families' perceptions of care? *Academic Pediatrics*, 14(2), 159–166.

26. Klein, M., Kahn, R., Baker, R., Fink, E., Parrish, D., and White, D. (2011). Training in social determinants of health in primary care: Does it change resident behavior? *Academic Pediatrics*, 11(5), 387–393.

27. RCGP. (2017). *GP curriculum: Overview.* [Online]. 2017. Rcgp.org.uk. Available at: http://www.rcgp.org.uk/training-exams/gp-curriculum-overview.aspx. [Accessed: 5 September 2017].

28. Mehay, R. (2012). *The Essential Handbook for GP Education and Training.* London: Radcliffe Publishing.

29. Mercer, S.W. et al. (2016). The CARE Plus study – a whole-system intervention to improve quality of life of primary care patients with multimorbidity in areas of high socioeconomic deprivation: Exploratory cluster randomised controlled trial and cost-utility analysis. *BMC Medicine*, 14, 88.

36

Examples of Innovative Service Models Across the UK

GABI WOOLF AND MILENA MARSZALEK

The patients that need it the most are offered services most tailored to their complex needs'

Clinicians will always face the challenge of contextualising the care plans they provide for patients within their environment. Unfortunately, the model of brief consultations will not always effectively deal with the most pressing priorities in a patient's circumstance. This has led to a variety of developments in new ways to provide more holistic healthcare services. Based on the rise of Focused Care in Manchester, practices across the UK have demonstrated the effective use of coordinating different service sectors to tackle health inequalities. Five different case studies are discussed below.

CASE STUDY

Case Study One: Social Prescribing in Bromley By Bow

The benefits of adding social prescribing to traditional GP services are outlined in the interview below with Dan Hopewell, director of knowledge and innovation at the Bromley by Bow Centre, and Dr Selvaseelan Selvarajah, GP at St Andrew's Health Centre. They work in the Bromley by Bow Centre, opened in 1984 in east London as a charitable organisation with the aim of creating an integrated social provision for the local population that suffers with high levels of deprivation.

The service was provided by GPs who were familiar with the relationship between the health and socio-economic needs of the patients in this deprived area, in a centre built and rented back to the local health authority. Initially started in the Bromley by Bow Health Centre, it has now been expanded to other practices in the surrounding area. It works on the principles of well-being and health predominantly being socially and economically determined, therefore needing to be addressed with social prescribing to prevent further ill health. GP surgeries act as a point of access for the population for information and programmes that meet their social and economic needs. They are a frequently under-utilised resource in tackling health inequalities given that 90% of patient contact is within general practice.

The services provided by the centre not only include social prescribing, but the additional services mentioned here:

- Proactive programmes that involve informing patients of non-clinical options as they wait for their clinical appointments.
- Self-referral services for advice regarding social welfare, debt, skills and employability, offered either via the health centre or the community centre's connection zone.

The Principles of Social Prescribing

Patients are referred to a social prescribing coordinator for hour-long appointments, in which they have the opportunity to discuss their social and economic needs. Patients are then directed to appropriate services within the centre or third sector organisations.

There are 150 staff, the majority of whom started as volunteers; they are employed to programmes provided by the centre and work in the following areas:

- Healthy lifestyle and weight management advice;
- Community gym;
- Advice on managing debt and benefits;
- English courses;
- Digital inclusion courses;
- Vocational skills development;
- Support gaining employment;

Activities that target social isolation are also provided:

- Community café and gardens;
- Walking;
- Cooking and gardening groups;
- Arts and volunteer programmes.

Consistent contact is maintained with their coordinator. Although the services represent ethnic diversity both through staffing and location to try to ensure universal access, patients may not always be able to fully access the services due to the following:

- Lack of confidence;
- A lack of trust towards professionals;
- Feeling overwhelmed by the multiple issues faced;
- Mental health problems;
- Drug/alcohol issues.

Expanding Social Prescribing

The School of Integrated Solutions is run by the centre to provide visitors with the knowledge and experience to set up similar establishments. Factors to consider include determining the scale of the service – whether it serves one or multiple GP practices, providing proactive advice to patients coming for appointments and coordinating with other services such as the voluntary sector, health trainers, children's centres, schools and housing associations.

Although robust and longitudinal data on the combined effects of the integrated services on the local population have not yet been collected, social prescribing is recommended in the NHS's five-year forward plan for general practice and a multi-year review is being initiated by PHE and the Wellcome Trust.

CASE STUDY

Case Study Two: The Deep End Group and Links Practitioners

To create a strong supportive network between GPs working in the most deprived areas of Scotland, the Deep End Group was established by RCGP Scotland as part of a working group on health inequalities. This group is intended to help clinicians to improve their practice when working with complex multi-morbidity, drug and alcohol problems and social isolation. Support is provided from the Glasgow Centre for Population Health, RCGP and the Scottish Parliament to ensure that GPs in the group have time to attend the 6–8 weekly meetings.

The Deep End's GP group in Scotland works on providing support by using a 'links practitioner', a member of staff funded by the Scottish Government assigned to a single practice. They aim to provide knowledge about local primary care, social care, voluntary and community services which may benefit patients presenting with psycho-social complaints i.e. depression or back pain. These patients commonly need a more holistic approach to their treatment, with non-clinical support. Frequently, they will have been referred on to services but may not have attended due to personal trust issues with healthcare professionals. Links practitioners provide a flexible and supportive service that aims to break down such barriers, taking into account initial adherence issues by proactively communicating with patients by using more informal methods instead.

The Deep End Group has subsequently produced a report highlighting six ways of working as part of their collective vision:

- Spend more time with patients.
- Improve use of repeat consultations to create strong patient narratives and increase patients' knowledge and confidence as they live with their conditions and access services.
- Develop local health systems around practice hubs, developing and nurturing all of the relationships that involves, including the community workers who assist with the practice.
- Establish better connections between practices, sharing experiences, views, learning and activity.
- Establish better support for the front-line staff from central organisations
- Improve leadership at every level, sharing power, resources and responsibility.

Other branches of the service include:

- Alcoholic outreach workers;
- Adult and child social workers as part of the Govan Integrated Care Project to improve the integration between health and social care in accordance with the Low Commission's suggestions in *Getting it Right in Social Welfare Law.*

The Deep End Project acts as an effective method of linking GPs working with the most deprived members of society, to pool their knowledge and experiences to make long-term changes at a grassroots level. This work is being extrapolated to Yorkshire and Humber, Greater Manchester as well as to Irish GPs and the Welsh Government Inverse Care Law Programme.

CASE STUDY

Case Study Three: HealthWORKS

Providing an establishment that houses the variety of services needed to provide a holistic approach to healthcare was the basis of the HealthWORKS project. Professor Chris Drinkwater, a retired academic GP and emeritus professor of primary care development at Northumbria University, aimed to provide services that tackle health inequalities in a wider sense, all under the same roof. As part of the City Challenge Newcastle regeneration project, an old shopping centre that was initially to be demolished was used to house the project. It then expanded

between two sites due to tender processes for changes in funding, now using the local authority's Children's Centre as a replacement tenant. Sir Michael Marmot is the acting patron of the organisation.

The centres include the following:

- GP practice;
- Gym;
- Exercise facilities;
- Community room;
- Creche;
- Community-based coronary rehabilitation programme;
- Breastfeeding peer support;
- Food and nutrition services with weaning, healthy cooking and food hygiene classes;
- Health trainers;
- Social prescribing;
- Falls prevention service;
- Change4Life Health Champions in schools
- The Living Well, Taking Control programme for type 2 diabetes sufferers includes 5 educational sessions, regular reviews of management and lifestyle habits. (The service was audited over 18 months and had a 40.5% compliance rate, with an average 6.75mmol/mol drop in HbA1C.)

These services can be accessed either through GP or through self-referral. In terms of funding, 70% comes from contracts with the City Challenge, the regional health authority primary care development budget, Public Health England, the local authority and CCGs, with the remaining 30% coming through grants i.e. from the National Lottery.

CASE STUDY

Case Study Four: BRICSS

SUPPORTING THE MOST MARGINALISED POPULATIONS AROUND BRADFORD

Although Public Health England works on a broad premise of general health improvement, targeted services that focus on improving non-clinical issues that vastly affect medical outcomes have been shown to be very effective.

One third of Bradford's population live in areas that are in the most deprived 10% of the country, with unemployment rates at 8.6% – above the national average of 5.4%. It also houses a high

Middle Eastern refugee and homeless population. This marginalised population has frequently found it difficult to access primary healthcare services and therefore requires a more targeted approach to their healthcare. Asylum seekers, vulnerably housed patients, sex workers and victims of domestic violence also fall into this population.

Bevan House Practice opened in 2003 to cater for this population, which has steadily increased with the economic crisis and welfare changes linked to the homeless. Its funding has been provided by a range of sectors, with the Right to Request scheme allowing an expansion of services, as well as the Social Enterprise Investment Fund and Public Health England.

It offers the following services:

- 15-minute appointments that can be booked on a flexible drop-in basis;
- Sexual health and family planning clinics;
- Primary care mental health team clinics;
- Benefits advisory service;
- Social prescribing;
- A weekly evening clinic for sex workers;
- A volunteer and patient engagement coordinator;
- Specialised counselling for female trauma victims;
- Links with the local drug and alcohol services;
- Tuberculosis screening for the homeless and new arrivals, as well as guaranteed health screens and four-week follow ups for all new registrations;
- Programmes that focus on refugee relocation – these include the Vulnerable Persons Relocation Scheme and the Gateway Protection Programme, run by the Home Office and United Nations High Commissioner for Refugees;
- A specialist migrant Nurse;
- Outreach services such as the Street Medicine Team – GPs, nurses, mental health workers and volunteers who attend drop-ins, shelters and churches in a camper van to provide healthcare.

Another vital part of this service is BRICSS: Bradford Respite and Intermediate Care Support Service. Horton Housing runs this inpatient facility to provide intermediate care to homeless patients who are being discharged from hospital with ongoing health needs and housing issues. It includes the pathway team: two nurses, a housing support worker and a care support navigator who ensure that homeless and vulnerably housed patients admitted to hospital receive adequate tailored support on discharge. To improve service adherence, appointments are not booked more than a week in advance and consistency of patient-support worker contact is provided. This ensures patients can always be followed up.

The services provided by Bevan Healthcare have been expanded by collaborations with Deep End Yorkshire, the northern hub of the Faculty for Homeless and Inclusion Health and Pathway, the national homeless health charity.

As well as countless case studies of improved re-admission and treatment compliance rates, the valuable work of the organisation has been recognised through receiving an 'outstanding' CQC assessment and the BRICSS team being shortlisted for the BMJ Awards as the primary care team of the year.

CASE STUDY

Case Study Five: Pathway: A Haven for the Homeless

One of the biggest breakthroughs for providing support for the management of homeless patients has been the establishment of Pathway. Dr Nigel Hewitt and Professor Aidan Halligan – Director of Education at UCLH – explored the factors that affect the quality of care received by homeless patients. The homeless population is much more challenging to treat (the average life expectancy of a homeless person is 47) and if they are admitted with a drug-related problem they are seven times more likely to die in the next five years compared to those with a permanent residence. Their A & E attendance rates are five times higher than the general population, admissions are 3.2 times more frequent and the incurred secondary care costs are therefore eight times higher than with the general population.

This inquiry sparked a collaboration between the two and Professor Barry McCormack, chief economist at the Department of Health, along with other healthcare professionals, to develop a model of integrated care. This was a multi-disciplinary work lead by GPs for managing homeless patients in hospital. It eventually led to the concurrent development of the Pathway charity. It is used in four other London hospitals as well as in Bradford, Leeds, Manchester, Birmingham and Brighton.

GPs are seen as the most suitable leads for this project due to their experience in managing physical health, mental health, drug and alcohol problems in the same consultation. This constellation of issues very much characterises long-term homelessness. The members of the multidisciplinary (MDT) team that work alongside the GP include 'care navigators'– people who have experienced homelessness and exclusion – who provide advocacy, mentoring and support during hospital admission and discharge.

The team's input begins right from the start of a hospital admission. A comprehensive MDT assessment is made on each admitted homeless patient. This will include information regarding the following:

- Their physical and mental health;
- Drug and alcohol history;
- Financial and housing history;
- Ongoing care needs.

As part of the ongoing initial assessment, the team can give advice regarding the following issues:

- Administering the Hep B vaccination;
- Cognitive assessments for patients with a long history of alcohol dependency;
- Identifying any communication issues the patients may face during their hospital admission e.g. the need for a translator.

Throughout the admission patients are given regular support and the time they need to discuss their concerns. This has been shown to dissuade patients from early discharge. The team involved with the patient have regular multi-agency meetings with drug and alcohol teams, housing and social services, mental health and primary care services, and outreach services for the homeless. This links the necessary services together to effectively plan for the patient's discharge.

The patient's key worker can then be closely involved in the usual discharge planning process that includes liaison with the occupational therapy and physiotherapy teams. Input is maintained following discharge – teams can take the patient to a housing appointment, provide access to intermediate care beds, help them settle into new accommodation and aid them with registration at a new GP practice.

Support in this post-discharge period is vital, as this is when a lot of patients experience complex issues with housing. Difficulties arise when patients have uncertain eligibility for housing either within an area or within the UK. Under the Housing Act 1996, an individual can only be entitled to social housing in a given area if they can show proof of a local connection to said area. In reality, this is a lot harder for a patient to produce, especially for homeless migrants who have uncertain rights within the UK and for those with previous rejections for asylum requests. Pathway teams offer funding for legal advice around these issues.

A quantitative and qualitative evaluation of Pathway at one of its roll-out centres was published in 2015. There was a 30% reduction in the number of days spent in hospital by patients within this population, without significant reductions in the numbers of admissions. Qualitative feedback reflected the impact the services have had on the lives of these patients.

Comparison of these various services shows a strong running theme between them – focus on social prescribing, integration of community and voluntary sectors and deviating away from the traditional condensed patient consultations. The patients that need it the most are offered services most tailored to their complex needs.

37

Widening Participation in Medical Education

CHARLOTTE AUTY

Many students from lower socioeconomic backgrounds find themselves defined by their background.

Widening participation (WP) is an educational initiative to increase the number of disadvantaged students and students from under-represented groups who attend higher education.

Students from the least deprived areas still make up the largest group that go on to study medicine, while those from the most deprived areas make up the smallest group. The proportion of the general population in each indices of multiple deprivation (IMD) ranking has remained static over time and is evenly distributed. Socioeconomic classification (SEC) is a major determinant factor in medical school applications [1]. Students from LES backgrounds are less prone to apply and to succeed in medical school applications [2–3]. These students are also the most debt averse which is a major barrier to higher education studies [4].

Homes of a lower socioeconomic status often lack adults who attended higher education. Having not been exposed to such possibilities means children brought up in these homes may never consider higher education as an option. In addition, schools and their teachers in these areas will also tend to be less aware of medical school application processes, and therefore not in a position to guide and motivate their students. For example, students will be deprived of extra-curricular activities and work experience which is valuable for medical school applications [5]. It is important to highlight the effect of peers and family upon a students' expectations of what they themselves can achieve. Many students from lower socioeconomic backgrounds find themselves defined by their background, having no peers or family members who have attained higher education. This leads to students from more disadvantaged backgrounds establishing a social identity in which they self-define as a person who does not belong in higher education, let alone medicine [6]. Families with a parental background of managerial occupations and traditionally higher paying professions generate the highest proportion of medical students and this trend has been increasing [7]. Proportionally, lower SEC groups access medical and health services more due to poor housing, diet and poverty [8] and WP clinicians can also help these patient groups feel less secluded from the NHS, which happens when they encounter these cultural barriers in their physicians [9]. When examining the demographics of the population of students attending medical school in the UK, whilst socio-economic factors are exceptionally important to consider, it is important to examine other protected characteristics. For instance, data from UCAS 2011 shows a true disparity between the proportion of the population who define as Afro-Caribbean or African and people who define in the same way in medical school, with these students being heavily under-represented. More provision for those with registered disabilities at GCSE and A-level has allowed the proportion of students entering medical school who have a declared disability to increase, however there is still work to be done [7].

WHAT IS THE IMPACT OF WP?

WP hopes to address social inequality, social mobility and improve diversity and equality in higher education. The outcomes of WP initiatives for graduates have demonstrated several positive outcomes in the areas of employment, social mobility and wider economic growth [10, 11]. The British Medical Association (BMA) celebrates diveristy in its statement, 'recognising that we are all different, and celebrating and valuing these differences' and the right for any individual to be granted equal opportunity regardless of disability, gender, ethnicity or age [12, 13]. The Medical Schools Council states the population of medical students and doctors graduating to serve the NHS should be demographically representative of the UK population, claiming medical schools should be working towards their students having the 'social, cultural and ethnic backgrounds…(which) reflect broadly the diversity of those they are called upon to serve' [7]. Despite multiple widening participation initiatives around the country working to achieve this aim, there is still clear work to be done. A report by the Social Mobility and Child Poverty Commission in 2012 highlighted the medical field in particular as in dire need of diversity, stating 'medicine lags behind other professions both in the focus and in the priority it accords to these issues. It has a long way to go when it comes to making access fairer, diversifying its workforce and raising social mobility' [7].

So why is it so important that the medical profession is as diverse and representative as the population it serves?

Studies from both sides of the Atlantic Ocean have illustrated that such diversity in the medical workforce creates better clinicians. Studies from both the UK and the US have consistently shown that students from WP backgrounds perform better in medical school. Not only this, but students from WP background are most likely to remain working in the same country and to work in rural and in disadvantaged neighbourhoods [15, 16]. It is not just grades of medical students on which this research has focused, but the attributes of what makes a good clinician too. Studies utilising questionnaires on medical students throughout their careers highlight that students learning within a more socioeconomically diverse medical school score higher on questions relating to feelings of empathy and empathic behaviour towards their patients in later medical school and after graduation.

BEST PRACTICE

Several strategies have been identified and trialled to improve WP for medical schools [7]. The Higher Education Funding Council for England (HEFCE) provided funding supplements to institutions enrolling disadvantaged students such as the Office for Fair Access, incentivising them to generate WP aims and strategies, as well as special WP projects [17]. Currently, most UK medical schools have provision for those from disadvantaged backgrounds, usually culminating in outreach programmes, four more WP courses were added between 2016 and 2018 [17]. Whilst this is an excellent step forward, there is a flaw in this strategy. This strategy leads to 'cold spots' where outreach does not extend, as much of the widening participation work will be focused in the areas surrounding the medical schools. Whilst this is valuable, it should be highlighted that most medical schools are in university cities, which, by nature, tend to be more affluent and have higher achieving schools. Attempts to avoid this and create outreach programmes which hit the cold spots too are of utmost importance.

Another factor which can be more easily modified when it comes to underperforming schools is entrance criteria. The General Medical Council highlighted simple changes to interview formats.

SUGGESTIONS FOR PRACTICE

- *Switch from a traditional panel interview to multiple mini interviews (MMI).*
  This has been seen to moderately increase WP and should therefore be utilised across all medical schools.
- *Use of situational judgement tests (SJTs).*
  These were were found to have a similar effect on the success of WP applicants [9].

One reason for the success of these may be that applicants are less able to predict what will be on these interviews and tests and therefore there is less scope for coaching, something which will only be open to the more economically fortunate. A handful of medical schools have now begun to utilise contextual data (CD) in order to identify candidates from lower socioeconomic backgrounds using criteria such as home postcode, school or if applicants are the first generation in their family to attend higher education [9].

SUGGESTIONS FOR PRACTICE

- *Use contextual data holistically.*
  This could be used to provide a balance with the qualitative criteria such as the UKCAT score or amount of work experience an applicant has had. Alternate suggestions include lowering the grade entry requirements for candidates who meet enough CD criteria.

Types of Widening Participation Programmes

Programmes vary in nature and can be delivered in a variety of forms to different age groups. The most common way of classifying is based on their intensity. The lowest intensity programmes have minimal time commitment and focus. They are usually delivered in the evenings or during open days. High intensity projects usually deliver information to students over a weekend or require a long-term commitment from both mentors and mentees, forming a tutoring relationship over a series of activities, often in the form of summer schools or weekly tutoring sessions [2]. Whilst the latter type are often hailed as having a more positive impact on students, they can be difficult to deliver, with a difficulty in recruiting tutors, and

the long-term nature of these projects leading to high costs [19]. For this reason, many institutions prefer to hold multiple low-intensity projects and activities [9].

Student initiatives run by those who have just undergone the application process successfully are useful, with the addition of the expertise of clinicians who help with the selection process in universities lending insight. There is value in collaboration between clinicians of different grades and medical students but time, availability and excessive workload should be considered. A current barrier to WP is limited funding for societies at medical school and a lack of engagement by schools who need WP initiatives most [19]. Last year, the British Medical Association began work on lobbying medical schools to incorporate WP work into student selected placements, allowing students to participate without sacrificing their studies. Student societies should also collaborate with those who have connections with local schools, such as councils and the Social Mobility Foundation (SMF), a charity working towards implementing positive change to social mobility and Reach Scotland, a charity aiding Scottish children who are struggling in school. One of their ultimate aims is to boost the confidence of young people to help them succeed in all aspects of life, including higher education.

One example of student societies collaborating effectively with third-sector organisations in order to make an impact on WP in their area is Manchester Outreach Medics (MOMs). The idea was conceived by a medical student at the University of Manchester in 2015. A team of medical students who were passionate about supporting young people interested in medicine was created with the goal to inform and inspire those who didn't have any friends or family in the medical profession. MOMs began holding free events for those from disadvantaged backgrounds, equipping them with the tools, information and skills needed to ace the application to medical school.

The main challenges to societies like MOMs are finding venues which are affordable for a society running free events. Funding can be very difficult for initiatives like these and learning how to navigate grants and bursaries for widening participation projects was difficult.

SUGGESTIONS FOR PRACTICE

- *By forming collaborations with local organisations, barriers can be overcome with support in finding venues, covering costs and providing expertise. This allows for the smooth running of projects without passing any cost on to those who need the help.*

The most important and telling indicator of this WP project's success is the sixth formers themselves. Students who are now on the committee for MOMs attended MOMs events as sixth formers and are now first-year medical students. It is doubtful they would have got into medical school without the opportunity widening partipation projects offer.

REFERENCES

1. Seyan K, Greenhalgh T, Dorling D. The standardised admission ratio for measuring widening participation in medical schools: Analysis of UK medical school admissions by ethnicity, socioeconomic status, and sex. *BMJ.* 2004;328(7455):1545–1546.
2. Brown G, Garlick P. Changing geographies of access to medical education in London. *Health & Place.* 2007;13(2):520–531.
3. British Medical Association. Equality and diversity in UK medical schools (Internet). London; 2009 p. 13. Available from: http://www.nhshistory.net/bmastudentreport2009.pdf
4. Callender C, Jackson J. Does the fear of debt deter students from higher education? *Journal of Social Policy.* 2005;34(04):509.
5. Hill N, Castellino D, Lansford J, Nowlin P, Dodge K, Bates J et al. Parent academic involvement as related to school behavior, achievement, and aspirations: Demographic variations across adolescence. *Child Development.* 2004;75(5):1491–1509.
6. Maras P. 'But no one in my family has been to University' aiming higher: School students' attitudes to higher education. *The Australian Educational Researcher.* 2007;34(3):69–90.
7. Selecting for Excellence Executive Group: Medical Schools Council. Selecting for excellence final report (Internet). London; 2014. p. 15–26. Available from: https://www.medschools.ac.uk/media/1203/selecting-for-excellence-final-report.pdf
8. Angel C. Broadening access to undergraduate medical education. *BMJ.* 2000;321(7269):1136–1138.
9. Selecting for Excellence Executive Group. How can greater consistency in selection between medical schools be encouraged? A mixed-methods programme of research that examines and develops the evidence base (Internet). Medical Schools Council; 2014. Available from: https://www.medschools.ac.uk/media/2447/selecting-for-excellence-research-professor-jen-cleland-et-al.pdf
10. Guide to Widening Participation — Causeway Education (Internet). Causeway education. 2019 (cited 25 March 2019). Available from: https://causeway.education/guide-to-widening-participation
11. Patterson R, Price J. Widening participation in medicine: What, why and how? *MedEdPublish.* 2017;6(4).
12. British Medical Association. BMA corporate equality, diversity and inclusion strategy 2016–2021. London; 2016 p. 3.
13. Young M, Razack S, Hanson M, Slade S, Varpio L, Dore K et al. Calling for a broader conceptualization of diversity. *Academic Medicine.* 2012;87(11):1501–1510.
14. Whitla D, Orfield G, Silen W, Teperow C, Howard C, Reede J. Educational benefits of diversity in medical school. *Academic Medicine.* 2003;78(5):460–466.
15. Dowell J, Norbury M, Steven K, Guthrie B. Widening access to medicine may improve general practitioner recruitment in deprived and rural communities: Survey of GP origins and current place of work. *BMC Medical Education.* 2015;15(1).
16. Selection Alliance 2017 Report. *An Update on the Medical Schools Council's Work in Selection and Widening Participation.* London: Medical Schools Council; 2017.

17. Lewis B. Widening participation in higher education: The HEFCE perspective on policy and progress. *Higher Education Quarterly*. 2002;56:204–219.

18. Kamali AW, Nicholson S, Wood DF. A model for widening access into medicine and dentistry: The SAMDA-BL project. *Medical Education*. 2005;39:918–925.

19. Sartania N, Haddock G, Underwood M. The challenges of widening access to the medical profession: How to facilitate medical careers for those at a genuine disadvantage. *MedEdPublish*. 2018;7.

Index

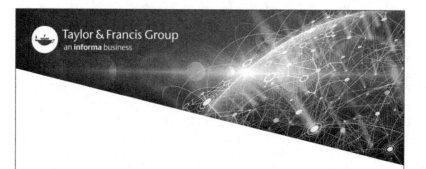

Printed in the United States
by Baker & Taylor Publisher Services